"The editors' starting point was the surprising discovery that love has been little explored and conceptualised in the literature of psychoanalytic work with intimate couple relationships. Gathering together the thinking and practice of experienced psychoanalytic clinicians from around the world – from South America, North America, Australia, China, Poland and the UK – this collection certainly makes up for that absence! Utilising psychoanalytic and link theories, it explores love in all its complexities, personal, interpersonal and social. It explores issues of attachment, sexuality and the impact of culture. It examines the experience of love in more disregulated couples, in cross-cultural partnerships, in same-sex and in non-monogamous relationships, and its fate in later life. Matters of love, hate and curiosity, or the lack of curiosity, about the otherness of the other, are all variously addressed by every author. Each chapter is grounded in conceptual considerations, richly informed by clear clinical illustrations. As a result, practitioners arc invited to keep in mind that however vulnerable, or even absent, feelings of love might be for couples in conflict and distress, who come into treatment, rediscovering the developmental potential of a loving relationship might still be possible."

Stanley Ruszczynski, Psychoanalyst, former Clinical Director, Portman Clinic, Tavistock and Portman NHS Foundation Trust

"Without knowing it we have been waiting for this book! Morgan and Friend have assembled a unique collection of rich and beautifully written papers addressing the subject of love and its vicissitudes in the couple relationship and clinical work. Addressing various psychoanalytic perspectives, cultural themes, developmental registers and diverse populations, this book will remain an invaluable resource for years to come."

Rachael Peltz, Psychoanalyst, Former Co-Director Community Psychoanalysis Track, Psychoanalytic Institute of Northern California

"This timely volume returns love to the center of psychoanalytic couple therapy, where it belongs. Edited by two deeply experienced clinicians from different backgrounds, it offers a rich range of theoretical, clinical, and cultural perspectives, deepening our understanding of love's complexities, transformations, and vulnerabilities in intimate relationships. Essential reading for clinicians working with couples and for thoughtful readers interested in love."

Elizabeth Palacios, Psychoanalyst, Chair COFAP (IPA Couple and Family Committee)

"Love and couples. They go together. Yet love has been relatively neglected as a focus in couple psychoanalysis. This book brings love in from the cold with a brilliant collection of papers from around the world, evidence that couple psychoanalysis has arrived as an international discipline. Including cutting-edge thinkers and many analytic perspectives, the editors have created a remarkably coherent, insightful, and much-needed book, bringing fresh thinking to our understanding of love and of our attempts as clinicians to help those who come to us with developmental injuries in their capacities to love and be loved."

Andrew Balfour, Consultant Clinical Psychologist, Adult & Couple Psychotherapist; Chief Executive at Tavistock Relationships

Love, its Meaning and Exploration in Couple Therapy

Love, its Meaning and Exploration in Couple Therapy explores essential questions about love in couple relationships and couple therapy.

The respected international contributors assembled here consider a range of topics in relation to love: its place in the consulting room, what love means to couples and whether this can be problematic, specific challenges for same-sex couples, love in non-monogamous relationships, and the impacts of cultural difference. Each chapter considers an aspect of love and psychoanalytic practice or theory with openness and curiosity, providing a valuable and vibrant perspective on this essential topic. The contributing authors offer a variety of perspectives on love reflecting different theoretical perspectives and conceptual frameworks.

Love, its Meaning and Exploration in Couple Therapy will be essential reading for all clinicians who want to understand, and find new ways of working with, love in intimate adult relationships.

Mary Morgan is a psychoanalyst and consultant couple psychoanalytic psychotherapist. She is a leading figure in the field of couple psychoanalysis and is author of several books, chapters and articles in the field, including *A Couple State of Mind: Psychoanalysis of Couples and the Tavistock Relationships Model* (2019) and *Couple Relations: A Contemporary Introduction* (2025), both published by Routledge.

Julie Friend is a psychoanalytic psychotherapist serving individuals and couples and offering professional consultation. A founding member of the Psychoanalytic Couple Psychotherapy Group of the San Francisco Bay Area, she is past director of their Intensive Study Program and current core faculty. She also sits on the editorial board of *Couple and Family Psychoanalysis*. Her publications (2013, 2021) have explored creative engagement and love in couple relationships.

The Library of Couple and Family Psychoanalysis

Series Editors: Christopher Clulow, Brett Kahr, Elizabeth Palacios and David Scharff

The library offers the best of psychoanalytically informed writing on adult partnerships and couple psychotherapy. A full list of the titles in the series can be found at https://www.routledge.com/The-Library-of-Couple-and-Family-Psychoanalysis/book-series/KARNLCFP.

Recent titles in the series:

Interpretation in Couple and Family Psychoanalysis: Cross-Cultural Perspectives
Edited by Timothy Keogh and Elizabeth Palacios

Marriage and Family in Modern China: A Psychoanalytic Exploration
David E. Scharff

Same-Sex Couples and Other Identities: Psychoanalytic Perspectives
Edited by Damian McCann

Sensate Focus and the Psyche: Integrating Sense and Sexuality in Couple Therapy
Susan Pacey

Couples as Parents: Explorations in Couple Therapy
Edited by Kate Thompson and Damian McCann

Life and Death: Our Relationship with Ageing, Dementia, and Other Fates of Time
Andrew Balfour

Love, its Meaning and Exploration in Couple Therapy
Edited by Mary Morgan and Julie Friend

Love, its Meaning and Exploration in Couple Therapy

Edited by
Mary Morgan and Julie Friend

Routledge
Taylor & Francis Group
LONDON AND NEW YORK

Designed cover image: Rachel Davis, racheldavisstudio.com.

First published 2027
by Routledge
4 Park Square, Milton Park, Abingdon, Oxon OX14 4RN

and by Routledge
605 Third Avenue, New York, NY 10158

Routledge is an imprint of the Taylor & Francis Group, an informa business

British Library Cataloguing-in-Publication Data
A catalogue record for this book is available from the British Library

Library of Congress Cataloging-in-Publication Data
A catalog record has been requested for this book

ISBN: 978-1-032-85425-0 (hbk)
ISBN: 978-1-032-85423-6 (pbk)
ISBN: 978-1-003-51812-9 (ebk)

DOI: 10.4324/9781003518129

Typeset in Times New Roman
by Taylor & Francis Books

To Philip Stokoe and Philip Dreyfus, and to our families with love

Contents

Contributors

Rachel Cooke, PsyD, is a clinical psychologist in private practice in Oakland, California, in-person and via Zoom. She sees couples and individuals and provides consultation to couple therapists. She is a founding member, faculty and current board president for the Psychoanalytic Couple Psychotherapy Group (PCPG), which is the Bay Area's training program for psychoanalytic couple therapists. She presented two papers for IPA Couple and Family Psychoanalysis Committee (COFAP) in 2020. Her discussions of two visiting scholars' papers, given at PCPG's annual lecture, are published in the volumes edited by Shelley Nathans, titled *Couples on the couch* and *More about couples on the couch* (Routledge, 2017 and 2022).

Julie Friend, LCSW, BCD, is a psychoanalytic psychotherapist working with individuals and couples and offering professional consultation to individuals and groups. A board and founding member of the Psychoanalytic Couple Psychotherapy Group, she was director of its three-year Intensive Study Program from 2010 to 2022 and she continues to serve there as core faculty and on its curriculum committee. She is a member of the editorial board of the journal *Couple and Family Psychoanalysis*, invited faculty at William Alanson White's Couple Therapy Training and Education Program, and an associate member of the San Francisco Center for Psychoanalysis. She has presented her work and teaches at various institutes and groups nationally and internationally. Her previous publications include "Love as creative illusion and its place in psychoanalytic couple psychotherapy" (2013) and "Creative illusion in couples: Thoughts about the value of transitional experience for couple relationships" (2021).

Gary Grossman, PhD, is a clinical psychologist and psychoanalyst in San Francisco with a career spanning more than four decades. Dr Grossman is a volunteer clinical professor in the Department of Psychiatry & Behavioral Sciences, University of California, San Francisco. He is a training and consulting analyst for the San Francisco Center for Psychoanalysis, and personal analyst for the Psychoanalytic Institute of Northern California. He has taught and presented locally, nationally and internationally on psychoanalysis and psychotherapy with queer and gay men. Dr Grossman chaired the American Psychoanalytic Association's Committee on Gender & Sexuality from 2000 to 2005. He is on the editorial board of the *Journal of Gay & Lesbian Mental Health* and a co-editor of the "Sex & gender" section of *Psychoanalytic terms & concepts* (Auchincloss & Samberg, eds, 2012).

Timothy Keogh, PhD, is a training analyst and past president of the Australian Psychoanalytical Society, an adjunct associate professor (University of Sydney) and a visiting professor (Tongji Medical College, Huazhong University of Science & Technology, Wuhan, China). He is also founding president of *Penthos*, a psychoanalytic charity for couples, co-chair (Asia-Pacific) of the IPA Committee on Couple and Family Psychoanalysis (COFAP) and newly appointed chair of the IPA Scientific Committee (SCIPA). He co-edited *Psychoanalytic approaches to loss: Mourning melancholia and couples* (Routledge) with Cynthia Gregory-Roberts and *Interpretation in couple and family psychoanalysis: Cross-cultural perspectives* (English edition Routledge; Spanish edition Psimatica) with Elizabeth Palacios. He is a member of the international editorial board of *Couple and Family Psychoanalysis.*

Dr Ortal Kirson-Trilling, PsyD, is a personal and supervising analyst trained at the Psychoanalytic Institute of Northern California. Dr Kirson-Trilling is on the editorial board of the *Journal of Couple and Family Psychoanalysis* and is the director of the Intensive Study Program for the Psychoanalytic Couple Psychotherapy Group (PCPG). She is a faculty member of PCPG and the San Francisco Center for Psychoanalysis (SFCP). She teaches analytic couple theory, practice and technique locally, nationally and internationally. She maintains a private practice in Oakland, California.

Dr Tao Lin is a psychoanalyst and a full training analyst of the International Psychoanalytical Association (IPA) and a couple psychoanalytic psychotherapist trained at Tavistock Relationships, London. He is a direct member of the IPA, a member of the IPA China Study Group, a member of Tavistock Relationships Association of Psychotherapists and Counsellors, and a guest member of the British Psychoanalytical Society (BPAS). He currently works in private practice in Beijing and teaches psychoanalytic theory and clinical practice in China. His main areas of interest are psychoanalysis – particularly Kleinian and Bionian thought – couple psychoanalytic psychotherapy, and their dialogue with Chinese philosophy and cultural narratives.

Damian McCann, DSysPsych, is a psychoanalytic couple psychotherapist working as a visiting clinician at Tavistock Relationships, London; adjunct faculty member of the International Psychotherapy Institute (IPI) Washington, DC; an associate of Queen Anne Street Practice, London;

and an editorial board member of *Couple & Family Psychoanalysis.* He is also a consultant systemic psychotherapist with many years of experience working with children, adolescents and their families. He has a particular interest in working with gender and sexual diversity in psychoanalytic practice and has published and taught widely on this topic. His doctoral research was concerned with understanding the meaning and impact of violence in the couple relationships of gay men and he is involved in developing approaches to working with couples more generally in which there is violence and abuse. He is the editor of *Same-sex couples and other identities: Psychoanalytic perspectives* (Routledge, 2021) and co-editor of *Couples as parents: Explorations in couple psychotherapy* (Routledge, 2024).

Perrine Moran is a psychodynamic psychotherapist and a couple psychoanalytic psychotherapist. She is a visiting lecturer and supervisor at Tavistock Relationships. She is the arts editor for *Couple and Family Psychoanalysis*, and a member of the editorial board of the *Revue Internationale de Psychanalyse de la Couple et de la Famille.* She is bilingual, works with individuals and couples in English and in French, and has a private practice in London. She is the author of *Love songs: Listening to couples* (Karnac Books, 2025) and co-editor of a special issue of *Couple and Family Psychoanalysis* on "Couples and families in film" (Spring 2025).

Mary Morgan is a psychoanalyst, consultant couple psychoanalytic psychotherapist, and a writer. She is fellow of the British Psychoanalytical Society, senior fellow of Tavistock Relationships and honorary member of the Polish Society for Psychoanalytic Psychotherapy. She is a consultant member of the International Psychoanalytic Association's Committee on Couple and Family Psychoanalysis (COFAP), a member of the editorial board of the *International Journal of Psychoanalysis* and a member of the international advisory board of the *Journal of Couple and Family Psychoanalysis.* At Tavistock Relationships, London, she was the reader in Couple Psychoanalysis and head of the MA and PD in Couple Psychoanalytic Psychotherapy. She has been part of developing couple psychotherapy training programmes in Sweden, the USA (San Francisco and New York) and Poland. Along with Andrew Balfour and Chrisopher Vincent, she co-edited *How couple relationships shape our world: Clinical practice, research and policy perspectives* (Karnac Books, 2012). Her book *A couple state of mind: Psychoanalysis of couples – the Tavistock Relationships model* (Routledge, 2019) is available in several languages. Her latest book *Couple relations: A contemporary introduction* was published by Routledge in 2025.

Dr Shelley Nathans is on the faculties of the Psychoanalytic Couple Psychotherapy Group, the Psychoanalytic Institute of Northern California, and the San Francisco Center for Psychoanalysis. She is the director/producer of the film, *Robert Wallerstein: 65 years at the center of* *psychoanalysis.* Her article, "Oedipus for everyone: Revitalizing the model for LBGTQ couples and single parent families", was published in *Psychoanalytic Dialogues*, 2021. She is co-editor, with Milton Schaefer, of *Couples on the Couch: Psychoanalytic Couple Psychotherapy and the Tavistock Model* (2017) and the editor of a second volume of collected papers about psychoanalytic couple psychotherapy titled, *More about couples on the couch: Approaching psychoanalytic couple psychotherapy from an expanded perspective* (2022). Dr Nathans is in private practice in Oakland, California.

Dr Judith Pickering is a psychoanalytic couple therapist, psychotherapist and Jungian analyst. She is author of *Being in love: Therapeutic pathways through psychological obstacles to love* (Routledge, 2008); *The search for meaning in psychotherapy: Spiritual practice, the apophatic way and Bion* (Routledge, 2019; winner of the 2020 American Board & Academy of Psychoanalysis clinical book award); *Transformation in love: Bion and the couple* (Routledge, forthcoming); and co-editor of *Recycling madness: Clinical writings of Giles Clark* (Routledge, 2025), as well as author of numerous articles on couple therapy, psychoanalysis and psychotherapy and musicology. Her PhD was on "Love and couple therapy". She is on the editorial boards of the *Journal of Analytical Psychology* and *The Journal of Couple and Family Psychotherapy.*

Karolina Pniewska is a psychotherapist of the Polish Society for Psychoanalytic Psychotherapy and board member of the Couple and Family Psychotherapy section. She has for many years been engaged in a wide range of professional and organizational initiatives dedicated to the advancement and promotion of psychoanalytic couple and family therapy in Poland, including the co-organization of the annual Warsaw conference, "Working psychoanalytically with couples". She is the scientific editor and initiator of the Polish edition of Dr Judith Pickering's *Being in Love.* She also convenes the literary-clinical seminar "On love", addressed to professionals specializing in therapeutic work with couples.

Philip Stokoe is a psychoanalyst in private practice working with adults and couples, and an organizational consultant, providing consultation to a wide range of organizations. He has been a senior manager in a range of health and social care settings since 1978, finally working in the adult department of the Tavistock & Portman NHS Foundation Trust between 1994 and 2012, where he was responsible for a wide range of successful innovations. He was the clinical director from 2007. He was a member of the European Psychoanalytic Federation Forum on Institutional Matters for 10 years (since 2015), which studies the nature of psychoanalytic institutions. His book, *The curiosity drive: Our need for inquisitive thinking*, was published by Phoenix Publishing in November 2020 and short-listed for the Gradiva® Award for Best Psychoanalytic Book in 2021.

Christopher Vincent, MA, BPhil, MPhil, is a couple psychotherapist, now retired from clinical practice. He has been a staff member and visiting lecturer at Tavistock Relationships and visiting lecturer at the Tavistock Clinic, London. His current interests are twofold. He writes, and helps others write, about the interface between the meaning of serious illness, couple functioning and couple psychoanalysis. In this endeavour, he is particularly interested in the bridges that may be made between phenomenology, psycho-social perspectives and psychoanalysis. He also offers consultations to colleagues who seek help in writing for publication.

Monica Vorchheimer is a training and supervising psychoanalyst at the Buenos Aires Psychoanalytical Association (APdeBA). She has a private practice in psychoanalysis with adolescents, adults, families and couples in Buenos Aires, Argentina. She teaches and lectures locally and abroad as a guest professor in several countries. She was co-chair for Latin America on the IPA Committee on Couples and Family Psychoanalysis (COFAP) and is currently a consultant member. She has published articles and chapters in books, and co-edited *Clinical dialogues on families and couples* (Karnac Books, 2017) with David Scharff.

Acknowledgements

We begin with our appreciation and heartfelt thanks to the contributors, without whom this book would not have come to fruition. Their inspiring and scholarly chapters offer a range of perspectives on love and expand our understanding of the complexity of love in the life of the couple and in relation to our therapeutic work.

Thank you to Routledge Press, and to publishers Susannah Frearson and Saloni Singhania, for their skilful oversight in bringing this book to life. We also wish to thank the editors of the Library of Couple and Family Psychoanalysis, Christopher Clulow, Brett Kahr, Elizabeth Palacios and David Scharff for supporting this project and including it in the series.

Additionally, we would like to thank Rachel Davis (racheldavisstudio.com) for the book's cover image. Finally, our thanks to Andrew Balfour, Rachael Peltz, Elizabeth Palacios and Stanley Ruszczynski, whose generous endorsements of this volume are much appreciated.

Mary Morgan

My warmest thanks to Julie Friend for collaborating with me on this project. It has been a creative and greatly enjoyable partnership.

I would like to thank the many colleagues who have encouraged my writing and teaching over the years and given me the inspiration to be part of bringing together a book such as this on couples and love. There are too many to name fully, but here I would like to acknowledge and thank those I have worked closely with in recent years in London, Warsaw, Poznan, Krakow, New York, San Francisco, Athens, Helsinki and Vienna. Listening to the different theoretical and clinical perspectives of others is central and has been an important part of editing this book. Thus, I would like to thank colleagues who have provided this opportunity through seminars and conferences – those from Tavistock Relationships, the IPA Committee on Couple and Family Psychoanalysis (COFAP) the International Association of Couple and Family Psychoanalysis (IACFP), the International Psychotherapy Institute, and the Couple and Family Section of European Federation of

Psychoanalytic Psychotherapy (EFPP). My thanks to Stanley Ruszczynski, Andrew Balfour, Vivian Eskin, Anna Nicolo, David Scharff, Elizabeth Palacios, Daniella Lucarelli and Cristina Călărăşanu. Finally, I would especially like to thank my family, for their unfailing patience, and encouragement.

Julie Friend

I begin with my heartfelt thanks to Mary Morgan. Bringing together our different perspectives on love, a subject of great interest to each of us, has made our collaboration on this book a great pleasure.

I have appreciated the opportunity to think with and learn not only from Mary, but from other scholars from Tavistock Relationships including Andrew Balfour, Christopher Clulow, David Hewison, Stanley Ruszczynski, Chris Vincent and the late James Fisher. Their thinking has deeply inspired me, as has my participation on the editorial board of Couple and Family Psychoanalysis.

It would be impossible to identify everyone who I would like to thank for their contribution to my clinical thinking, and thus to this project. Particularly noteworthy are my colleagues of several decades, Leora Benioff, Rachel Cooke, Shelley Nathans, Sandra Seidlitz and Milton Schaefer. Together we co-founded the Psychoanalytic Couple Psychotherapy Group training program in analytic couple therapy, which has grown into a stimulating intellectual community. Thanks to Ruth Kalb, Nancy Kaplan, Ortal Kirson-Trilling, Shelley Nathans, Rachael Peltz, Joan Sarnat and Milton Schaefer for their helpful critiques of my writing, to Leora Benioff and Elizabeth Palacios of COFAP, to Shelly Goldklank and Ethan Graham of William Alanson White CTTEP, to the seminar members connected with the Polish Society for Psychoanalytic Psychotherapy, to Perrine Moran, and to Vivan Eskin of CPCPNYC for enriching discussions. The ongoing challenge and privilege of clinical work, and of consultation and teaching, inspire and necessitate the continual rethinking that has gone into the editing of this volume. My thanks to all.

And finally, my deepest thanks to my husband Philip Dreyfus and to our family, for their love and support.

Introduction

Love cannot be captured in a singular definition. Most often it is experienced as a feeling, strong and passionate or deep and enduring but also fragile and evanescent. Couple therapy clinical experience sheds a bright light on the different perceptions and apperceptions of love. Here, the unique meaning of love for each couple as that love evolves and changes in the relationship can be seen. Thus, this book is relevant not only to couple therapists of all persuasions, but to all therapists seeking to understand the meaning of love for those they encounter in their work. Moreover, some of the authors in this book define therapy as love in action and thus this book potentially contributes to thinking about best therapy practice.

One of the important themes in this book is the challenge of facing the active process of loving another person over time, which involves recognizing, accepting and being curious about valuing their differences as well as their similarities. Several chapters refer to the illusion of "oneness", which helps to create the couple's bond, and the need for this to give way to disillusionment that allows for differentiation. As a relationship develops over time in older age and with mortality on the horizon, an essential question arises – can the loving bond contain each partner's vulnerabilities and dependency needs?

There are different assumptions underpinning some of the chapters. While most ideas originate within a Western cultural framework that supports heterosexual monogamy, there are cultural issues that impact upon identity and the realization of love both within and outside families. These are evident in the LGBTQ (lesbian, gay, bisexual, transgender and queer) and polyamory chapters, and also in those that address sociocultural factors impacting on couples and their legacies. These differences challenge some theoretical assumptions, and this is an area that merits further exploration and conceptualization.

As editors we are curious about what happens to love, both its development over time and the ways in which to love can be a challenge and may be turned away from. Love can feel uncertain or lost. Couple therapists know their work is not about encouraging the members of the couple to love each other, but its perceived absence may be one reason for the relatively spare appearance of the topic of love within the analytic couple therapy literature. This volume reflects our interest in an exploration of various ways couples think about and experience love and the meaning of love in the therapeutic encounter.

Love has been addressed to some extent in the broader realm of psychoanalysis. Freud, strongly influence by Plato, saw love as a life force, underpinning his view that the goals of treatment were to have the capacity to love and to work. Ethel Spector Person (1988) explored the phenomenology of love, with a particular interest in romantic and transference love, and noted that psychoanalysis, like "most academic disciplines either ignore[s] love or treat[s] it in accordance with the rationalist tradition" (Person, 1988, p. 16). Otto Kernberg (1995) detailed what he viewed as the multiple component psychological capacities he considered necessary for a mature love relationship. From a relational perspective, Stephen Mitchell (2002) asked the question "Can love last?", in which he described romance in a relationship as "a sandcastle for two" that requires continual rebuilding. Judith Pickering explored a wide range of definitions of love in various iterations, and underscored love's power as an agent of change and development (Pickering, 2008). More recently, Michael Parsons (2024) situates love as central to the psychoanalytic endeavour.

As colleagues we have previously each approached the topic of love from different perspectives. Julie Friend, taking a middle-school perspective and enlisting the thinking of Winnicott and Bollas, has explored love's potential as a context of transitional experience, in which creative engagement with life can be fostered. Mary Morgan has taken Bion's notation of L, H & K and explored the creative interrelationship between love, hate and curiosity in the development of creative couple relating.

This volume includes a variety of perspectives on love, reflecting different theoretical perspectives and conceptual frameworks. The contributing authors, all experienced psychoanalytic clinicians, address key aspects of love in relationships stemming from their experience of working with couples. They draw our attention to vital aspects of love seen in couple relationships of which the couple therapist can be cognisant. These include love's changing nature over time, for example: the "in love" state and its development into mature love; the transformation of couple love as it develops into family love in Chinese culture (or, in Taoist philosophy); the relationship between love, attachment and sexuality over time; different phantasies of love that stem from the most primitive layers of psychic development; and the impacts of ageing on love. Several authors elaborate the creative and transformational potential of love. Explorations of the impact of societal and cultural norms on the different forms love relationships can take and how they are experienced are described. These include, same sex couples, interracial and intercultural couples, and non-monogamous love relationships. The belief that love is foundational in couple relationships within Western culture is questioned and seen as problematic if it cannot be transformed from its narcissistic foundation into a love that is object-related and can accommodate difference and uncertainty.

Love: its presence, absence and meaning

In the opening section, Morgan, Friend and Pickering each offer their perspectives on love – its presence, absence and meaning in couple relationships.

In Chapter 1, "The fate of love in intimate relationships", Mary Morgan asks the question "What has happened to love?", both in the course of the couple's relationship and in the therapeutic encounter. Drawing on the work of Bion, in which he formulates the minus forms of L, H & K as a turning way from love, hate or wanting to know another, she explores what might lead a couple to a minus L form of relating, a state that Bion sees as indifference, leading to apathy. One idea, familiar in the couple analytic literature, is the difficulty in managing disillusionment in moving from the "in love" state to the mature love state. In addition, she explores the complex relationship between love and hate, the fear of being loved and loving, love as part of a merger, internalized prohibitions on love stemming from the world outside, and the idea that a mature love, or depressive position love, can sometimes become an uncreative retreat.

In Chapter 2, Julie Friend explores the question "Does love matter in the consulting room?" within the couple relationship and within the treatment relationship. She argues that in addition to the importance of helping couples tolerate ambivalence and the reality that one person cannot completely know another, we also remain aware that love can evoke moments of confluence between reality and imagination, a creative experience of idiomatic aliveness. Placing love at the heart of the therapeutic endeavour, Friend asserts that, in addition to the importance of understanding the projective dynamics that structure couple relationships, we should be cognisant that our clinical attention is in itself a form of love – a vital substrate for emotional growth and development.

In her encyclopaedic and wide-ranging chapter, Chapter 3, "A question of true love?", Judith Pickering brings a broad view of the numerous fluid and inherently creative potentials of love. Grounding her chapter in the premise that love relationships offer a context for "transformation into our true selves", she describes multiple definitions and perspectives on the meaning of love over time and through different philosophical lenses. Love, she says, can enable us to confront, work through and heal relational lacks, losses and traumas that have constrained our full potential. She emphasizes the developmental significance of moving from the "in love" state, through inevitable disillusionment, to a fuller relational intimacy grounded in recognizing and appreciating the alterity of the other. In agreement with Levinas, she sees this developmental path as holding the potential for an increased sense of sanctity, wonder, compassion, altruism, and gratitude.

Love, attachment and sexuality

Shelley Nathans asks whether erotic desire and attachment are incompatible, as is often assumed in popular culture and in much psychoanalytic literature. In Chapter 4, "The dialectics of attachment, sexuality, and love in couple relationships", she interrogates the common presumption that the need for security on the one hand and erotic desire on the other are separate and mutually negating forces. She questions the limitations that result when such an assumed opposition is enlisted to explain – and simplify – the many complexities and challenges inherent to adult romantic relationships. In contrast, she proposes that, as love is a complex experience, it is better understood from a perspective that recognizes the dialectical relationships between attachment, sex and love, rather than their opposition to one another.

Love and transformation

With the increasing emphasis on the interpersonal and relational aspects of psychic life over the past few decades, several chapters focus on the value of contributions by Winnicott, Bollas and Bion looking at love as holding, transformative, and containing developmental potential.

In Chapter 5, "Love is where we start from", Ortal Kirson-Trilling places love at the heart of relational and psychic life. She demonstrates the developmental potential in an individual's willingness --and ability – to encounter the alterity of their partner, and she addresses the challenges in doing so, especially as a consequence of relational trauma. In Kirson-Trilling's view, love is learned and psychic growth is generated through the process of learning about the other. It is through this complex process, more challenging in the context of relational trauma, that we come to understand, and love, the needed other, creating and strengthening our senses of both self and other.

Karolina Pniewska, in Chapter 6, "You make me feel …", invites us to consider how love sometimes distorts in order to transform. Exploring Bollas's concept of transformational object in love relationships, she describes couple relationships as operating in an oscillation between what could be described as an experience of the other in terms of Winnicott's transitional object and that of Bollas's concept of the transformational object. She suggests that (re-)finding and acknowledging the transformational function in the other person forms the foundation of falling in love, and of mature love in general. Pniewska expands our understanding of love, emphasizing the power of the experience of the other as possessing transformational possibility, which she sees as holding enriching potential for the relationship and the individuals within it. In so doing, she invites us to reconsider our clinical focus, shifting our understanding of familiar couple dilemmas and our measure of healthy couple-relating and offering an additional frame to include in our work.

Love in primitive states

Philip Stokoe, in Chapter 7, and Timothy Keogh, in Chapter 8, each enrich our understanding of the impacts on love of the needs and dynamics in couples when the other is required for their psychic survival and thus not experienced as a separate other. Each of these chapters outlines the developmental challenges to love in the context of primitive mental states, as well as giving technical recommendations in relation to working with such couples.

Stokoe notes that, for borderline couples or individuals, merger is misperceived as love. Such couples often appear in our consulting rooms experiencing the loss of the desired experience of merger, which is felt as catastrophic. How, then, do we help? In Chapter 7, "Helping borderline couples find love", Stokoe details the profound impacts to the sense of self in the face of difference, and details various "solutions", such as sado-masochistic bonds that are activated between the members of the couple to escape the terrors of feeling utterly alone and disintegrated. Through case examples he delineates the clinical perspective and interventions that address the underlying fears that underpin demands for merger, offering a thoughtful clinical framework for helping such couples.

Timothy Keogh also asserts that the capacity for mature love, exemplified by a capacity for a mutual and reciprocal relationship, is inextricably linked to the level of psychic development exemplified in the couple relationship. In Chapter 8, "Primitive layers of love", Keogh discusses couples whose love and associated sexuality is rooted in the most primitive layers of psychic development. In these couples, the other is experienced as a means of psychic necessity, rather than wanted as a desired other. Keogh shows that the capacity to bear separation and to be able to think about the state of mind and feelings of another, without feeling one's own existence is erased or at too much risk, is challenging for such couples. This can result a compromised ability to love, including the exploitation of sexuality in defensive ways. Through clinical vignettes, he demonstrates the technical considerations in working with this primitive form of relating.

Love and same sex relationships

In Chapter 9, "On love, loss and longing in lesbian couple relationships", Rachel Cooke describes how certain lesbian couples often seem to impose on each other a host of demands to be "seen and understood" that, when met, produce the most fulfilling loving states. When these go unmet, however, the feeling is one of near catastrophic disappointment, and the partners lurch between feelings of being deeply connected and a correspondingly torturous disconnect. The impacts of these painful vacillations are explored in terms of the lost connection with the mother. An unconscious pressure to restore something akin to the earliest infantile symbiotic experience can result. She sees this as expressing itself as a tendency in lesbian women to look particularly closely at the ebbs and flows of emotional relating. This need for precise attunement strains the capacity to sustain love and demonstrates in various ways the old adage that 'perfect is the enemy of the good'.

In Chapter 10, "Obstacles to love in gay male coupling", Gary Grossman explores the impacts of "growing up in a society that values other sex eroticism and relationships" while devaluing those between members of the same sex. Drawing on his extensive experience of working with gay men individually and in couple relationships, he illustrates the impacts of such ongoing misrecognition, particularly throughout oedipal development, for boys whose erotic and relational desires are different from those expected by their parents. Grossman describes the consequent shame and humiliation that such misrecognition can engender, and the complicating subsequent effect on their adult relational and sexual life. While increasing diversity in relationships may enable more empathic connection by parents with children who have same-sex desires, the individuals and couples presenting for help now have usually not had this experience.

Love and the influence of culture

In Chapter 11, "All you need is love?", Monica Vorchheimer interrogates the common assumption in Western culture that love is enough as a foundation for couple relationships. She explores what she sees as wide discrepancies between our cultural assumptions about love in contrast with the realities of couple relationships. Vorchheimer grounds her enquiry through the lens of link theory, demonstrating both its relevance and its distinction from more familiar psychoanalytic approaches. From the perspective of link theory, what binds the couple together is not only reciprocal love between two individuals, but the unconscious structure that emerges in the encounter itself. This unconscious structure, created by them, also constitutes them. This representation of their togetherness – the "we" – is vulnerable to collapse when confronted with difference. This may be experienced not only as the loss of love but as the loss of identity as a couple.

In Chapter 12, "The evolution of love through psychoanalytic and Daoist perspectives", Tao Lin enlists both psychoanalytic theory – from Winnicott, Bick and others – and ancient Chinese philosophy, describing the evolutionary path of love "from narcissism to Da Ai (Great Love)". Drawing on philosophical analysis, literary examples and psychoanalytic theory, including Morgan's conception of "creative couple" functioning, he interrogates the origins of love, which he states are always intertwined with the theme of "sad beauty". The acceptance of "life in its entirety" includes facing the disillusionment that lovers inevitably encounter, and the acceptance of which he sees as holding the potential for a path to enlightenment. The author believes that understanding the meaning of love is deeply linked to understanding the meaning of our lives.

In Chapter 13, "Somewhere there's a place for us …", Perrine Moran explores the challenges – and opportunities – of difference in intercultural relationships from the perspective of her understanding that "difference is on the side of life". She considers various factors that might draw individuals from different backgrounds together, as well as exploring the efficacy and limitations of our customary theoretical tools in relation to cultural difference. Moran considers it important to include link theory in our thinking with intercultural and interracial couples to help us understand the challenges such couples face in developing their unique relationship, a new creation, rather than being bound to inherited models of relating.

Damian McCann, in Chapter 14, "Open and polyamorous relationships", notes that non-monogamous relationships are often negatively contrasted with the assumed advantages of monogamy and fidelity, implicitly questioning the quality of love within open and poly affiliations. How do we begin to think about the needs of individuals within a couple when relating romantically or sexually to others outside that relationship? Yet some studies show non-monogamous couples feeling able to maintain their primary relationship, as the strongest source of comfort, reliability and security, alongside emotional and sexual intimacy with others. For others the primary relationship can come to feel under threat and the needs of each partner may not easily be brought into alignment. McCann argues that the complexities of open and polygamous relationship points to the need for a greater awareness and openness in the therapist, in order to fully engage with and understand the conscious and unconscious processes at work.

Love in later life

We close our exploration on the meaning of love in couple relationships with Chris Vincent's rich and wide-ranging chapter on love and older age. In Chapter 15, "Love as a containing function in later years – or its victim", he considers several interrelated questions about love itself, and what we mean by old age. He highlights distinctive opportunities and stresses experienced by couples in later life and considers how couple psychotherapists have responded to them. He addresses the material effects of ageing, whether healthy or marked by constraining and life-altering illness, societal attitudes, available support services and the lack thereof. Ageing, especially (but not only) if it includes infirmity, brings dependency and the feelings about it take centre stage in couple relationships, sometimes altering long-established relational patterns. Discussing the alterations that ageing, illness and increased dependency have on couple relationships, he frames our work as – optimally – helping couples develop a "love that tolerates each partner's vulnerabilities, foibles and differences in a shared experiential world where each partner knows, consciously or not, that time is running out and that one will outlast the other".

Love's relatively spare appearance in the psychoanalytic literature on couple therapy inspired us to explore how others in the field think about love. Love has historically appeared in the context of drive theory, or as a repetition of early relationships. We felt that the complexity and creative potential of love, and of love's fuller importance psychically, had not been fully developed. Our vision for this volume was to expand the meaning of love through its exploration in analytic couple therapy. This collection draws from clinical experience, various theoretical perspectives and cultural observations to help illuminate how love operates in the consulting room within the couple relationship as well as in the therapeutic relationship.

Alongside the many issues that are brought to the attention of couple therapists, we consider that love itself is indeed important to recognize, explore and understand. The thoughtful contributions herein of different experiences of and perspectives on love in couple relationships can expand our thinking, helping us consider more fully how we understand and address love in our therapeutic work.

References

Person, E.S. (1988). *Dreams of Love and Fateful Encounters.* New York: Penguin.

Kernberg, O. (1995). *Love relations: Normality and pathology.* Yale University Press.

Pickering, J. (2008). *Being in love: Therapeutic pathways through psychological obstacles to love.* Routledge.

Mitchell, S. (2003). Review of *Can love last? The fate of romance over time. Psychoanalytic Psychology,* 20 (2): 395–399.

Parsons, M. (2024). Practice and praxis: Psychoanalysis as an act of love. *Psychoanalytic Quarterly,* 92 (2): 219–248.

Chapter 1

The fate of love in intimate relationships

Mary Morgan

Love is widely considered both within and outside psychoanalysis as a basic human drive. For most couples it is through love that they form a bond. When a couple present for help with their relationship they are often struggling with issues that seem a long way from love, for example with managing difference, depression, betrayal, anger and anxiety. A question in my mind, is what has happened to love? What path has love taken in the course of the couple's relationship and how is this manifested in the analytic session in its present or absent forms.

Some couples do bring love as their concern. As the relationship has evolved and love has become represented in many different ways – emotionally, physically, sexually and concretely and in the couple's beliefs about their unique bond – the meaning of love for each partner may cause disharmony. One partner's felt expression of love may not be felt as love by the other and vice versa. Evidence of being loved on one's own terms might not be forthcoming from the other and anxiety may ensue about whether they still love and feel loved by the other.

In this chapter I explore the fate of love – some of the problematic paths that love can take in couple relationships. As couple analysts we might be curious about what has happened to love and what is curtailing it now and, further, whether we might incorporate an understanding of this within our work. Analytic work in this area might turn out to be an important and unexpected part of couple analysis.

Minus L

I'd like to begin this exploration of the fate of love with Wilfred Bion and his thoughts about minus L. Bion fruitfully conceived of a system of symbols to describe different forms of emotional links in relating. He was referring to the emotional key of a psychoanalytic session, which I also consider but expand to include the couple's relationship over time. Bion used the letters K (for knowing), H (for hate) and L (for love), each with a positive (+) or negative (–) prefix. L, H & K are states of mind but they are also drives, which are a

DOI: 10.4324/9781003518129-1

healthy part of relating to another and to life (Bion, 1962). Bion essentially reformulates and expands the three basic human instincts that had so far been devised by psychoanalytic theory: the life and death instincts described by Freud (Freud, 1920) and the epistemophilic instinct, described by Melanie Klein (Klein, 1928).

The experience of a drive being activated in one is a feeling, the intensity of such depends on one's capacity to manage the feeling. Thus, the positive of the loving drive is a loving urge. Taken together L, H & K seem fundamental in human relating and are thought about by Ronald Britton as follows, "Human beings have an urge to love, to hate, to know, and a desire to be loved, a fear of being hated and a wish to be understood" (Britton, 1998).

However, it is important to note that for Bion "*–L is not the same as H, nor –H the same as L*" *(* Bion, 1962, p. 52) In the minus key L, H & K turn away from or deny these drives. Minus L is the switching off of the loving urge. I find this a very interesting way of thinking about problems with love, i.e. that there is a turning away from something that is fundamental to our being. It makes me think about why one might turn away from love.

Thus, although most couples do not present for therapy in loving states, if thought about in this way, we could consider that love is in fact very present in couple therapy, though often in Bion's minus L form. Reflecting on my own clinical practice I noted that I sometimes see loving gestures from one partner to the other that are not noticed, ignored or turned away from, or that cannot freely be expressed.

Several analysts have explored K and minus K, which can also be thought about as the curiosity drive as elaborated by Philip Stokoe (2021). An important part of this elaboration of K is a consideration of what it is that closes down curiosity and turns instead to a minus K state of mind, one of certainty, which is also described as a fundamentalist state of mind (Stokoe, 2021; Fisher 2006). I mention this here as I think K and minus K are linked to love and to a turning away from love.

Less has been written about minus L and, actually, it seems that in Bion's work, minus L itself was not elaborated very fully. Freud had, in 1915, observed:

> Loving admits not merely of one, but of three opposites. In addition to the antithesis "loving–hating", there is the other one of "loving–being loved"; and, in addition to these, loving and hating taken together are the opposite of the condition of unconcern or indifference.
>
> (Freud, 1915, p. 133)

For Bion minus L was not just about the absence or repudiation of love but also how apathy can result through the mechanism of indifference. Thus, minus L is, in my view, inextricably linked to minus K in Bion's thinking. This is because activating interest and curiosity must be some sort of antidote to minus L.

The state of indifference leading to apathy is very different to the linking up of L with a K state of mind. This, Fisher evocatively describes as being, "a very powerful experience, whether it be a nursing mother and her infant or two adults 'falling in love'". He continues,

> We experience this when we (re-)discover the coming together of our infantile capacity for both "*K*-impulses" and "*L*-impulses". Think of Count Almásy in *The English Patient* wanting to know the geography of his lover's body, the hollow at the base of her neck (Ondaatje, 1992, p. 162). Having someone genuinely curious, wanting to know you, can be a very erotic experience.
>
> (Fisher, 2006)

Does Bion's understanding of L and minus L help us in our work with couples? Couple therapists know their work is not about encouraging the couple to love each other, which unfortunately would not work, but about bringing into our couple analytic thinking an understanding of what has happened to L and is happening to L in their encounter with each other and their analyst.

So, what is it that causes individuals in a relationship to turn away from love, or to repudiate the emotional link of L? And what forms can minus L take in intimate couple relating? In what follows I explore the disillusionment in the relinquishment of the "in love" state, the relationship between love and hate, fear of love, love as merger, prohibition on love and depressive position love sometimes becoming a retreat.

Love lost through disillusionment

The move from the "falling in love" state or "romantic love" to a more "mature love" state is the most fully explored problem with love from a couple psychoanalytic perspective. Falling in love and then being in love is usually temporary and often encompasses heightened emotional states, intense sexual feelings, merger and illusion. This intense state is powerful and can enable one to take the risk of making a committed bond to another person.

Once in love there might be no impetus (at least for a while) to test reality. Engaging in the fantasied "in love" universe is preferable yet reality, wanted or not, usually intervenes. It is not usually a total illusion – the "psychoses" Freud refers to – but positive aspects of the other may be exaggerated, similarities may be sought and less pleasing aspects of the other ignored or downplayed.

The loss of this heightened state may not be what the couple present as their problem, in fact the couple rarely present it in this conceptualized way. However, the analyst may witness their disappointment and their struggle with the disillusionment of the fantasy of the relationship they had once had. What had bound them together effortlessly, and now requires increasing effort as reality intrudes, is coming apart. The magical feeling of having found "the one", is replaced by the work of love.

One could say that in the "in love" state H and K do not have a strong presence. The loving connection between the pair is not yet one that incorporates hate and the illusion of oneness means K – in the sense of getting to know the other as they really are – is not needed. The disillusionment paves the way for love to come into connection with the drives and emotional linking of H & K.

For many this developmental change is accepted and the idea of having found "the one" becomes an exploration of finding "the other". This involves giving the object its freedom from one's omnipotent phantasy of knowing them completely or needing them to fulfil the needs of the self.

Fisher describes it thus,

> Knowing held in tension with the emotional links of love and hate requires that the object remain always outside the orbit of either the impulse to possess or to control and destroy. Meltzer describes this as the "enigmatic" quality of the object.
>
> (Fisher, 2000, p. 972)

For some, feelings one had before do not feel entirely lost but a more reality-based version of the other comes into being. For others it may feel a real stumbling block, that love is in fact lost. The disappointment and anxiety that this creates can interfere with a natural process of allowing a different kind of love to develop. At this point one might say real love is just beginning, but having mistakenly identified idealized love as real love, there may be a turning away from love, a minus L state in one or both partners.

It is also interesting to consider why this becomes a crisis for some. One way of thinking about this is that, as Freud put it, "The finding of an object is in fact a refinding of it" (Freud, 1905, p. 222).

The loss of, and re-finding of, the intimate connection that was experienced earlier in life with one's primary object may be a powerful component of the in-love experience. However, this kind of primitive love in the infant is fused with dependency on the primary object for survival, which is not the same as love that develops between two adults – in which it is not only about one's own needs but about care and concern for the other. The unresolved earlier loss of the primary object may be painfully reactivated. Futile attempts to reconstitute the other as an ideal may in some cases lead to a depressive withdrawal, or a seeking of the ideal object outside the relationship.

Another reason that this step can be so hard to make is that relinquishment of the idealized state is a loss, requiring mourning of what can no longer be, and this can throw the couple into a state of "not knowing". Now there is a different mindset of having to get to know "an other" as they really are, and this means encountering difference, otherness and aspects of the other that are hated as well as loved. The feeling of oneness departs as the experience of never being able to fully know an other emerges and no one knows where this is going to lead. Uncertainty and unpredictability, while potentially creative, can create intense anxiety (Puget, 2010).

It may be, however, that aspects of the in-love state of mind are not completely given up. In a healthy relationship in which there is safety, states of unintegration in the relationship are re-encountered as the couple continue to reconfigure their relationship creatively. According to Angela Joyce:

> As a couple relationship gets established, there are regressive pulls to the illusory state of merger and one-ness, which might be dangerous if in the two individuals this is predicated on the collapse of the paradox that allowed the illusion to be experienced originally. This is the paradox of one-ness and two-ness, with mother and infant as one, although, in objective reality, they are two. I would say that this collapse *is* the state of disintegration, a disaster that heralds the possibility of annihilation and ushers defences with which to fend off this catastrophe. This is not the same as un-integration, which is a creative, generative state of possibilities.
>
> (Joyce, 2019, p. 161)

To be able to return to states of illusory unintegration rather than disintegration in an adult couple relationship, Joyce points out that there needs to be a sufficient sense of safety to contain this regression. Julie Friend also explores these regressive and potentially creative states in couple relations. She believes that even in more mature love, illusion remains including the aspects of idealization, fantasy and merged boundaries. She argues:

> Illusion is indispensable as a form of vitalising engagement with life, and it is often through an experience of love and merger with another that it is refreshed and re-created.
>
> (Friend, 2013, p. 12)

John Steiner suggests that in mature love the couple may still continue to believe the illusion, even though they now know it is not true.

> Perhaps here, in the cradle we find the earliest appearance of irony in our lives, which may then be established as a critical step on the path to mature love. It enables us to enjoy an illusion while remaining aware it is not quite real.
>
> (Steiner, 2024, p. 569)

The illusory state may be returned to at different times in the couple's life cycle, or in the to and fro of their daily interaction without the reality of separateness and difference being lost. But without the playful capacity to move between reality and illusion the development towards mature love might be curtailed.

Love and hate

> The part played by love may escape notice because envy, rivalry and hate obscure it, although hate would not exist if love were not present.
>
> (Bion 1962, p. 10)

Following Bion's notation of L, H & K as the main drives and keys of emotional relating, it is useful to consider how they sometimes interact. Can love be hidden or defended against by hate? Referring to the work of Melanie Klein, which takes us into the complex arena of depressive position love, one can see why loving feelings may be avoided. Steiner writes:

> Once we recognize that love is not simply romantic and libidinal, but carries a deep burden of sorrow, guilt, and anxiety, in relation to loved and endangered objects, we can better understand that patients may find love too painful, and will try to avoid and deflect loving feelings, sometimes by increasing hatred and grievance. This means that love is sometimes buried beneath hate and is only released as the hate is analysed.
>
> (Steiner, 2017, audio presentation)

Members of a couple can sometimes hold onto a grievance, as it can give the aggrieved one a sense of agency, control and power in the relationship. Some couples describe events that occurred earlier in their relationship, often a betrayal, an abandonment or a perceived injury, which are brought up and felt as if they were happening in the current moment. The offending partner is rendered powerless to undo what cannot be undone. Thus, when the grievance takes hold, the power dynamic in the relationship can feel reversed. However, the grievance might operate as protection from the vulnerability that comes with loving another.

As well as hate hiding love, especially in a grievance, hate can interact more creatively with love and the wish to know another. We can also see how these interact, for example, as described above, K being an important part of L. Elsewhere I have written about L and H interacting in a potentially creative way, whereas minus L leading to apathy or minus H denying hate is not creative in any sense (Morgan, 2019, 2026). However, some couples can feel alarmed to discover the hatred in their minds and as manifest in their relationship, and thus for some it goes underground (minus H). Couples in therapy sometimes verbally deny their hatred of the other and yet it is palpably in the room. There is a belief that this has no place in a loving relationship and yet it is part of the essence of a real connection with an intimate other.

Without allowing room for hate, it can then be acted out in destructive behaviour or have an ongoing, insidious effect on a relationship, including a couple's sexual relationship. Suppressed hate or unacknowledged hate may block love and liveliness, and it may also lead to a turning away from the other. Knowing about hate, alongside love, leads to development in the relationship.

In Kernberg's view:

> The ambivalence of all relationships implies that events of mutual aggression are unavoidable in the course of a life lived together but, by the same token, the possibility of their clarification and resolution carries with it the possibility of further strengthening and deepening the relationship.
>
> (Kernberg, 2011, p. 1512)

According to Stephen Mitchell:

> A love that has endured episodic aggression has a depth and resilience obtainable in no other way. Because of love's profound risks, hatred is its inevitable accompaniment, and, paradoxically, the survival of romance depends not on the skill in avoiding aggression but on the capacity to contain it alongside love … the inhibition in hating a potential object of desire can serve as an obstacle to the development of romantic passion.
>
> (Mitchell, 2002, p. 120)

The complications of loving – the ambivalence that accompanies it and the risks in loving and allowing oneself to be loved – picked up by these two authors highlight some of the complexities of loving over time. Some individuals become defeated by these difficult times in their relationship and may give up on love. Others find the strength to continue, and, in that process, they build up their relationship as stronger container.

Fear of love – being loved and loving

For those who have had a good-enough early experience that has enabled them to develop basic trust and an internal sense of security, it feels much more possible to love and allow oneself to be loved in an ordinary and non-idealized way. I have described earlier the wish to return to an earlier idealized state of love in which one was contained by a loving other. This is clearly not everyone's experience. If there has not been sufficient containment, an absence of reliable holding earlier in life, an experience of insecure attachment, or if the person has suffered trauma or abuse, then they may find it very difficult to trust an other. Love may feel dangerous as loving another and allowing oneself to be loved by another, makes one vulnerable to hurt, rejection and abandonment.

Joe & Lucy

A heterosexual couple in their 30s, each from different European countries, Joe and Lucy met in London while undertaking postgraduate study. This couple seemed to have experienced a lack of ordinary maternal containment and considerable disturbance in relation to the primary object. Joe's mother had a psychotic illness. He described how as a child he felt he could not penetrate his mother's mind and was fearful of what lay behind what he perceived as her "glazed eyes". Lucy described how she often could not get the response she needed from her deeply depressed mother, and when she did get a response, she was not sure what belonged to her and what belonged to her mother.

The couple said they wanted to feel loved by the other, but these difficult, disturbing and confusing emotional experiences had had an impact on their capacity to give and receive love, often throwing them into a state of minus L and apathy. As their analyst I had my own experience of it too, as they moved from feeling overly guarded, a state in which I could not make contact with them, to overly exposed. In either emotional state they were very wary of taking anything in from me. I thought it was hard for them to trust my link to them through K, as minus K was always threatening. The idea that I might hold something for them and/or try to contain what they were unable to, was not something they were familiar with. They felt much more familiar with an object projecting into them.

I felt therefore that I had to be very careful in sharing any potential understanding with them. It was difficult to find a way of connecting at a deeper level that did not also feel threatening them. In relation to each other, they struggled enormously to find a way of managing the paradox of being seen and heard by the other, without at the same time feeling unsafe in opening themselves up too much. This couple illustrates how linked knowing and being known by another (K) is to feeling loved (L), but for them this was a very risky process because of their fear of intrusion.

Often, and for quite a long time, I felt I couldn't help them. However, we kept going. The regular weekly sessions and managing the breaks were fundamental for them – over the five years of the therapy I do not recall them ever missing a session. Looking back, I could see that they were slowly building up trust based on my reliability and consistency. This seemed to allow their paranoid anxiety about my intent to gradually give way and to allow them a feeling of sufficient safety to develop for me to be able to help them.

The fear of love, whilst often having its roots in difficulties in the care giving relationship early in development, may also have a cultural dimension. A notable example of this is the British tradition – one that has a long history – of the affluent sending their children to boarding school, sometimes at a very young age. It is seen as a privilege, but in recent years the emotional damage of this, particularly in the cases of those sent to boarding school as young children, has caught the attention of psychoanalysts and therapists who see the repercussions of this experience in adults coming for individual or couple therapy.

Joy Schaverien has coined the term the "boarding school syndrome" (Schaverien, 2011). She evocatively describes the experience of the child's experience of being left at school by the parents when the child is too young to manage this. The love of the parents can be felt to be lost, and care from the parents is replaced by care from the staff, who, even if caring, do not love them. The developmental needs of the child, which in ordinary circumstances are accommodated within a family setting, are met by an institutional setting to which the child has to accommodate.

Quite quickly any form of relating through love can feel like a weakness that is dangerous and has to be turned away from in order to survive. According to Schaverien, "There are no words to adequately express the feeling state and so a shell is formed to protect the vulnerable self from emotion that cannot be processed" (2011, p. 141). Minus L, a state of indifference, becomes the survival strategy. Stokoe, drawing on his own experience of being sent away to boarding school says,

> I was deeply distressed at finding myself in this institution, away from my mother. In my experience, the only way to survive this sort of experience is to disconnect from your loving self, otherwise the loss is too unbearable.
>
> (2021, p. 45)

Schaverien argues that boarding as a young child is often a traumatic experience that has a lasting psychological impact on the core of the personality.

> The sudden loss of attachment figures (parents, siblings, pets and toys) causes the child to protect itself. For the first time in their life the child may be in a situation where there is no intimate contact; no love. Even when not mistreated, being left in the care of strangers is traumatic.
>
> (Schaverien, 2011, p. 141)

What happens, then, when someone with this early trauma is in a potentially loving intimate relationship later in life? For some individuals the expectation of intimacy, being able to talk about feelings, may feel threatening, as this part of the self, the loving part, may have been split off in order to protect it. Stokoe describes how there may be a masquerading of love in which good etiquette can feel like being cared for. He suggests this is an expression of minus H; "I don't hate you" but that this is ultimately suppressing any loving contact, something that may come crashing in on a couple's seeking of true intimacy.

Love as merger

Referring to a patient of his, Bion said, "If he means by L that the two objects are linked by strong feelings of love, he will not use K for a causal tie such as may be expressed by an impatient 'yes I know'" (Bion, 1962, p. 45).

In a relationship that is a merger there is a strong correlation between L and minus K. It is as if one does not need K, the curiosity drive, because one already knows the other, as in Bion's statement above. Love is hard to define but in such relationships an aspect that figures strongly is the need to be seen, heard and accepted all the time and in every way. Love is equated with an experience of perfect attunement. This is the emotional experience of being in a love merger. The need to be seen, heard and accepted may be especially acute for those who did not experience this as a child, or those who have been subjected to discrimination, especially homophobic responses towards same-sex couples.

In a merger being "in love" can feel like being "one", knowing the other from the inside. It is hard to come to terms with the fact that one can never perfectly know, or be known by, an other, though an important element in a loving relationship is the wish to know the other and be known by the other, not completely but sufficiently to create a loving bond. As a consequence of the primitive feelings that are stirred up when finding oneself part of an intimate couple in a relationship, some struggle to feel separate and allow the other to be separate from the self. The couple may instead re-create, each in their own mind, a version of the "other" in their own image, or an image of another shaped by their own preconceptions or a version of what they need the other to be. Fisher argues that it is only by engaging with the separateness of the other that genuine intimacy can occur. The alternative becomes a narcissistic form of relating (Fisher, 1999). I have described one version of this narcissistic form of relating as a "projective gridlock", a projective system in which the partners, through the process of mutual projective identification, psychically live inside one another and maintain a feeling of oneness (Morgan, 1995).

It can be difficult for a couple who have enjoyed the merger – a merger that had felt like the foundation of their relationship – when one of them develops beyond this need. One partner tries to hold onto the merger, while the other needs to relinquish something that had felt like real love and certainly felt loving. Yet the other no longer feels that way, as the merger erodes the K drive and what once had felt like being known by the other (K) starts to feel the opposite (minus K). In my experience it is often one of the partners who needs to break free first, yet perhaps within the couple's projective system they deal with a shared anxiety about this development, by one guarding the merger as the other tries to break free of it.

This is paradoxical, since merged couples can look like they are remaining in and maintaining the in-love state. However, as Mitchell observes, "Total safety, predictability, and oneness, permanently established, quickly become stultifying" (Mitchell, 2002, p. 51).

I would say it may not be quickly, but usually eventually. In a sustained merger the relationship does not develop, love and hate do not interact creatively, and curiosity is kept at bay. The following is a brief exchange between a couple who have been in a merger.

Joanna & Eddie

Joanna and Eddie are a couple in their late 20s. They met at the gym, where Joanna worked as a personal trainer. Eddie started sessions with her and from the beginning they felt an intense connection – physical and sexual. They fell in love quite quickly, which was felt to be a very special and new experience for each of them. At the time they came for therapy they had been together for two years. In one session they arrived having just come back from a trip to the United States to see Joanna's sister. Their flight had been delayed, and feeling tired and frustrated, Joanna had had an argument with one of the airline staff. The following is a brief extract from their next session:

EDDIE: When we were talking yesterday about what happened at the airport it was difficult because we thought about it differently. I know we usually think the same way and I like that.

JOANNA: Yes, that is part of who we are, what point are you making?

EDDIE: I don't know, I like the feeling, you know, of feeling one, but at the same time I am starting to realize, sometimes I see things differently to you.

JOANNA: I'm not sure that is true, perhaps you are not being honest with me or with yourself about how you feel?

EDDIE: No, I don't think that's it, I think I am trying to be honest, with myself and with you. I think it's just that sometimes I see things differently from you. Maybe not that differently, but a bit. You felt it was necessary to complain to the person at the desk, I felt more resigned to the situation and there wasn't any point. I mean, it was a bit embarrassing Joanna!

JOANNA: I don't really know what you are talking about.

EDDIE: Look it doesn't mean I don't want us to be together, and I still like that feeling of being one, which is most of the time isn't it?

In this interchange we can see that although this couple enjoyed their merger, a merger that felt like true love, and in one sense it was, one of them feels the need to break free of the merger and make room for some difference. The other is left with anxiety about difference destroying their link, a link based on being one, that is felt to be vital within their coupling. The merger can be thought about as an extended version of the in-love state described earlier, but for the merged couple it becomes part of their valued identity as a couple – sometimes as a feeling of specialness that eludes others. Breaking free of the merger, usually driven by the developmental needs of one or both partners, can severely challenge the relationship. Turning away from the merged love can feel like turning away from a very special love.

Prohibition on love

Sometimes love is shut down because of a superego prohibition that may stem from the internalization of societal norms, as in internalized homophobia or the internalization of other social, cultural, racial or religious beliefs.

Leezah Hertzmann has theorized that:

> Internalized homophobia, functioning as an unconscious introject, acts as host for aggressive aspects of the superego potentially resulting in a very punitive attitude towards the homosexuality of the self and of others. In lesbian and gay couple relationships where internalized homophobia exists unconsciously in one or both partners, and therefore in their shared unconscious world, it can act as host for the couple's superego. Consequently, one's sexuality is repeatedly and persistently called into question not only by others, but inevitably by oneself.
>
> (Hertzmann, 2011, p. x)

The resulting belief that one's sexuality is wrong may contribute to difficulties for some same-sex couples in sustaining their relationship. In internalized homophobia there is the love of the other and at the same time the horror of the love of the other – the more that one loves the other, the more one has to turn off one's loving drive. It may be that this internal conflict underlies the feelings of endless frustration and despair in some same-sex couples as loving contact is repeatedly turned away from. A painful state of "stuckness", or apathy may result – as Bion describes in minus L. Moss poignantly states: "One hates oneself for wanting what one wants, and therefore for being what one is. Object love is transformed into object hate" (Moss, 2002, p. 30).

According to Poul Rohleder, in gay love:

> A pervasive message may dominate that "you are not one of us". Gay love is not the same as straight love, it seems. So, one is left grieving for what one does not have and is not able to have.
>
> (Rohleder, 2025, p. 637)

Thus, internalized homophobia and shame may become a problematic obstacle in some same-sex relationships where the feeling of "there is something wrong with me" becomes "there is something wrong with you, and with us" (Hertzmann, 2011; Moss, 2002).

As part of their research into the experience of gay men, Poul Rohleder and Julie Walsh looked at the experience of holding hands in public. They found that:

> Some participants struggled to work out whether only they prevent themselves holding hands with their partner out of shame, or whether they are prevented from doing so by the hostile gaze of society. The two, of course, are intertwined. While there was a wish to hold hands with their partner, without fear and anxiety, this seemed risky and somehow perceived as prohibited – the simple ideal of a loving couple that seemed foreclosed to them.
>
> (Rohleder and Walsh, 2025, p. 640)

Holding hands for many couples is an easy declaration of love and a sense of acceptance of that love within society. The *felt* accepting gaze of others, along with many other societal confirmatory experiences, are internalized and support the couple's loving connection. The feelings of gay men identified in Walsh and Rohleder's research, must represent the many ways in which non-normative love can be undermined and reinforce a sense of "wrongness". This can affect couples not only in same-sex relationships but those who defy other societal, cultural, racial and religious norms. These injunctions on relating can thwart the loving drive leading to a minus L state.

Perrine Moran, in a paper on cross-cultural couples (Moran, 2017), describes the case of Michael and Bashirah, a couple in their 30s. Bashirah had come from Ghana to the United Kingdom with her parents when she was a few months old and Michael came from a white, middle-class, British background. Bashirah, who feared dependence, had agreed that she and Michael should live together for a few years if they had a child, but she was adamant that the relationship would not last and that one day she would leave, and they could then have joint custody of the child. According to Moran, "Bashirah felt very guilty for 'selling out' and betraying her class and her race by choosing a white partner". In Bashirah's mind it seemed that the loving connection to Michael, symbolized by an imagined baby, would never be able to be sustained.

Too much depressive position love?

Kernberg describes several elements of mature love – an ongoing curiosity and interest in the other, the presence of basic trust, mutual empathy and capacity for honesty, the capacity to forgive and ask for forgiveness (especially after aggression), and gratitude for the existence of the other person and the love received (Kernberg, 2011). But of course, relationships, however mature, cannot function like this all the time. Can these positive developments in a couple's relating also become a kind of stagnant retreat?

Britton, developing Bion's view of the fluctuations between the paranoid-schizoid and depressive positions describes a continually evolving movement between the two, necessary for development. He suggests that Kleinian theory, as it has developed,

> [i]mplies that the depressive position is no final resting place, that leaving the security of depressive-position coherence for a new round of fragmented, persecuting uncertainties is necessary for development. The only alternative to continuous development is regression; in a world of flux an attempt to stand still produces a retreat. Yesterday's depressive position becomes tomorrow's defensive organisation.
>
> (Britton, 1998, p. 73)

The idea that the depressive position is no final resting point seems an important one. Life does not stand still, nor can a couple relationship. Each partner is affected by the impact of the world outside them and changing internal worlds. Take for example the impact of having a baby or losses through illness or ageing. Changes occur interpsychically in the couple's shared inner world and interpersonally in their couple dynamics. Events act in a way that has been described from the link perspective as an "interference" between them and on them as a couple (Berenstein, 2012). The capacities that can be seen to exist in mature love are not necessarily stable and certainly not absolutes – trust, empathy, forgiveness and curiosity may be challenging to maintain and be tested out in the relationship many times, sometimes failing.

Thus, another aspect of mature love, which is not often highlighted, is a capacity to be aware of what is not working now (even though it might have been before), along with the security of allowing it to come apart and be reconfigured between the two. Without this capacity there may be stagnation and a turning away from L, as Bion described and which I believe is closely linked with K, curiosity and wish to know, and without which states of apathy, minus L may develop.

L and minus L in couple therapy

Might we consider that, although L is not often the issue a couple bring to therapy, minus L is quite often present and having an impact on the relationship. Instead of L interacting creatively with H and K, it is turned away from; and, in this chapter, I have suggested some of the paths it may have followed, affected by internal anxieties, prohibitions, trauma, loss and the inability to mourn, as well as difficulties in integrating love and hate and a shutting down of curiosity.

It is possible to trace the fate of love not only in the individual and couple histories but also, and perhaps most importantly as Bion had in mind with L, H and K in their positive and negative forms, in the to and fro of each session. The analyst can, for example, observe when loving gestures are risked but not noticed, or are turned away from by the other, or when hate is there but avoided and, in that process, continuously obscures love, often in a grievance. The wish to be truly known and loved appears alongside the fear of actually being seen and accepted with all the good and bad attributes one has. Some individuals feel the fragility of love almost constantly, or there is an ambivalent love that comes and goes, or even that love has never been allowed to fully come into being. Some couples feel they have lost the passionate idealizing love they had at the beginning of their relationship and that what follows feels like a poor substitute that cannot be allowed to develop. Others feel fundamentally unlovable, fear a loving connection with another or feel conflictual or shameful feelings about their loving impulses. For those couples for whom love feels enduring and secure, there may still be times that a loving connection feels threatened, suddenly fragile and in danger of being lost. These are all complex dynamics, but perhaps a focus on love, particularly including minus L along with hate and minus H, can be part of our exploration with a couple in K – in other words led by curiosity.

References

Berenstein, I. (2012). Vínculo as a relationship between others. *Psychoanalytic Quarterly*, 81 (3): 565–577.

Bion, W.R. (1962). *Learning from experience.* Karnac Books.

Britton, R. (1998). Introduction. *Belief & imagination; Explorations in psychoanalysis.* Routledge, p. 3.

Fisher, J. (1999). *The uninvited guest. Emerging from narcissism towards marriage.* Karnac Books.

Fisher, J.V. (2006). The emotional experience of K. *International Journal of Psychoanalysis*, 87: 1221–1237.

Fisher, J.V. (2000). A father's abdication: Lear's retreat from 'aesthetic conflict' 1. *International Journal of Psychoanalysis*, 81: 963–982.

Freud, S. (1905). *Three essays on the theory of sexuality.* In J. Strachey (ed. and trans.), *The standard edition of the complete psychological works of Sigmund Freud* (1953–74), Volume 7. Hogarth Press, pp. 123–246.

Freud, S. (1915). *Instincts and their vicissitudes.* In J. Strachey (ed. and trans.), *The standard edition of the complete psychological works of Sigmund Freud* (1953–74), Volume 14. Hogarth Press, pp. 109–140.

Freud, S. (1920). *Beyond the pleasure principle, group psychology and other works.* In J. Strachey (ed. and trans.), *The standard edition of the complete psychological works of Sigmund Freud* (1953–74), Volume 18. Hogarth Press, pp. 1–64.

Friend, J. (2013). Love as a creative illusion and its place in psychoanalytic couple psychotherapy. *Couple and Family Psychoanalysis*, 3 (1): 3–14.

Hertzmann, L. (2011). Lesbian and gay couple relationships: When internalised homophobia gets in the way of couple creativity. *Psychoanalytic Psychotherapy*, 25 (4): 346–360.

Joyce, A. (2019) The couple, the self, and the problem of the other. *Couple and Family Psychoanalysis*, 6 (2): 181–193.

Kernberg, O.F. (2011). Limitations to the capacity to love. *International Journal of Psychoanalysis*, 92: 1501–1515.

Klein, M. (1928). Early stages of the Oedipus conflict. In: *The writings of Melanie Klein*, Volume 1. Hogarth Press, pp. 186–198.

Mitchell, S. (2002). *Can love last: The fate of romance over time.* W.W. Norton & Company.

Moran, P. (2027) "Somewhere (there's a place for us) …": A cross-cultural approach to psychoanalytic psychotherapy with cross-cultural couples. *Couple and Family Psychoanalysis*, 7: 153–167.

Morgan, M. (1995). The projective gridlock: A form of projective identification in couple relationships. In: S. Ruszczynski and J.V. Fisher (eds.), *Intrusiveness and intimacy in the couple*. Karnac Books, pp. 33–48).

Morgan, M. (2019). Love, hate, and otherness in intimate relating. *Couple and Family Psychoanalysis*, 9: 15–21.

Morgan, M. (2026) *Couple relations: A contemporary introduction*. Routledge.

Moss, D. (2002) Internalized homophobia in men: Wanting in the first person singular, hating in the first person plural. *Psychoanalytic Quarterly*, 71: 21–50.

Ondaatje, M. (1992) *The English patient*. McClelland and Stewart.

Puget, J. (2010). The subjectivity of certainty and the subjectivity of uncertainty, *Psychoanalytic Dialogues*, 20 (1): 4–20.

Rohleder, P. (2025). Homophobia, heteronormativity and melancholia: A psychoanalytic essay on the film all of us strangers. *International Journal of Psychoanalysis*, 106: 630–644.

Rohleder, P. and Walsh, J. (2025) Gay men's experiences of holding hands in public: Psychosocial dilemmas and the discourse of homophobia. *Psychoanalysis Culture and Society*, 30: 298–319.

Schaverien, J. (2011). Boarding school syndrome: Broken attachments, a hidden trauma. *British Journal of Psychotherapy*, 27 (2): 138–155.

Steiner, J. (2017). Melanie Klein's technique then and now. *Institute of Psychoanalysis UK Audio Video Project*, 1: 15.

Steiner, J. (2024). Differentiating between romantic and mature love: Revisiting the three caskets. *The International Journal of Psychoanalysis*, 105: 564–575.

Stokoe, P. (2021) *The curiosity drive: Our need for inquisitive thinking*. Phoenix Publishing House.

Chapter 2

Does love matter in the consulting room?

Julie Friend

Does love matter in our understanding and treatment of couple relationships? Or does the rather limited mention of love in the otherwise rich body of psychoanalytic couple psychotherapy literature accurately reflect the scope of love's clinical relevance in working with couples? Does love's transience, along with the multiplicity of its expressions and meanings, bring it closer to a mood than to a reflection of the interplay of projection and projective identification? If love is closer to a mood, how does this bear on its clinical relevance, and on our customary lenses through which we view couple relationships? Is an awareness of love enriching to our work, or is the relative absence of the topic in the literature an indication of love being clinically beside the point?

From one perspective, these might seem odd questions, since there is generally a shared assumption that people long for and seek couple relationships because of love or at least hoping for love. There may be an expectation that one hopes to be "in love" with one's partner and falling "out of love", or even adjusting to different intensities of connection, can be a worrisome and disillusioning experience, one that often brings couples to our consulting rooms for help. Couples come to us in distress, not infrequently when love feels lost to them or betrayed or occluded, a distress strong enough to override their sense of privacy about what is likely their most intimate relationship. In addition, unlike in individual treatment, in couple psychotherapy the members of a couple face the very real possibility that their partner may speak about something that they themselves would not have wanted to disclose or even to think about. The challenges to love in a couple relationship can feel compelling enough to undertake such a risk. In what follows, I consider the place of love in the context of analytic couple psychotherapy, including its relevance and utility in our clinical approach with couples. I will say at the start that I come to this question with considerable bias, as I believe love indeed matters.

Theoretical perspectives represent a lens through which we organize our thinking, essential in the highly complex context of analytic work with couples, in which there are the interactions of three people – and their internal

DOI: 10.4324/9781003518129-2

worlds – in the field. In the principally post-Kleinian theoretical frame that has been the main context for much of the literature regarding couple analytic psychotherapy, the fundamental organizing matrix with which to think about what couples are doing with and to one another emphasizes projection and projective identification as central structuring elements with which to think about and work with couple relationships (Ruszczynski, 1993; Morgan, 2005, 2019a). While of undeniable clinical utility, thinking about love merits greater attention, and so an expansion of our theoretical frame.

I will consider love's place in our work from two vantage points. First, I review love's place in psychoanalysis as a foundational element of our work. Second, I consider experiences of love in relation to Winnicott's thinking about creativity and transitional experience (Friend, 2013, 2021) and explore the clinical significance of weaving his alternative ideas about psychic functioning into to our approach to working with couples.

Love in psychoanalysis

Many who have written about love in psychoanalysis (Bergmann, 1987; Green & Kohon, 2005; Person, 1988) have noted that it is a topic usually left for the realms of poetry, music and art. Ceccoli, in her essay exploring the notion of chemistry between people, noted that "affect … resides in the senses (the gaze, voice, smell, and touch), which are experienced as powerful because of their unmediated (through language) intensity and which attain a magical (read 'alchemy' or 'chemistry') status (like sex)". She stresses that such experiences are "activated through object use" (Ceccoli, 2004, p. 346).

It is difficult to capture such unrepresented experiences as love in words, particularly with enough clarity and specificity to render them clinically useful. What is it we are talking about when we speak of love? What sorts of love? And what of love, if anything, is relevant to how we orient our work with couples? The multiple contexts and definitions of love complicate clarity and thus discussion, no doubt one factor in its infrequent mention in our field's literature until recently.

The word love is both a noun and a verb, its meaning sometimes mundane and sometimes transcendent. Love can refer to a range of emotions, from simple and transitory pleasures to profound and transformative rapture. Never having been easy to define, the ancient Greeks designated at least seven words for love, describing its various qualities in different contexts and registers of relationships. Of most obvious relevance regarding couples is the expression of love we know as "eros". Although we now generally consider eros in reference to sexual passion and erotic love, Socrates described eros differently, as an emotion that helps the soul recall its inherent knowledge of ideal beauty and spiritual truth. Similarly, Plato stated that "Love is simply [*sic*] the name for the desire and pursuit of the whole" (Symposium, c. 385–370 BCE). Whilst worded plainly, paradoxically, Plato's words carry profound implications. Love is seen here as something that leans us towards, unites, pulls us to something – or someone – expresses a longing for connection, and, perhaps, of an imagined experience of wholeness,[1] alluding to something beyond the sense of an individual self.

Freud was quite influenced by Plato's writings and described psychoanalysis as "a cure effected through love" (Freud, 1974), considering love as "a basic developmental force in nature" (Lear, 1990, pp. 12–13). Loewald, in his classic paper "On the therapeutic action of psychoanalysis" (1960) stated that psychoanalysis "requires an objectivity and neutrality the essence of which is love and respect for the individual and for individual development", thereby describing love as the context in which "the organization and reorganization of ego and psychic apparatus take place" (p. 20). Loewald situated love as the foundational ground in which psychic development and structural change unfolds, reflected also in the recognition of love within the transference as a central force and fulcrum of change in analytic treatment of individuals. Others share this view. For example, Oliver (2002, p. xxv) summarizes Kristeva's view that "psychoanalysis is a love relationship that builds spoken spaces through transferential love", love considered here as the context in which the capacity for representation takes place. She adds that "transference and countertransference *are love relations that can spark the imagination* and open up the possibility of re-imaging and thus re-signifying affects". There is agreement that "finding fulfillment of our deepest potentialities takes place within the fabric of loving relationships" (Pickering, 2008, p. 7).

In a recent paper, Parsons (2024) situates love as integral to psychoanalysis and describes our most essential tools – reverie and evenly suspended attention – as forms of love in action (p. 228). He introduces us to a late twentieth-century philosopher, Ruddick, whose conception of "attentive love" aligns with Bion's concept of reverie:

> Attention is at once an act of knowing and an act of love … Attentive love, or loving attention, represents a kind of knowing that takes truthfulness as its aim but makes truth serve lovingly the person known.
>
> (Ruddick, 1990, pp. 119–20)

Parsons offers that "As well as an emotion, love is a capacity: one that analysts hope their work will help patients to develop and become more able to exercise" (Parsons, 2024, p. 234).

The core importance of love in psychoanalysis is also reflected in an ontological perspective, attending less to prioritizing the interpretation of the interplay of internal objects, and more oriented towards supporting the patient's experience of idiomatic aliveness (Ogden, 2024). In this context the frame, the setting in which we work, carries a quality of emotional contact via "the feel of the couch depressed against one's body … the inflection of tone of the analyst's voice … the impression made by the experience – when not excessive, doesn't only 'mean' love, as Winnicott put it – it *is* love" (Blum et al., 2023, p. 126). Markman (2022, p. 23) describes our love for our patients as expressed via:

> our desire to know, understand and recognize the singularity of the patient in a deep way that fosters intimacy … involves communicating in various modes – words, rhythms, gestures … love manifest in our desire to know the patients as fully as we can and communicate that … in the patient's idiom.

From various theoretical vantage points, love is recognized as integral to the analytic endeavour and as an essential and transformative component of the experience of containment. The fundamentals of psychoanalysis, including reverie, our capacity for holding our minds and bodies in suspended, receptive openness as we listen, and our thoughtful, considered honesty represent "expression(s) of love … evoked by the need of another human being" (Parsons, 2024, p. 245). From this perspective, the act of creating meaning with another person can be seen as an act of love, making love central to our work. It is expressed in our thoughtful attention, qualities of containment, honesty, attuned presence, in our rhythms of relating, our modulated tones of voice and in our gaze. The emotional connection between analyst and patient includes love, itself foundational for emotional growth and development.

Love and psychoanalytic couple psychotherapy

What about the place of love specifically in relation to psychoanalytic work with couples, and within couple relationships?

Some years ago, an experience with a couple caught in a painful and urgent stalemate regarding the fate of their relationship jolted me – heart pounding – to explore the place of love in our work (Friend, 2013). At that time, I was surprised to find that the otherwise rich body of psychoanalytic literature specifically on couple relationships included rather little about love itself but instead emphasized attention on the patterns of projection and projective identification that are seen to structure couple relationships, aiming to support a realistic view of one another. Although useful, I find this perspective incomplete, as I have previously noted:

> Psychoanalytic couple psychotherapy emphasizes building depressive position capacities, aiming to help couples to think more clearly about each other, and strengthen their ability to perceive each other more realistically. And yet love, at the very heart of couple relationships, is a state that is often far from realistic – it can be full of idealization, blurred boundaries, fantasy, and illusion.
>
> (Friend, 2013, p. 5)

The music – the non-verbal, embodied, implicit and imaginative aspects of relating – has been insufficiently included in the literature until comparatively recently (Abse, 2022; Clulow, 2023; Moran, 2025; Pickering, 2008), and there may be good reasons why love has not been more of a focus. Love is mercurial, hard to define with clarity and takes many forms. We also know that there is more to a couple relationship than love – even the closest couples do not always feel loving – and, in fact, have times when they might hate one another. There are the mundanities of the tasks of life: balancing work, raising children and other interests within the couple relationship; the social network and extended family in which the couple is embedded; financial realities; differing rates and directions of development; the impacts of ageing; and changes in health of the couple – multiple factors affect the couple relationship and require some kind of adjustment, hopefully ones that feel well enough coordinated and reflective of each partner's needs. My point here is not to idealize love; rather to attempt to illuminate its enlivening, creative and even healing potential, as well as how including a consideration of love affects our clinical approach. I begin by reviewing some of the central thinking about love in couple life through a psychoanalytic lens.

Kernberg (1995) linked ego psychology and object relations theories, extending psychoanalytic thinking to explore the complexities of love in couple relationships. Outlining the interweaving ego capacities that he considered necessary for sustaining what he called "mature sexual love", he included the ability to transform one's embodied sexual excitement into sexual desire for the other, tenderness that results from the capacity to integrate both libidinally *and* aggressively invested self and object representations – love and hate – resulting in love predominating over aggression, an ability to tolerate what he termed normal ambivalence, and an ability to identify with the partner – including a capacity for reciprocal gender identification – and what he called "mature idealization". Kernberg highlighted "the passionate character of the love relation in all three aspects: the sexual relationship, object relationship and the superego investment of the couple" (1995, p. 32), emphasizing various ego capacities he sees as necessary to sustain functioning love relationships.

Fisher (1999) contrasted what he called "marriage", which he defined as "the passion for and dependence on the intimate other" with narcissism, "a longing for an other that is perfectly attuned … and thus not a genuine other at all" (Fisher, 1999, pp. 1–2). Fisher chose the word marriage to describe "perhaps the most complex and difficult encounter with the beauty of the object". Notably, while he referred evocatively to "passionate intimacy with another human being" (Fisher, 1999, p. 11), he did not call it love. Pickering (2008, p. 7) speaks of love directly and, like Fisher, describes love relationships as representing "a marriage of altruism and alterity", highlighting the importance and developmental potential for the partners to have the capacity to recognize and be curious about one another.

Elaborating on Bion's theoretical conceptions of L (love), H (hate) and K (curiosity) in relation to couple relationships, Morgan (2005) highlights the importance for couples to develop the capacity to accommodate experiences of both love and hate, the integration of which "is what gives the relationship life and creativity". Morgan emphasized the importance of a capacity for curiosity (K), which we know can be especially challenging in the context of disturbing difference, and of crucial importance in couple relationships, expressed in "the wish to know" the partner "imaginatively, and to engage with their difference from oneself", even – to some degree – when the other represents something feared, hated or dreaded. She further describes the stultifying and destructive impact on a relationship when "the phantasy that the other is known from the inside" prevails, occluding both difference and the actual, complex reality of the other, making curiosity irrelevant. We see couples who cannot bear difference or uncertainty, and witness the strangulating atmosphere that can ensue, a lifeless connection and one that I would say is emptied of love. The wish to make the other the same can result in the nullification of a generative, dynamic, "creative couple" relationship (Morgan, 2005).

The influential body of thinking about couple relationships that has emerged from Tavistock Relationships has predominantly emphasized attending to the patterns of projection and projective identification of internal objects that are seen to structure couple relationships, for good and ill. Partner choice, for example, has been described as an outcome of "the other's receptivity to projected parts of the self" (Ruszczynski, 1993, p. 27) and consequently our clinical focus tends to be on identifying and understanding these patterns that connect the couple. This process of mutual projective identification is seen as a central mechanism in the establishments of a couple relationship (Ruszczynski, 1993). To the degree that couple relationships are seen as structured largely in relation to projection and projective identification, it follows that we formulate interpretations to illuminate the projective patterns connecting the couple. We hope that, as these projective systems can be recognized and thought about, the couple's capacity to see one another more clearly and tolerate difference will be strengthened. We hope, too, that the outcome of treatment will be a richer relational matrix, as well as increased individual development of each partner.

Thinking in terms of the impacts of patterns of projection and projective identification provides a useful matrix in which to organize our thinking. In the treatment of individuals, the field of information is already dense, layered and highly complex, with "just" two people in the room. When a third person is present, the possible relational connections, conscious and unconscious, expand exponentially (Nathans, 2017, p. 8) and include not only our relationship and responses – conscious and unconscious – to one person, but to two people, as well as to the relationship they construct. Likewise, each member of the couple brings their own conscious and unconscious emotional response to the therapist, their responses to their partner, and also to the relationship they experience between their partner and the couple therapist. In the context of such a dynamic, multifactored and highly complex experience, a structured way of organizing one's experience is undeniably useful.

Yet Colman raised important questions about the implications that ensue from an emphasis on viewing projective identification as the central, structuring element in couple relationships, asking "if partner choice is based on projective identification and the developmental aim of couple relationships involves the withdrawal of projections, what need would anyone have for a relationship if all projections could be withdrawn?" (Colman, 1995, p. 60). While much of our work is geared to helping couples see one another more realistically, and to addressing the deforming impacts of forceful projections, it is also true that when we love another, we also have an internal experience of them which does not align perfectly with a realistic perception of the actuality of the partner, and so this model, while useful, is incomplete.

Love, creative illusion, and transitional experience

Some years ago, I wrote:

> ... love, at the very heart of couple relationships, is a state that is often far from realistic – it can be full of idealisation, blurred boundaries, fantasy, and illusion ... How do ... couple psychotherapists hold a place for both, and help couples build their capacity to hold a tension between more mature, reasoned kinds of relating on the one hand, with the creative potential of less rational, more aesthetic qualities of relating on the other?
>
> (Friend, 2021)

The emotional currents that we experience and that can pass between us can enrich us, change us and challenge us. There is more to couple relationships than projection and projective identification alone. Winnicott's (1953) conception of transitional experience offers a perspective that more fully elaborates the creative potential of love in couple relationships.

Green (2005) commented "Ultimately the experience of love teaches us that it is linked to illusion" – love in this context existing within a tension between imagination and objective reality. We sometimes hear an example of the shimmering between realistic perception and imagination in the stories couples tell of their first meetings. They can offer a glimpse of a dream they had once had about their relationship, about who they were, and who and what they were hoping to become. Such recollections are often very moving to hear and are typically marked by acute sensory detail, as if it happened yesterday rather than years ago. Here is an example, an amalgam of many such moments I have heard. Describing her feeling when she met Steve, Louisa said: "I don't know why, just something about the way he was standing, maybe his seriousness when he spoke. It stands out. I remember it all so clearly, what he was wearing, the light in the room … his face was so serious as he was listening to the person he was speaking to … I can't explain it, but that was it for me. I just knew in that moment that we could build a good life together."

How can we think of such transformative experiences, and are they relevant to our work with couples? From the perspective of internal objects, we could imagine Steve as a transference object of a kind to Louise, perhaps reminding her of an earlier object of love. Alternatively, moments like Louisa's meeting of Steve can exemplify Winnicott's conceptualization of transitional phenomena, in which "what is objectively perceived is to some extent subjectively conceived of" (Goldman, 2012). Such an experience seems to include both reality and imagination, a transitional arena in which the "interplay between inner dreams and outward reality" (Goldman 2012) can add to a feeling of being idiomatically alive, as love can do. Bollas described similar experiences as carrying an "illusion of deep rapport between subject and object" (Bollas, 1978, p. 385), endowing the desired object with transformational potential, promising an experience in which "the unintegrations of self find integrations through the form provided by the transformational object" Bollas, 1978, p. 385). In falling in love with Steve, Louisa experienced him as a vision of her future, right there, perhaps a dream of a version of herself and a life waiting to be – a moment of creative illusion.

> We are always making an imaginative connection with the world around us as we make contact with it, especially other people; both inanimate objects and other people come to have meaning for each individual person as we become engaged with them. This is the place of illusion. Without this, the world may well be lifeless and flat.
>
> (Seligman, 2018, p. 263)

In contrast to projection, illusion constitutes "a more flexible and bidirectional transactional linkage" (Seligman, 2018). There is an ongoing tension inherent in maintaining a relationship between internal fantasy and external perception, keeping them distinct yet connected, so that meaning can arise naturally from what is both created/discovered, encountered/imagined.

Thinking in terms of projection and projective identification as the main avenues of emotional communication between couples can overlook the importance of the creative engagement that illusion adds. What I wish to emphasize here is that experiences of love, enriching and potentially transformative as they are, can exceed a solely realistic view of the other. Addressing problematic projections and patterns of projective identification in couple relationships, while essential, does not sufficiently recognize the importance of other valences of emotional connection, nor how our interventions at these different moments may vary. So, while much of our work is geared to helping couples see one another more realistically, and to addressing the deforming impacts of forcefully imposed projections, it is also true that when we love "an other", we have an internal vision of them that may not align perfectly with a realistic perception of the actuality of the partner. It is important to register such moments and consider the clinical utility of making such recognition explicit.

Along with love, for a couple relationship to thrive there must also be recognition of the other as separate – not only a dream or an extension of oneself – and differences must be accepted with some curiosity, thus retaining the potential of enriching the couple relationship. Many couples that come to us are disturbed by difference, or fear that disliking or hating parts of their partner means the loss or destruction of love. Sometimes differences are denied, blinding the ability to see the other as real and separate, and generating pressured attempts for alignment that constrain the vitality of the relationship and of each partner. A feeling of falseness or a claustrophobic atmosphere can ensue, constraining creative engagement. For a creative experience of love to thrive, the inevitability of some hate must also be accepted by the couple.

In "Object relating and object usage" (1969), Winnicott made clear that it is via the experience of hatred and destructive feelings that have been met and contained by a primary object, who can continue to care and stay relationally alive, that objective reality is established and that the other is experienced as real.[2] Taking liberties with Dodi Goldman's discussion of Winnicott's ideas about creative aliveness I have changed the pronouns in his statement, transposing his mother/infant context into the couple realm:

> The (couple's) psychic health – creative meaning making – is contingent, in other words, upon (each partner's) capacity to survive (their own and the other's) emotional reactions – remaining (themselves) without losing connection to what (the other) needs them to be. Only then can (they) be enriched rather than shocked by (their) difference.
>
> (Goldman, 2012, p. 18)

In Winnicott's (1953) terms, it is particularly via the object's survival of the subject's hatred and destructive feelings that both the creative potential of transitional space as well as a sense of external reality are established, because the object's resilient survival of destruction places it outside of the subject's control, and they become more "real" (Winnicott, 1969). Along with the strengthening of the capacity to recognize the other as real, outside of subjective control, and separate, comes the possibility of another triadic representation – that of the self, the other, and a less differentiated area in between, where the question of "were you there or did I create you" is not to be asked. This different representation of a triangular configuration can be another "angle" of a "creative couple state of mind" (Morgan, 2005), in which it can become more possible to think feelingly about oneself, one's partner, and about the relationship as a joint creation, as well as to confront differences and hatred, without feeling the relationship is at unbearable risk.

The two following vignettes – each disguised amalgams of couples with similar dynamics – illustrate differing capacities for sustaining a loving connection and the consequent different clinical implications.

Alan and Gloria spoke more to one another than to me in response to my asking about their beginning, smiles lighting their faces as they shared the recounting of their first meeting; they had clearly captured one another's attention and enjoyed revisiting the experience. The attraction between them was evident. Alan had been widowed several years before, leaving him to raise his young son from that marriage. He described his previous marriage as having been difficult, and was delighted to have met someone as compelling, and competent, as Gloria. While he loved Gloria and felt lucky to have met her, he was nervous about committing himself. Afraid of conflict, he withdrew in the face of any disagreement, which evoked anxiety in Gloria, who then doubted his commitment to her. We came to understand that her reaction to his anxiety had its roots in her relationship with her unpredictable and self-involved parents with whom she never felt secure. In the room I could see that when Gloria was more anxious or pressured, Alan could become quite frozen. Gloria in turn could experience this as ominous. Her upset frightened him in turn, increasing his withdrawal.

Sometimes couples speak of love, yet the atmosphere in the room does not match the words. With Gloria and Alan, the words and the music aligned. They listened with focused interest to one another, were generally warmly curious to learn more, and usually responded thoughtfully to one another. They made each other laugh – sometimes even during a tense interchange – and clearly found pleasure in one another's presence. In general there was room to think. I found it easy to speak freely about my observations of their interactions, which were generally accepted as constructive or modified and built upon comfortably. While there could certainly be a sense of tense urgency and anxiety as they talked, and they could get quite upset with one another, they were generally able to return to thinking about the other's experience to some degree, without persistent worry that own perspective was being ignored or subsumed. I felt a calm confidence in the strength of their love for one another and in their capacity for a broad area of inquiry, thought, and connection.

Randall and Jim, in contrast, seemed to need to be loved *by* the other. They had met at work and gone on to build a business a together, and for a time their relationship carried an experience of optimism and creativity; they were in step. Once their business was successful and they were no longer in synchronized collaboration, things began to break down between them. Jim could hear any request or separate feeling of Randall's as criticism and control and felt devalued by him. Over time, they had become more cautious, distant and angry with one another, leaving them each feeling doubtful about being loved. The capacity to feel love – if we can call it that – *for* the other seemed to rest on feeling in step and admired. When this was not the case, the sense of rage, anxiety and painful abandonment was profound. Their capacity to think about and empathize with one another vanished.

Jim could be controlling of Randall, which I saw as an effort to bring them back into a more merged arrangement, in which he felt they were in step. He would "suggest" what Randall should wear, for example, which elicited a rageful response. There was sometimes a quality of scorn in his inquiries about Randall's separate activities and achievements, and he regularly asserted that something might have been done differently, projecting his own feelings of shame and insecurity onto his partner, who needed ongoing reassurance that he was good and lovable. Jim seemed to feel safer being critical, and Randall's sense of self could fall apart in the face of Jim's displeasure, so for a time he tended to comply with Jim's "requests". The capacity to think about one another often seemed out of reach; despair, hopelessness and rage gathered in the room like weather. They would lament the loss of the idealized beginning of their relationship, an experience that had provided each of them with a sense of redemptive escape from their traumatic pasts, as neither had felt seen or loved in their families.

The work with Randall and Jim was quite different from that with Alan and Gloria. In the room with two people, each of whom desperately need to feel recognized and valued, interpretation alone often falls short or lands like an accusation. It falls to us to provide a sense of care and containment, demonstrating the capacity to keep them each in mind, and survive their emotions. I was mindful not only of what I said, but how I said it, attending carefully not only to the words I chose, but to my tone of voice, the speed and rhythm of my words, the accompanying expression on my face – in an effort to reach out to them and to generate a containing atmosphere. Addressing the destructive impacts of the more hostile aspects of the way they related to one another needed to be direct, yet it also needed to communicate my understanding of the emotions underpinning the hostility and control. Couple interpretations were often experienced as an abandonment or erasure of one of them and, in the absence of careful, nuanced attunement to each of them, separately, observations and explorations were likely to be experienced as attacks. Randall would be plunged into his experience of being unloved, angry and bad; Jim would become even more emotionally removed, intellectualized, cold and contemptuous. They could feel "loved" when seen as good, but it vanished, turning into abandonment or rage if the emotional alignment, conveyed by tone, posture, rhythm or gesture, was not precise. This left little room for curiosity, to see each other wholly, to accept things about one another they didn't like, to hear each other, or certainly to work together to address each of their needs as best they could.

For some time, the tasks with Randall and Jim were less in the realm of interpretation, and more in that of recognition and containment, and in surviving the emotional intensity without withdrawal, retaliation or intellectualization. Witnessing their anguish and rage, their conviction – each of them – that they were unlovable, I had to palpably survive and offer recognition not only by what I said, but through my gaze, tone of voice and the pace of my speech. Communicating my awareness of what they might be experiencing and not making light of their pain – recognition as forms of love in action – were my focus. Over time, they each developed a greater capacity to empathize with one another, accept some difference, and indeed constructed a more loving relationship.

With Alan and Gloria, we see a couple who usually possessed the capacity to view one another as separate, be curious about difference, and – with help – tolerate some hatred as well. Work with them corresponded comfortably with a model that emphasizes interpretation and, by implication, the capacity for secondary process thinking. When their experience was received and recognized by the other, they were reflective and able to think about the other's experience, even when it was different from what they wished from one another. Difference, disagreement and uncertainty, while stressful, did not usually equate to an experience of abandonment or erasure by the other. There was a creative atmosphere between them and between the three of us. They could link their current concerns with their pasts meaningfully, making interpretation an effective way of reconsidering their experience of the current relationship.

In contrast, Randall and Jim, neither of whom had felt lovingly kept in mind by their carers, needed a demonstrable experience of my survival and continued care for them, and for their relationship. For much of the treatment, recognition and attunement, rather than interpretation, were essential in creating a setting in which each of their emotional experiences could be registered and held. Connecting their current experience with their early lives was not helpful, as it was experienced as a forceful refusal to accept their feelings, a convex response rather than containing receptivity, the opposite of love. Randall would begin to sob, a lost and unloved child in the room, and Jim would become more remote and intellectualized. In witnessing the experience of the "absence of a maternally preoccupied presence, our primary task is to ... establish such a presence in the space we share" (Peltz, 2023, p. 269). With Randall and Jim, consistent, empathic recognition of their emotional experience was necessary, an experience of love in action.

Slowly, it became possible for Randall and Jim to develop a more nuanced understanding of each other's feelings. The couple setting in which this transpired contributed to the establishment of a greater capacity to think about the other's experience without feeling obliterated, the fragile beginnings of a triangular internal space and depressive position capacities in which they could hold concern for themselves, the other, and for the relationship (Morgan, 2019a, Ruszczynski, 1993).

Does love matter in the consulting room?

Love matters, both within the couple relationship and as part of our clinical thinking.

Most couple relationships begin with love, or with the hope of it, and couples often come to us when it seems to have faded, failed or is in peril. Couples do not always, or only, love one another. Love can be more or less palpably present at different times. People differ in their capacities to love, to be vulnerable, to navigate the varied and sometimes unpredictable terrain of relationships. Partners develop at a different pace and can become out of step. The material conditions of life – children, finances, ageing, illness – impact the experience of connection and can cause strain. Love, even if there, can be hard to feel or believe in. Working psychoanalytically, while we do not explicitly direct or encourage feelings or expressions of love between the couple, we do demonstrate love though our sustained, thoughtful attention to and survival of their emotional experience.

We do this in a multitude of ways. Our reliable presence and focused listening, our emotional receptivity and attunement, our silence, playfulness, our honest and thoughtful confrontations of destructiveness when we see it – all of these are ways we communicate love to our patients, whether individuals or couples. Our ability and willingness to be receptive to each member of the couple, and to think deeply about what they are creating between them and evoking in us, are ways of witnessing and presence that are not only profoundly affecting but are forms of love.

> The fundamental activity of psychoanalysis, which goes by many names – free-floating attention, evenly suspended attention, freely associative listening, reverie – is an expression of love, inspired by hope and dependent on faith … evoked by the need of another human being.
>
> (Parsons, 2024, p. 245)

This is true for analytic work with couples as well as individuals.

A greater consideration of love and the impediments to it enriches our clinical approach to couples. Especially with couples under strain, or where one or both partners have not been well met in their early life, the need for precise attunement can be exacting, constrain creative relating and generate an atmosphere in which it feels as though there is only room for one. The capacity to tolerate, no less be intrigued by, an other who is both known and not known, is essential for a couple to relate creatively and flexibly and is much more difficult.

Our demonstrable recognition of their experience, reaching towards them with emotional resonance, is essential to support a setting in which development can ensue, and this recognition is an expression of love. This is also consistent with holding a couple state of mind (Morgan, 2019b), as we endeavour to understand and relate to each member of the couple, and to what they create between them. The enriching potential of different theoretical perspectives is also evident in "the reconceptualization of the idea of projective identification as *both* an intrapsychic and an interpersonal process" explored in the Italian relational school (Zavattini et al., 2015, p. xiii), in which they also identify that "the therapist's function is to become involved in the intersubjective relation, available through [their] engagement to offer a new, alternative experience" (Zavattini et al., 2015). These are forms of love in action.

The numerous intersecting vertices of relationships, connections, transferences and countertransferences in the room are a great deal to hold and to think about. I have previously suggested (Friend, 2021) that integrating theoretical approaches is useful and enriching in our work with couples. This includes the importance of internal objects, psychic structures, projection, and projective identification – which helps organize our thinking and identify patterns of connection and difficulty in couple relationships, as well as attention to the idiomatic, less representational, but deeply life-affirming qualities of emotional experience are equally important to recognize and include in our thinking about couple life.

Capello describes that "development happens through micro-experiences of being on the same wavelength rather than by decodifying interpretations … The function is to create a new transformative relation" (Capello, 2015, p. 83). Such emotional resonance – receptivity and attention to the other – can be considered love in action. Our focused listening, tones of voice, our silence or our humour, our attentive receptivity to what is being communicated to us, our offering connections to consider, our firmness – all of these are ways we communicate love to our patients, whether individuals or couples. Our capacity to embody a couple state of mind (Morgan, 2001) is itself a profound example of our loving care, and thus carries transformative potential, aiming to support the health and vitality of the couple relationship, with all its emotional vicissitudes. Our receptivity to each member of the couple, while also thinking deeply about what they are creating between them and evoking in us, is a quality of witnessing and attention that I believe is not only clinically useful, but is itself a form of love.

Notes

1 Although beyond the scope of this chapter, Plato's statement raises a number of questions regarding the distinctions, for example, between merger – eliding the self – and a sense of deep connection, which includes the maintenance of some distinct sense of self and recognition of the other.

2 For example, Ogden (2016) usefully elaborated the importance of the child's experience of the object's survival of destruction in creating an object to use and a robust relationship with reality.

References

Abse, S. (2022) *Tell me the truth about love: 13 tales from the therapist's couch.* Ebury Press.

Bergmann, M.S. (1987). *The anatomy of loving: The story of man's quest to know what love is.* Columbia University Press.

Blum, A., Goldberg, P. & Levin, M. (2023). *Here I'm alive: The spirit of music in psychoanalysis.* Columbia University Press.

Bollas, C. (1978). The aesthetic moment and the search for transformation. *The Annual of Psychoanalysis*, 6: 385–394.

Capello, M. (2015). The therapist at work: Technical matters. In: G.C. Zavattini et al. (eds), *Talking with couples: The psychoanalytic psychotherapy of the couple relationship.* Karnac Books, pp. 61–88.

Ceccoli, V. (2004). Finding home in (an)other: Relational chemistry and its psychoanalytic derivations. *Psychoanalytic Dialogues*, 14 (3): 337–348.

Clulow, C. (2023) Interpretation viewed through the lens of attachment informed couple psychotherapy. *Attachment: New Directions in Relational Psychoanalysis and Psychotherapy*, 17: 173–184.

Colman, W. (1995). Gesture and recognition: An alternative model to projective identification as a basis for couple relationships. In: S. Ruszczynski and J. Fisher (eds), *Intrusiveness and intimacy in the couple.* Karnac Books, 59–74.

Fisher, James (1999). *The uninvited guest: Emerging from narcissism towards marriage.* Karnac Books.

Freud, S. (1974) Letter from Sigmund Freud to C.G. Jung, December 6, 1906 (41). In: W. McGuire (ed.), *The Freud/Jung letters: The correspondence between Sigmund Freud and C.G. Jung*. Princeton University Press, pp. 11–13.

Friend, J. (2013). Love as creative illusion and its place in psychoanalytic couple psychotherapy. *Journal of Couple and Family Psychoanalysis*, 3 (1): 3–14.

Friend, J. (2021) Creative illusion in couples: Thoughts about the value of transitional experience for couple relationships. *Couple and Family Psychoanalysis*, 11: 158–169.

Goldman, D. (2012). Weaving with the world: Winnicott's re-imagining of reality. *Psychoanalytic Quarterly*, 81 (1): 1–23.

Green, A. & Kohon, G. (2005). *Love and its vicissitudes.* Routledge.

Kernberg, O. (1995). *Love relations: Normality and pathology.* Yale University Press.

Lear, J. (1990). *Love and its place in nature: a philosophical interpretation of Freudian psychoanalysis.* Yale University Press.

Loewald, H.W. (1960). On the therapeutic action of psycho-analysis. *International Journal of Psychoanalysis*, 41: 16–33.

Markman, H. (2022). *Creative engagement in psychoanalytic practice.* Routledge.

Moran, P. (2025). *Love songs: Listening to couples.* Karnac Books.

Morgan, M. (2001). First contacts: The therapist's "couple state of mind" as a factor in the containment of couples seen for initial consultations. In: F. Grier (ed.), *Brief encounters with couples.* Karnac Books, pp. 17–32.

Morgan, M. (2005). On being able to be couple: The importance of a "creative couple" in psychic life. In: F. Grier (ed.), *Oedipus and the couple.* Karnac Books, pp. 9–30.

Morgan, M. (2019a). Love, hate, and otherness in intimate relating. *Couple and Family Psychoanalysis,* 9: 15–21.

Morgan, M. (2019b). *A couple state of mind: Psychoanalysis of couples and the Tavistock Relationships model.* Routledge.

Nathans, S. (2017). Introduction: Core concepts of the Tavistock couple psychotherapy model. In: S. Nathans and M. Schaefer (eds), *Couples on the couch.* Routledge, pp. 1–29.

Ogden, T.H. (2016). Destruction reconceived: On Winnicott's "The use of an object and relating through identifications". *International Journal of Psychoanalysis,* 97 (5): 1243–1262.

Ogden, T. (2024). Ontological psychoanalysis in clinical practice. *Psychoanalytic Quarterly,* 93: 13–31.

Oliver, K. (ed.) (2002). *The portable Kristeva.* Columbia University Press.

Parsons, M. (2024). Practice and praxis: Psychoanalysis as an act of love. *Psychoanalytic Quarterly,* 92 (2): 219–248.

Peltz, R. (2023). Discussion of "Love as creative illusion and its place in couple psychotherapy". In: S. Nathans (ed.), *More about couples on the couch.* Routledge, pp. 47–56.

Person, E.S. (1988). *Dreams of love and fateful encounters.* Penguin Books.

Pickering, J. (2008). *Being in love: Therapeutic pathways through psychological obstacles to love.* Routledge.

Plato. (1999). *The symposium* (C. Gill, trans.). Penguin. (Originally published 385–370 BCE.)

Ruddick, S. (1990). *Maternal thinking: Towards a politics of peace.* Women's Press.

Ruszczynski, S. (1993). *Psychotherapy with couples.* Karnac Books.

Seligman, S. (2018). Illusion as a basic psychic principle: Winnicott, Freud, Oedipus, and Trump. *Journal of the American Psychoanalytic Association,* 66 (2): 263–288.

Winnicott, D.W. (1953). Transitional objects and transitional phenomena: A study of the first not-me possession. *International Journal of Psychoanalysis,* 34: 89–97.

Winnicott, D.W. (1969). The use of an object. *International Journal of Psychoanalysis,* 50: 711–716.

Zavattini, G.C., Bianchini, B., Capello, M., Lupinacci, M.A., Monguzzi, F. & Vitalini, L. (eds) (2015). *Talking with couples: The psychoanalytic psychotherapy of the couple relationship.* Karnac Books.

Chapter 3

A question of true love

Judith Pickering

Introduction

Love is a central issue in couple therapy, dealing as it does with matters of the heart: longing for love, fear of love, love gone sour or off the rails. The one word "love" has manifold meanings, including romantic love, passion, sexual desire, friendliness, affection, altruistic love, compassion, and less interpersonal forms of love such as love of wisdom, art or nature. Couple relationships embrace many facets of love in various shades at different times as well as a host of other emotions.

Love as an emotion is dynamic, shifting from erotic passion to the humdrum, from peaks of excitement to boredom and irritation. It is inherently evanescent and unstable. The bliss of falling in love fades. The orgasm lasts a few moments. An experience of sublime felicity is mutable. Yet we can enjoy each phase of loving without artificially trying to prolong it or pin it down like a butterfly. We can welcome the ecstasy of a moment of beauty, despite its impermanence and the mundane aspects of life that inevitably intrude. Emotional life is also polyvalent: we can feel overwhelming desire followed by irritation, boredom, jealousy, possessiveness, all for the one person, in varying degrees at varying times.

Love relations may potentially be a place for transformation into our truer selves, enabling us to confront, work through and heal relational lacks, losses and traumas that have disabled us from fulfilling our potential. This depends on a capacity to work through an array of psychological obstacles to love towards relational intimacy based on appreciation of alterity, a sense of sanctity, altruism and gratitude.

For Freud the goal of psychoanalysis is to work and to love, for Jung it is individuation. Psychotherapy may aim towards self-realization, yet self-realization is inherently interrelational and interdependent. It requires not only other-realization but a transcending of such dualities. When, in 1996, I began a PhD on the topic of love and psychoanalytic couple therapy (Pickering, 2004), psychoanalysis was mostly cast as an individual affair. Many "methodologies" of human development – the Socratic goal to "know thyself" and

DOI: 10.4324/9781003518129-3

lead the examined life, spiritual and psychological growth, the pursuit of enlightenment, to search for wisdom, individuation, "being fully analysed" – tended to focus on individual work rather than a more relational approach. One became analysed, individuated or enlightened in spite of one's relationships, not within them. Yet psychoanalysis takes place within a relationship and the emergence of relational psychoanalysis and intersubjectivity theory has seen a seismic shift towards recognition of inherent intersubjectivity and relationality. Couple therapy also involves a deeply connected and committed relationship with the therapist. The couple therapist's *agápē* love is an intrinsic curative element. The promise a therapist makes is to be there for the couple through the labyrinthine passages of darkness and despair, to plumb the depths of caverns of relational trauma, hurts and disappointments, where angels fear to tread, opening out to new vistas of healing and transformation.

Despite numerous difficulties, "being in love" may challenge us to face, work through and heal relational lacks, losses and traumas that obstruct us living and loving fully. The work of love, including both couple therapy and the relationships themselves, may lead towards more fulfilling, creative and authentic lives. This depends on a capacity to overcome many obstacles to love, moving through processes of disillusionment to relational intimacy based on appreciation of alterity, a concept refined by Levinas. Other "servants" of love include Bion's K and L links, a capacity to tolerate unknowing and Bion's (1970) advice to eschew memory, desire and understanding, all of which I will be applying to couple therapy in this chapter.

In following philosophical and theoretical explorations of love, there is the question of its relevance to couple therapy. How might these love themes be located in the intersubjective, embodied, confusing and difficult field of psychoanalytic couple therapy? In our own love lives?

Love indefinable

"One of life's deepest mysteries and most powerful emotions has remained one of the darkest corners of history", writes Stephen Kern (1992). Innumerable books on love deal with the topic from a historical, cultural, anthropological, philosophical and psychological perspective. Yet many authors point out that the topic of love has been sadly neglected in both philosophy (Singer, 1966, p. xi) and psychoanalysis (Friend, 2013). Nussbaum comments on how philosophers are suspicious of love and would have it removed from the ethical life altogether (Nussbaum, 2001, p. 463). Mann observes that there is "a notable scarcity of references to love" in psychoanalytic works (Mann, 2002, pp. 2–3). Lear wonders whether psychoanalysts "dismiss love as cosmological speculation" (Lear, 1990, p. 156). Solomon observes that analytic literature tends to concentrate on negative emotional states such as "hatred, envy, jealousy, perverse and violent feelings, anxieties, depressions and psychotic states" (Solomon, 2002). Little is said about love "as a driving emotive force … propelling much of the self's psychological development … a primary emotion at the core of object relating" (Solomon, 2002, p. 53).

What remains striking, given the universality and power of love, is how little we understand its full meaning in our lives. "The language of love is impossible, inadequate, immediately allusive … a flight of metaphors", writes Kristeva (1987 (1983)). The philosopher John Armstrong asks:

> "What is it to love another person?" This is to raise one of the deepest, and most puzzling, questions we can put to ourselves. Love is a central theme in the autobiography we each write as we try to understand our lives; but we may feel that we become only more confused the more we reflect upon it.
>
> (Armstrong, 2002, p. 1)

Love's many facets

The Ancient Greeks had numerous words for love, including *érōs, philía, agápē, storgé, xenía* and *nómos* (Singer, 1966). Each term has a multitude of meanings in the Western tradition. *Philía* represents love as friendship as well as love of ideas, as in the word philosophy meaning love (*philía*) of wisdom (*sophia*). *Agapē* includes love of a spouse or family member as well as divine love. *Storgé* is familial affection such as that of parents for offspring. *Xenía* is the Greek word for love of the stranger and is linked to love as hospitality. *Nómos* means law, by extension, submission to divine law, a form of religious love in which we surrender ourselves to God's will. These six words by no means cover the lexicon of love nor other qualities that condition love, such as altruism, understanding, sympathy, generosity, loyalty, trust, care, kindness, fidelity. Nor do they acknowledge the many facets of love in non-Western cultures, a topic in its own right.

Authentic love relationships encompass a host of different forms of love: physical, erotic, psychological and spiritual aspects. Love involves reciprocally enjoying loving and being loved. In Compte-Sponville's words:

> lovers know well how sensual, voluptuous, and intense it is to make love in joy rather than want, in action rather than passion, in pleasure rather than suffering, in the fulfilment rather than the frustration of our capacity – in other words, to desire the love we are *making* rather than the love we dream of, do not make, and are obsessed by.
>
> (Compte-Sponville, 2001 (1996), p. 251)

A multidimensional spectrum of love in couple relationships may include many components: an intertwining of *érōs, agapē, philía, storgé, xenía, nómos*; love-making that is an experience of non-duality rather than fusion; appreciating each other's alterity; negotiating shifting tides of intimacy and solitude; a sense of thirdness, of the relationship as having its own teleology; unknowing (Bion's K link); "*heaven in ordinarie*" or appreciating daily life; qualities such as gratitude, trust, loyalty; loving each other through emotional and physical difficulty, imperfection, sickness, ageing and mortality; tolerating ambivalence; a capacity for forgiveness ... this list is as endless as the plenitude of love.

Love as érōs

From Aristophanes, a comic, we derive the myth of the severed whole that continues to influence ideas about finding one's soulmate, the notion that there is one person who is our "other half". Having found the "one and only", we are at last complete. Relational breakdown is attributed to misfit – inadvertently hooking up with the wrong mate.

In Western philosophy erotic love has been seen as an intense longing for a particular person. This longing may be displaced, sublimated, transformed into longing for other objects (art, beauty, god) but it begins with personal attachment to the beloved, who is seen as sublime, necessary for the lover's happiness. Erotic love includes sexual desire, whether such desire is enacted or not. For Socrates, Stendhal, Freud and many others, erotic love is based on a sense of lack. *Érōs* "involves an opening of the self toward an object, a conception of the self that pictures the self as incomplete" (Nussbaum, 2001 p. 461).

In the Tavistock model of couple therapy, a sense of incompleteness manifests in unconscious choice of partner. We are often attracted to someone who has qualities that are undeveloped in ourselves. The relationship has the potential to form a container in which such qualities can be engaged with. The shy, inhibited introvert is attracted to a boisterous extravert. Here it might be that the introvert needs to come out of their shell and become more relationally confident, the extravert to be more capable of quiet reflection. An anxious, preoccupied person ostensibly seeks closeness but is attracted to an anxious, avoidant partner who loves their own solitude and space. If both are able to engage with their undeveloped side, the preoccupied person might begin to develop a sense of self-containment, the avoidant might become more relationally connected, and both ultimately become more securely attached.

Perhaps there is a developmental element at work in the arrows of *érōs*, which engenders the yearning to overcome the gaping void between self and other. *Érōs* dismantles watertight constructs of ourselves as independent, impermeable, static entities. *Érōs* disturbs our ordered equilibrium, creates upheaval in our lives, sometimes for better, sometimes for worse.

Philía

In the *Nichomachean Ethics* Aristotle talks about *philía* as the quality of friendship of the virtuous "who wish well to their friends for their sake", desiring to do "what is good for the other not for one's own sake but for theirs" (Aristotle, 1941, VIII, 8 1159a25–34). They rejoice in their friend's happiness, grieve for their sorrows (Aristotle, 1941, IX, 116a7–9). Love as *philía* is integral in couple relationships, the sense that one's partner is also one's best friend. Sometimes couples seek therapy because friendship is lacking in their relationship. Alternatively, they have settled into a comfortable state of companionship, and erotic desire has all but disappeared.

Max and Mathew, both environmentalists, met on a campaign to stop the culling of native forests. They share their work and life together. At the end of an often-demoralizing day campaigning, they cuddle up in a tent together, giving each other moral support, feeling they have each other's back. They seek couple therapy because although they enjoy love as *philía*, erotic passion has ebbed away.

Agápē

Agápē (Latin, *caritas*) derives from the verb *agapan* and is found in classical Greek where it means to welcome in friendship, to love and to cherish. Love as *agápē* is generous, patient, kind, loyal, self-giving, full of joy, hope, peace and truth. *Agápē* is not possessive, envious or covetous. Psychoanalytic writers (Lambert, 1973) have seen non-possessive, altruistic forms of *agápē* of analysts towards their patients as a major therapeutic agent for healing psyche.

Storgé

Storgé referred to familial love between parents and children, between siblings, and between grandparents and grandchildren. Some couples struggle with a conflict between *érōs* and *storgé*, sexual desire and affection. Erotic passion becomes "outsourced" sometimes leading to an affair.

Minna and Bob came to see me because Minna had had an affair. Their two boys had just left home. Feeling empty and unfulfilled, she asked Bob to join her in a meditation course in the Himalayas, but Bob said he could not take time out from work. Minna went alone. On retreat she met the mysterious and alluring Bandhitra. She described feeling bathed in his gaze as he listened deeply to her in a way she felt Bob never had. She felt met on spiritual as well as erotic levels: a heady mix.

Discovering emails to Bandhitra after she returned home, Bob was devastated. Through therapy they came to realize they had both neglected the erotic and the "soul-making" creative elements in their marriage. Bob was worried about saving for retirement, which he hoped would be a time when they could enjoy life together and reignite their sex life.

During a short break in couple therapy, Minna returned to India ostensibly to attend a yoga retreat in Delhi but it was to see Bandhitra secretly. She was, however, aghast to discover how undomesticated he was, his tiny flat was filthy. The gleaming array of idealizing projections on retreat in the Himalayas fell from her eyes. She realized it was her own inner life that needed to be rekindled and asked Bob if they might consider going on the Camino de Santiago together. This time Bob agreed, both hoping it might be a pilgrimage of relational healing, forgiveness, spiritual and physical renewal.

Xenía

Xenía refers to love of the stranger. How do we embrace that which is strange and unfamiliar in another person, as well as within oneself? Kristeva writes that the face of the foreigner "bears the mark of a crossed threshold" (Kristeva, 1991 (1988), p. 4). How do we come to value difference without either seeking to assimilate it falsely or to eradicate it? The stranger can be fascinating and alluring, as Bandhitra was for Minna, a projection of her inner spiritual yearning. The stranger confronts us with our own unfamiliarity:

> To discover our disturbing otherness, for that indeed is what bursts in to confront that "demon", that threat, that apprehension generated by the projective apparition of the other at the heart of what we persist in maintaining as a proper, solid "us". By recognising our uncanny strangeness we shall neither suffer from it nor enjoy it from the outside. The foreigner is within me, hence we are all foreigners.
>
> (Kristeva, 1991 (1988), p. 192)

Xenía includes love of the "stranger within", our uncanny strangeness. As Laplanche states, "internal alien-ness maintained, held in place by external alien-ness; external alien-ness, in turn, held in place by the enigmatic relation of the other to his own internal alien" (Laplanche, 1999, p. 80).

The other may become the repository for what we find alien and disturbing in ourselves. Our perception of their strangeness can be a projection of what is strange and unacceptable within us. This is like a double layer of obscuration: not only are we incapable of acknowledging their opacity, but their alterity is covered with a layer of projections of our own uncanny strangeness. They may then identify with the casting of them as alien, becoming truly alienated from one another.

Love's shadow: love and hate

Love has its dark side, and a range of destructive emotions can curtail if not pervert love relations. Bion argued that the opposite of love was not hate, but what he called minus love (–L) (Bion, 1962, 1963). Love stirs up hate: we hate our dependence upon the other, our lack of control over them, our vulnerability, the pain and frustration love brings.

Love's work: working through obstacles to love

It may be a cliché to say that the path of true love never runs smooth, but a cliché that rings loud and clear in the area of couple therapy. Being in love entails risks, fear of rejection, vulnerability. It challenges our solid sense of identity, of who we were before we met. There are defensive as well as developmental elements in our unconscious love-choice, regressive aspects of falling in love. We bring our "malignant dowries" (Pickering, 2006), project internal figures and relational templates onto and into our beloved, recreate wheels of repetition compulsion. There are numerous obstacles to love: illusions, delusions, fusion or merger, over-idealization, paranoid-schizoid splits, shared unconscious phantasies (Bannister & Pincus, 1965), interlocking traumatic scenes (Pickering, 2006, 2008), projective gridlocks (Morgan, 1995), traumatic and relational complexes, fixed memories, covetous desires, misunderstanding … the list is as endless as the vicissitudes of love.

And the two become one flesh: merger and fusion love

The notion that love is perfect when two halves become one has beleaguered us since Aristophanes' myth of the severed whole. Given Aristophanes was a comic, perhaps he intended this as a joke – and, unfortunately, we have taken it too seriously. Fusion love can be due to separation anxiety, fear of solitude, a defence against difference. If we completely merged with our beloved, we would not only dissolve our own subjectivity but obliterate theirs. Pathological modes of fusion love involving adhesive identification may amount to a violent assault on the alterity of the other, a cannibalizing attempt to become the other. Yet as Levinas reminds us, "Two have a better time than one." Our relations with others are "*better* as difference than as unity … The very value of love is the impossibility of reducing the other to myself, of coinciding into sameness" (Levinas & Kearney, 1986, p. 22).

Idealization

Love, for Santayana, "is an imaginative search for unattainable ideal objects which do not exist and thus cannot be attained" (Singer, 1966, p. 29). Falling in love often involves an elevation of the beloved into an idealized figure, whose every quality is exalted. As the French writer Stendhal had it, the birth of love transforms the beloved into a shimmering object of great beauty, just as a bare "wintry bough" thrown into an abandoned salt mine might become "studded with a galaxy of scintillating diamonds" (Stendhal, 1957 (1822), p. 45). Idealization can be both defensive and developmental, as unnatural and illusory as Stendhal's gleaming display of salt crystals upon a leafless branch, or a natural stage of loving. Stendhal believed that true love is obscured by idealizing projections where one imbues the beloved with all one's own good qualities, emptying oneself in the process (Stendhal, 1957 (1822), p. 60). Freud felt that overvaluation of the beloved and denigration of oneself was a form of displaced primary narcissism. Freud (1921)) also argued that, through loving someone with qualities we value ourselves, we might incorporate and enrich ourselves with these very attributes. This reiterates the Platonic idea that idealization involves admiring in the beloved the qualities to which we aspire.

In our intimate love lives, idealized love can lead to the enhancement of ideals, values, a sense of beauty and harmony with the world. It can also be a defence against conflict, ambivalence and feelings of helplessness. Idealization in love thus has both anti-relational and relationship-enhancing qualities. On the one hand it can be anti-relational because it renders the beloved as an image, not a flesh-and-blood, complex person. We defend against the uncontrollable and unpredictable qualities of an actual relationship, replacing it with images, because images, being abstract and universal, are used to defend against the pain of losing "that" particular, non-replaceable person, that relationship. On the other hand, idealization can be based on a sense of awe, wonder and gratitude for the beloved's existence for their own sake, gratitude for our relationship, for being together in all our ever-changing vicissitudes.

Disillusionment as a joyful iconoclast

It is often argued that romantic love is erroneous, after the "honeymoon phase", limerence stage or love psychosis wears out, after the projections fall away, one becomes disillusioned, the real person obtrudes and, if we are well adjusted (and/or well analysed), we discover a deeper, more mature form of love based on active choice rather than compulsion. It is hard to realize that one's beloved is both ideal and not ideal, satisfying and disappointing, exciting and boring, and to realize such feelings are subjective. Disillusionment may be fortuitous, a falling away of illusions may reveal something more profound and enriching than the thin two-dimensional veneer of our projections, as C.S. Lewis discovered in his own marriage:

> All reality is iconoclastic. The earthly beloved, even in this life, incessantly triumphs over your mere idea of her. And you want her to; you want her with all her resistances, all her faults, all her unexpectedness. That is, in her foursquare and independent reality. And this, not any image or memory, is what we are to love still, after she is dead.
>
> (C.S. Lewis, 1961, p. 52)

"All reality is iconoclastic." Every system of falsifications, defences, illusions and projections may obscure the truth, but cannot obliterate it. Each encounter with one's beloved has a potential for revelation of reality in this moment, something never experienced before, hence requiring a great deal of existential courage as well as negative capability, that is, a capacity to dwell in a mode of being full of "uncertainties, mysteries, doubts, without any irritable reaching after facts and reasons" (Keats, 1817, as cited in Bion, 1970, p. 125).

Transformations in O in Love: being without memory, desire and understanding in couple relations

We all too often impute stale memories upon our partners, children, friends and colleagues, expecting them to be in this given moment in time how they *appeared* to be in the past. Possessive desire and misunderstanding also thwart love. Laying aside memories, egocentric desire and false understanding aids love's work, however difficult this may be. Here I am drawing on Bion's advice to eschew memory, desire and understanding and applying this advice in the realm of couple therapy.

Old memories, covetous desires and misunderstanding concerning our relationships clutter our awareness and need to be cleared away if we are to meet each other afresh. We often hold each other to ransom on the basis of our memory of our last meeting, not allowing the other who comes before us to reveal themselves as they are here and now. As Bion warns, memories, desires and understanding overlay our perceptions of one another, often serving as defences against unknowing.

Memoria *and Bion's K link*

When a couple first meet and begin to form a relationship, they "get to know" each other through sharing vital elements of their lives. A new relationship, like a co-created tapestry, is stitched together through telling each other vital stories of origins, narratives of personal history, memories of childhood, of family background. We were not there. But as we share with each other the landscapes of our past, it is as if we somehow vicariously enter this past and weave together a new shared history. The activity of "getting to know" is related to Bion's K link. Bion recognized that emotional experience is always embedded in a relationship: "An emotional experience cannot be conceived of in isolation from a relationship" (Bion, 1962, p. 42). He notates three emotional intersubjective links between human beings as Love (L), Hate (H) and Knowledge (K) (Bion, 1962, p. 43). Their negatives are –L, – H and – K.

The K link is an emotional link between two people wanting to know and be known while recognizing that they cannot ever fully know each other or themselves. There is a paradox between the compassionate engagement in seeking to know while tolerating the frustration of not knowing. No matter how long we might have been together in a couple relationship we do not ever truly know each other. A static piece of knowledge can overlay the emotionally engaged activity of searching to know, the K link, which is a dynamic interrelational link predicated on uncertainty.

Memory

Confiding memories may be a vital element of love relations, but if self is intersubjective, not solitary, multiple, not unitary, dynamic, not static, then who we are today is not who we were yesterday, let alone last week or last year. The assumption that we are the same today as we were yesterday, Bion warns, is "suspect", a "sign of a collusive relationship intended to prevent emergence of an unknown, incoherent, formless void and an associated sense of persecution by the elements of an evolving O" (Bion, 1970, p. 52). Remembering what *was* prevents us facing the unknown of what *is*. The emphasis is on the present, not the past or future.

Being "without memory" does not mean we do not try to remember our loved ones, whether on a mundane or a more far-reaching level: their values, tastes, birthdays, how they take their tea … Remembrance is a vital aspect of feeling we are held in the open heart and mind of a loving other. But who we were yesterday is not quite the same as who we are today. Being without memory is about reminding ourselves of this, to approach our next encounter as if for the first time.

Possessive desire

Desire is an intrinsic element of love relations – wanting to be with another, desiring to make love, to enjoy each other's company, desiring their body, mind, spirit, desiring their happiness and wellbeing, wanting them to be free from suffering, and find fulfilment in their lives. It is problematic when desire is overly egocentric and possessive, failing to acknowledge that our partners are not merely an extension of self, or there only to fulfil our needs. Egocentric desire refers to a "tormenting irrationality of possessiveness, acquisitiveness and selfishness based on self-aggrandisement and self-centredness" which thwarts true love from flourishing (Guenther, 1976, p. 42).

Understanding: knowing and unknowing

We seek understanding in our relationships, but there are tensions between the desire to be understood and to understand, to know and be known, and the incomprehensible alterity and what Winnicott (1984 (1963)) saw as the inviolable privacy of a person. Couples often defend against the pain of not knowing via positing a *piece* of knowledge, grasping it like a possession, in place of the emotional activity of seeking to know afresh. How many times have we sat with couples where one partner confides a precious memory, only to feel betrayed when the other partner later uses this confidence as a "piece of information" against them?

False knowledge can become a tyranny, a way of categorizing and thus controlling the other. What Bion calls minus K (–K) is a tyrannous imposition of a false "knowledge" fuelled by envy for the other being outside the sphere of one's epistemological control. Minus K is an evasion of the pain of not being able to know, predict and control the other. The emotional aspects of –K are envy and greed, a spoiling, destructive impulse where meaning is denuded of vitality, thus occluding against discovery.

Presuming we *can* know another fully, or, even more erroneously presuming that we *do* know, inhibits the K activity of *getting* to know.

Love and alterity: Levinas

> Love aims at the Other; it aims at him in his frailty ... To love is to fear for another, to come to the assistance of his frailty. In this frailty as in the dawn arises the Loved, who is the Beloved ... The epiphany of the Beloved is but one with her *regime* of tenderness. The *way* of the tender consists in an extreme fragility, a vulnerability. It manifests itself at the limit of being and non-being, as a soft warmth where being dissipates into radiance.
>
> (Levinas, 1969, p. 256)

How might couples begin to be able to intuit any inkling of an incomprehensible mystery beyond all the various ways we cloak the face of the beloved? Cultivating a capacity for negative capability and laying aside memory, desire and understanding is a vital element in the art of loving. So too, is alterity. Here I draw on the ethics of alterity of Emmanuel Levinas (1906–1996).

Alterity derives from the Latin *alteritas*, but for Levinas *alterité* means much more than otherness, difference. *Alterité* seeks to avoid casting the not-I as Other, making "I" the central, privileged term. It involves paying homage to the ineffable nature of the person who comes before me face to face (*le face à face*). Responsibility towards that person's inviolable, unknowable mystery is primordial. How does one respond to others, not as "another me", but as subjects in their own right, with vastly different ways of being and seeing the world?

According to Levinas, we exist in a world of things other than ourselves, yet our perception is self-centred. The other who comes before me is not a mere object to be subsumed under one of my categories. The face of the actual other transcends the mere idea I have of them: "the way in which the Other presents himself, exceeding *the idea of the Other in* me, we here name face" (Levinas, 1969, p. 50).

For Levinas there is a mysterious way in which our own subjectivity comes into being through recognition of the Other. We become substantial through being subject to the ethical call of the other for our solicitude and care. Subjectivity is not based on egocentrism but as "founded in the idea of infinity" (Levinas, 1969, p. 26).

> When in the presence of the Other, I say "Here I am!" This "Here I am!" is the place through which the Infinite enters into language, but without giving itself to be seen.
>
> (Levinas, 1985, p. 106)

Thomas Ogden also shows how the strangeness of another "I-ness" radically confronts our sense of static self-identity and does not "allow us to remain who we were". Encounter challenges our sense of self, and we "cannot rest until we have somehow come to terms with its assault on who we had been prior to being interrupted by it" (Ogden, 1994, p. 14).

Levinas is criticized by some for going too far in abnegation of self at the expense of the other. But for Levinas the face of the other does not threaten to negate our self, it bestows freedom. It grants the possibility of expansion beyond narrow strictures of egocentrism. The alterity of the other in fact frees us from the emotional cage of solipsism, showing us the other is beyond us, so much more than any figment of our fantasies.

Alterity is an ethical activity of love that is aimed towards overcoming the isolation of the self. It is a form of love predicated on a capacity for alterity that enables us to overcome solipsistic egocentrism moving towards a recognition of non-duality and the embodied, intersubjective and relational self.

Transformations in love in times of darkness

Mark and Michaela come to see me because they are expecting a child. Mark is ravaged by nightmares and Michaela is suffering post-traumatic stress disorder and depression. They are not confident that they are suited to each other as there so many cultural differences in their backgrounds.

They met at a refugee camp. Mark, an aid worker, saw a hand sticking up from under a pile of rubble. He gently took the hand in his. It was warm. A rare sign of life in a carnage of death. He carefully removed each piece of rubble, revealing Michaela's bloodied, bruised face. She was saved by a gesture of compassionate love from the stranger: *agápē, philía, xenía.* They fall in love, *érōs* being added to the mix, a mix possibly including a range of transference projections of the rescuer, the Nightingale, the saviour, the saved … Eventually, after much bureaucratic red tape and further hardship, Mark sponsors Michaela for a refugee visa to come to Australia and they marry.

Mark, however, continues to be haunted by images of the camps, piled up dead bodies, the stench of death, overwhelming feelings of despair and powerlessness at having been able to do so little. The image of Michaela's warm hand in his is a beacon of hope in his psychological hell realm. Yet Michaela is more than a beacon of hope. She has her own personhood, her mysterious alterity, her four-square reality beyond noble aspirations to save and be saved. Underneath it all, she wonders, what do they have in common? She feels dead inside. Australia is meant to represent a new start, a new life, a safe haven, but it feels alien. How can she contemplate being happy, in love, with so many left for dead? All her family had perished under the rubble from which she was rescued.

The cry of a baby taking its first breath, emerging fist first from the womb, a cry for life becomes their first cry of shared wonder and joy. It enables a subtle yet seismic shift from living with one foot in the grave to feeling perhaps life was worth living, that Mark could forgive himself for all the lives that could not be saved, Michaela can begin to mourn the dead. They name their baby Joy. But a beacon of hope, whether a hand waving or a fist fighting, and a name are still not enough.

Michaela now sometimes feels Mark loves little Joy more than she does. She still finds it hard to feel anything other than guilt that she survived and her family did not. She sits with a blanked-out stare like a death mask, staring into space, little Joy wriggling uncomfortably on her lap, mouth open searching for a breast. She does not respond, and Joy becomes increasingly distressed. Mark takes Joy, puts a dummy in her mouth but it slips off, it is mother's loving warm milk she wants.

I feel helpless and inadequate. What could therapy offer that might heal such devastating trauma? When little Joy squirms and whimpers on Mark's shoulder, I find myself aching to take her in my arms, to offer comfort, body to body. Any interpretation I make seems to fall like bits of rubble. Between sessions I too am swamped by images of atrocity. I feel my own profound despair that the human race has come to this, that the basic moral imperative "thou shalt not kill" seems all but forgotten. If only being a couple therapist and analyst could in some small way act as an instrument of peace, healing, restoration, for this couple, for others, just as Mark was a peacekeeper and aid worker. Was I getting too caught up in Bion's "desire" or is there also a place for bearing witness, care, love for our patients, for humanity, for the planet? My own reverie was caught up in personal preoccupations, but it was also related to this couple and their predicament. How could I lay aside Bion's desire, for healing, for redemption, for a better future for them? Should I?

I cannot do justice to their story any more than I can to any other couple. I cannot adequately relay the intricate threads of therapy work over several years of weekly sessions, as Joy grew on their lap, then played at their feet. Yet there was something intangible, mysterious at work. I would like to think it was the work of love, theirs, mine, ours, my own heart going out to them, a heart filled, not with possessive desire, but *érōs, agápē, philía, xenía*, bearing with them what was unbearable, taking into my heart horrendous beta elements, fear of annihilation, nameless dread, holding such *beta-confusa* (Pickering & Samuels, 2025, p. 99) and seeking to metabolize it in a state of reverie, as through a dark cloud of unknowing (Bion, 1963). It was about providing psychological and physical refuge, an inner and outer sanctuary, in which they could begin to mourn the dead, give themselves permission to live, allowing inklings of vivacity to grow without ignoring unspeakable horror. Mark became increasingly curious about Michaela's full personhood, in all her cultural and religious difference, as she told me the ancestral history of her family before the war, as she shyly confided her dream of learning to be a seamstress. She too listened deeply as he relayed his upbringing in a tiny outback town in Australia. He told us how he became an aid worker to give back just a little of what he had been given, as his own parents had also been refugees, albeit from a different war, a different culture, a different time. As well as cultural differences, they shared a history of trauma, displacement, survival. Slowly, imperceptibly, the ravages of trauma began to heal. Slowly, so slowly, transformation in O in love enfolded us all in its mysterious embrace. This may seem as overly idealistic as idealizing love projections. Was I merely clinging to beacons of hope in places of terrible darkness as Mark had done, not able to lay aside Bion's desire? I like to hope at least this was the work of love, the love the analyst has for the couple, the love between a couple, their love for their little ones, a love that can never be fully defined or understood.

Conclusion

Can we say love exists as a thing in itself? In the same spirit that Winnicott said there is no such thing as a baby without a mother, perhaps there is no such thing as love without lovers loving. Love is full of contradictions, vicissitudes, paradoxes. Lovers may desire to cross the intersubjective space, to unite with one's beloved, to realize a state of non-duality, but we are not ever as one. If our subjectivity is forever in flux, each encounter is a revelation of the limitless ever-becoming of each other as we are now.

A real person and a real relationship exceed mere ideals, ideas, mutual projections and assumptions. In love-making we may transcend egocentric limitations into an ecstasy of conjunction, while also retaining a separation-in-union. Our unfathomable alterity is always revealing itself as if for the first time, a shock and a delight. When one's desire does not destroy, incorporate, possess or cannibalize the other, we may find ourselves liberated into a joyful appreciation and gratitude for simply being alive and loving one another.

References

Aristotle. (1941). *Nicomachean ethics: The basic works of Aristotle* (R. McKeon, ed.). Random House. (Original c. 335 BC.)

Armstrong, J. (2002). *Conditions of love: The philosophy of intimacy.* Penguin.

Bannister, K. & Pincus, L. (1965). *Shared phantasy in marital problems: Therapy in a four-person relationship.* Institute of Marital Studies.

Bion, W.R. (1962). *Learning from experience.* Jason Aronson.
Bion, W.R. (1963). *Elements of psychoanalysis.* Heinemann.
Bion, W.R. (1970). *Attention and interpretation*. Tavistock.
Compte-Sponville, A. (2001). *A small treatise on the great virtues* (C. Temerson, trans.). Metropolitan Books. (Original work published 1996.)
Freud, S. (1921). Group psychology and the analysis of the ego. In J. Strachey (ed. and trans.), *The standard edition of the complete psychological works of Sigmund Freud* (1953–74), Volume 18. Hogarth Press, pp. 67–145.
Friend, J. (2013). Love as creative illusion and its place in psychoanalytic couple psychotherapy. *Couple and Family Psychoanalysis*, 3: 3–14.
Guenther, H. (1976). *The tantric view of life.* Shambhala.
Keats, J. (1817). *Letters.* (Edited by M.B. Forman), 4th edition. Oxford University Press.
Kern, S. (1992). *The culture of love: Victorians to moderns.* Harvard University Press.
Kristeva, J. (1987). *Tales of love* (L. Roudiez, trans.). Columbia University Press. (Original work published 1983.)
Kristeva, J. (1991). *Strangers to ourselves* (L. Roudiez, trans.). Harvester. (Original work published 1988.)
Lambert, K. (1973).Agape as a therapeutic factor in analysis. *Journal of Analytic Psychology*, 18 (1): 25–46.
Laplanche, J. (1999). *Essays on otherness.* Routledge.
Lear, J. (1990). *Love and its place in nature: A philosophical interpretation of Freudian psychoanalysis.* The Noonday Press.
Levinas, E. (1969). *Totality and infinity* (A. Lingis, trans.). Duquesne University Press. (Original work published 1961.)
Levinas, E. (1985). *Ethics and infinity* (R. Cohen, trans.). Duquesne University Press. (Original work published 1982.)
Levinas, E & Kearney, R. (1986). Dialogue with Emmanuel Levinas. In: R. Cohen (ed.), *Face to face with Emmanuel Levinas.* State University of New York Press.
Lewis, C.S. (1961). *A grief observed.* Faber & Faber.
Mann, D. (ed.) (2002). *Love and hate: Psychoanalytic perspectives.* Brunner-Routledge.
Morgan, M. (1995). The projective gridlock: A form of projective identification in couple relationships. In: S. Ruszczynski and J. Fisher (eds), *Intrusiveness and intimacy in the couple.* Karnac Books, pp. 33–48.
Nussbaum, M. (2001). *Upheavals of thought: The intelligence of emotions.* Cambridge University Press.
Ogden, T. (1994). *Subjects of analysis.* Jason Aronson.
Pickering, J.C. (2004). *The exogamous conatus: Ontophanies of love.* Doctoral dissertation on psychoanalytic couple therapy. School of Psychology, University of Western Sydney, Australia.
Pickering, J.C. (2006). Who's afraid of the Wolffe couple: The interlocking traumatic scene. *Journal of Analytical Psychology*, 51(2): 251–270.
Pickering, J.C. (2008). *Being in love: Therapeutic pathways through psychological obstacles to love.* Routledge.
Pickering, J.C. & Samuel, G. (eds) (2025). *Collected writings of Giles Clark: Recycling madness with Jung, Spinoza and Santayana.* Routledge.
Singer, I. (1966). *The nature of love: Plato to Luther.* Random House.

Solomon, H.M. (2002). Love: Paradox of self and other. In: D. Mann (ed.), *Love and hate: Psychoanalytic perspectives.* Brunner-Routledge.
Stendhal (M.-H. Beyle) (1957). *On Love* (G. Sale and S. Sale, trans.). Penguin. (Original work published 1822, *De l'amour.*)
Winnicott, D. (1984). Communicating and not communicating leading to a study of certain opposites. In: D. Winnicott, *The maturational processes and the facilitating environment*. Karnac Books, pp. 37–55. (Original work published 1963.)

Chapter 4

The dialectics of attachment, sexuality and love in couple relationships

Shelley Nathans

Introduction

"Making love" – the expression of love in sexual activity, is central to most modern, romantic adult couple relationships. Typically, sexual attraction is part of the initial excitement of falling in love. Over time, erotic desire and its expression in sex may provide a unique place for love to grow and form part of the bedrock of attachment between partners. Sexuality and the need for security – upon which attachment is based – are fundamental to the experience of love and the formation of adult couple relationships. Sustained, gratifying sexual activity over time rests on the integration of these needs, whereby safety provides partners' freedom for an erotic life and sex enlivens a sense of stability.

Yet, many couple relationships suffer from problems that interfere with or arrest their sexual relations, and this may raise uncertainty about their love. If the origins of romantic love lie in erotic desire and sexual connection, when a couple stop having sex does this mean they have fallen out of love, or does it signal an underlying problem that might manifest itself in the bedroom?

Popular media and couple therapy literature are replete with cases of the loss of sexual activity in couple relationships. They chronicle obstacles to sustained sexual excitement and propose myriad techniques for its restoration. The narrative explanation most frequently offered is that the biology of sex and attachment are incompatible (Bowlby, 1969; Fonagy, 2009); good sex requires novelty (Perel, 2006); and familiarity over time equates to death in the bedroom. Thus, attachment-based needs for security and erotic desire have been positioned as reciprocally negating (e.g. Ben-Ze'ev, 2022; Clulow, 2009; Eagle, 2007; Perel; 2006). From this viewpoint, a couple's inevitable drift towards predictability in the service of security also signals the decline of excitement and sexual activity and this must be countered by efforts to create novelty and opportunities for separateness. But when considering couple relationships, is it necessary to view attachment in direct competition with sexuality?

I propose that sustained sexual desire and connection in a couple relationship can be conceptualized as a complex relational experience that is best

DOI: 10.4324/9781003518129-4

understood as an integration of attachment needs, sexuality and emotional experience. In my view, attachment and sexuality are not easily or usefully separated into distinct behavioural systems in either infantile or adult experience, and love in adult sexual relationships is a complex emotional and interpersonal experience that originates and relies on the psychic integration of early attachment and sexuality. Love, attachment and sexuality develop and thrive in mutually influencing dialectical processes.

Love, healthy attachment and sexuality develop contemporaneously and conjointly in the relationship between the infant and primary caregiver(s). Secure attachment develops and is embedded in sensuality, in both the *emotional and bodily experience* of being reliably and responsively fed, held, rocked and soothed by the hands, body and voice of a loving caregiver. This occurs, in both the literal and figurative sense, as a *holding environment* (Winnicott, 1964), a setting constituted by a caregiver's consistent, loving attention, which is essential for healthy development and which foundationally locates security in the infant's sensual, bodily experience.

Similarly, healthy infantile erotic experience and sexuality emerge and develop within an experience of being literally and figuratively held, in an *emotional and body-based relational experience* that is filled with both sensual contact and potential symbolic communication. Contributions from infant research (Beebe, 2006; Stern, 1985) and contemporary psychoanalysis have expanded beyond traditional Freudian and Kleinian one-person theories of infantile sexuality, situating the emergence of infantile sexual experience instead in a relational context (Atlas, 2016; Benjamin, 1988). These frameworks characterize the symbolically rich and reciprocally communicative qualities intrinsic to the relationship between infants and primary caregivers, as well as the impact of the caregiver's mind on the infant's early acquaintance with sexuality (Kristeva, 2014; Laplanche, 1989).

For Laplanche, sexuality is transmitted to the child via "verbal, nonverbal, and even behavioural enigmatic signifiers which are pregnant with unconscious sexual significations and lay the foundation for unconscious infantile sexuality" (Laplanche, 1989, p. 126). Similarly, Kristeva's concept of maternal eroticism describes unconscious aspects of the caregiver's mind that infuse the atmosphere between mother and infant with erotic meaning and experience. A passionate psychosomatic state that defies rationality and is rooted in the mother's own libido, maternal eroticism is communicated by the mother who "deploys (or sprouts) its libidinal force as tenderness" (Kristeva, 2014, p. 75).

Within this type of relational experience, infused with passionate tenderness, repeated over time, the infant has the visceral experience of actively seeking and passively receiving sensual bodily pleasures, being soothed, receiving relief from physical discomfort and feeling loved. In healthy scenarios, from the start babies actively communicate their needs to a responsive caregiver and subsequently develop the blueprint for reciprocal dyadic relationships that can be rooted in the erotic realm. This is the ground upon which many aspects of adult sexuality, security and love rest.

As such, attachment and sexuality need not be understood in opposition to one another. Security, sexuality and love develop simultaneously, and thrive as intertwined, essential and mutually influencing cohabitants in both infantile and adult experience. These inevitably inform and stimulate many aspects of emotional and corporeal life, such as hunger, frustration, excitement, satiety, safety and desire – all of which are intrinsic to emotional and sexual experience and form the mutually influencing dynamics in which love is created and flourishes.

John Bowlby and psychoanalysis

Although all psychoanalytic theories of sexuality, as well as attachment theory, assume that early infantile experience shapes adult romantic relationships, they differ significantly in emphasis. Bowlby (1969), the originator of attachment theory, maintained that infants develop an internal working model of the self and others based on their experience of parental responses in the first years of life. In secure attachment, a child develops a dependency on an adult who sensitively and reliably responds to their needs for safety, security and protection. Attachment theorists emphasize the necessity of a secure base to foster healthy psychological development and adult coupling. In contrast, most psychoanalytic theories of erotic love highlight a range of unconscious experiences and psychological structures, as well as early childhood experiences, that lay the foundation for object relations matrices and subsequently influence adult sexuality.

These two models have evolved in separate silos over time and are often positioned in opposition to one another. But the alleged split between attachment needs and sexuality does not solely arise out of theoretical differences but may be located in political splits that have frequently plagued psychoanalysis and cast as outsiders those whose ideas do not conform to the dominant hegemony of the time (Schwartz, 1999). Unfortunately, Bowlby was relegated to this camp of outsiders (Kahr, 2015; Schwartz, 1999).

Throughout the 1920s to the 1940s, when Bowlby was training and working, the medical profession and lay population in the West advised the use of discipline beginning at birth. Psychoanalysis, owing to its roots in classical Freudian theory and its emergence within an ethos concerned with the overindulgence of children, did not place emphasis on the relational environment or emotional circumstances in which children were reared. Bowlby, a trained psychoanalyst who was supervised by Melanie Klein, was keenly interested in child development from the perspective of actual life experience and its impact on behaviour and psychological growth.

Bowlby's ideas were greatly influenced by his observations of children who were separated from their parents due to hospitalization or war. He was especially interested in the child's experience of separation and loss and observed the negative effects on children and their patterns of proximity seeking behaviour during times of stress and isolation. He noted how caregivers could provide comfort and security to the child, and advocated changes to public policy, child-rearing practices, and the theory of child psychosocial development.

Although his views were controversial, Bowlby's observations were bolstered by the support of colleagues such as D.W. Winnicott and Harry Harlow. Winnicott's observations of children also led him to depart from the then dominant viewpoint and, like Bowlby, he was subjected to profound criticism because he emphasized the quality of the actual relationship between a child and their caregiver, instead of unconscious phantasy and structures (Kahr, 2015; Schwartz, 1999). Now that Winnicott's ideas are widely accepted and early dyadic experience plays a prominent role in psychoanalytic theory, it may be forgotten that this was not always the case. Given the political zeitgeist of the time, in which he did not find widespread acceptance within psychoanalysis, Bowlby turned to another arena and sought empirical confirmation for his ideas about the importance of a secure base for children.

Harlow (1958), who experimented with rhesus monkeys reared in isolation, demonstrated the importance of an attachment bond between primate mothers and infants that went well beyond the need for basic nourishment. When separated from their mothers, infant monkeys exhibited unusual, distressed behaviours that, in Harlow's view, resulted from a deprivation of physical contact. In his well-known experiment, infant monkeys who were separated from their mothers and subsequently given a choice between surrogate wire or cloth mothers, chose the cloth surrogate. Their preference for soft, tactile comfort gave further support to the emerging evidence that children need bodily contact and comfort to feel secure and thrive. Attachment bonds flourish in such circumstances and in their absence, deprivation is injurious to development. Bowlby visited Harlow's laboratory, and they stayed in contact over many years and influenced one another's work (Van der Horst et al., 2008). There is little doubt that these experiments impacted and supported Bowlby's focus on the centrality of security in child development and also helped to place empirical research as a cornerstone of attachment theory.

Because both Winnicott and Bowlby had been scorned for highlighting the impact of the mother–child relationship on development, and because they shared concerns about childrearing practices and policies, in 1939 they collaborated on a letter to the *British Medical Journal*. In it they resolutely argued against the evacuation and separation of children from their mothers in London during the Second World War, a proposal that had been implemented to protect children from German bombardments. Their letter stressed the potential for lasting and severe emotional disturbance should children be separated from their mothers in such a manner (Bowlby et al., 1939).

One can only wonder what might have been if creative, original contributions had been welcomed and integrated rather than taken as heretical. If Bowlby, Winnicott and others whose ideas were disregarded had been embraced by mainstream psychoanalysis, the basic tenets of attachment theory might have become integral to our understanding of psychosocial development (although outsider status may have benefitted attachment theory), and a theory of attachment-based needs might have been permitted to flourish. Perhaps this would have allowed a dialogue, creating the possibility of integrating these concepts into a general psychoanalysis, including all aspects of unconscious and conscious psychic life. Had such an integration occurred, perhaps the assumption that attachment and erotic needs are at odds would not persist and would not be relied upon to explain the death of erotic desire in couple relationships.

Sexual experience and its place in psychoanalytic theory

The theory of infantile sexuality outlined by Freud locates the origins of erotic desire in the earliest phases of life: "the prototype of every love relationship is the child sucking at his mother's breast. The finding of the love object is in fact a 'refinding'" (Freud, 1905, p. 222). His theory assumes that unconscious phenomena underlie adult sexual experience; biology and conscious sexual attraction are only the manifest content – the surface – of sexual desire. Psychoanalytic schools of thought post-Freud have remained faithful to these ideas, but their focus has been the psyche of the individual – a vantage point that lacks the interpersonal dimensionality requisite to understanding the emergent unconscious and conscious phenomena that may enhance or dampen sexual desire and love.

The theoretical turn elaborated in object relations theory was a departure from Freud's focus on sexuality, marginalizing and relegating it to a less consequential status (Stein, 2008). In an important attempt to restore sexuality's prominence, André Green notes that the frequency of patients suffering from sexual problems has not lessened, but the central role of sexuality has been overtaken by "object relations, pregenital fixations, borderline pathology and theories and techniques drawn from observations of child development" (Green, 1995, p. 871).

Contributions from contemporary psychoanalysis

Along with Green, other contemporary theorists have attempted to restore sexual love to its previous prominence. Kernberg (1995) elaborated a model of "mature" sexual relations that employs a composite of Freudian drive and object relations theories. Kernberg positioned sexual desire in a dialectic of regressive and progressive psychic forces that activate aggression, libido, idealization and superego functions and arise from self and object representations – a welcome counterpoint to the Kleinian emphasis on the apprehension of reality and depressive position functioning (Friend, 2023). If aggression swamps love it can destroy eros; the inhibition of aggression can sterilize passion.

Another example can be found in the work of Wilkinson and Gabbard who examined the nature of enduring love from a contemporary Kleinian perspective. In this conceptualization, sustained sexual desire depends upon the oscillation between paranoid–schizoid and depressive modes of relating, between love and hate, fragmentation and repair, and separation and merger. They coined the term "romantic space" to describe the liminal intrapsychic and interpersonal space in both inner and external reality that "allows the lover and the beloved to offer each other a relatedness that is reassuringly familiar as well as abruptly fresh" (Wilkinson and Gabbard, 1995, p. 201).

Other developments in psychoanalytic theory have helpfully resituated sexuality within a two-person model that enables us to reconsider the fictive split between attachment needs and sexual desire. Relational theory re-orients psychoanalysis to the essential role of relationships in psychic life and illuminates an active dialogue between the sources of love and erotic desire, and the obstacles to maintaining sexual activity over time in couple relationships (Atlas, 2016; Benjamin, 1988; Davies, 2005; Goldner, 2004, 2006; Kristeva, 2004, 2014; Laplanche, 1989; Stein, 1998, 2006, 2008).

The relational psychoanalyst Stephen Mitchell challenged the assumption that familiarity necessarily leads to the loss of sexual desire: "[It] is not that romance itself has a tendency to become degraded, but that we spend considerable effort degrading it" (Mitchell, 2002, p. 28). Mitchell proposed a radical reversal: sexuality in relationships may suffer, not because they are filled with safety but rather because they are inherently risky – individual partners may unconsciously defend against the terrors associated with the alterity of the other by deadening erotic desire.

Mitchell's novel thesis generated an abundance of articles, both in support and contrast to his ideas (see Goldner, 2006). For example, Goldner challenged the contention that safety stands in opposition to love:

> In this context, the desire for adventure and the need for safety are not one-person affairs, driven solely by the internal dynamics of each partner. They are, rather, two-person experiences that co-evolve over the length of a long relationship, each framing the other, held in the tension of figure and ground. In other words, the risk of falling in love with the one you love is possible only in a context of safety – not the flaccid safety of permanent coziness, but a dynamic safety whose robustness is established via the couple's lived history of risk taking.
>
> (Goldner, 2004, p. 388)

Goldner further argued that safety is not present in all relationships – many are tormented by insecure or disorganized attachment patterns that result in unconscious repetition of detrimental dynamics. In such scenarios, it is more helpful to consider how destructive attacks on emotional security impact sexual intimacy, not the other way around.

Stein has critiqued Mitchell's ideas about the fate of romance in relationships, framing sexual experience as enigmatic, infected by unconscious components not easily reduced to the terrors of intimacy. She elaborated a model of passionate desire and love that is grounded in the earliest aspects of sexual experience, when the traces of longing, frustration, lack and loss accompany the pleasures of gratification, transgression and transcendence (Stein, 1998, 2006, 2008).

Sexuality in the psychoanalytic couple psychotherapy literature

In contrast to the popular misconception that practitioners are preoccupied with the topic of sexuality, many couple therapists seem to avoid the topic (Abse, 2009). Fonagy (2009) has commented on the irony that couple psychotherapists, the clinicians best positioned to study sexual relationships, have written so little about them. Whether this neglect is born out of training models that underplay sex in favour of other phenomena, or an internalized cultural discomfort and prudishness to which couple therapists are not immune, the result is that many couple therapists seem to be reluctant to directly address a couple's sex life in clinical practice (Kahr, 2009).

Most of the early psychoanalytic couple literature, especially that which emerged from the model developed at Tavistock Relationships in London, reflects a similar de-emphasis of sexuality. Due to their allegiance to object relations and Kleinian theory, a primary emphasis is placed on the couple's need to achieve depressive position functioning. Thus, sexual activity was not foregrounded, and the central focus was placed on the ways in which couples, through projective identification, unconsciously choose one another, influence one another, and develop shared unconscious dynamics that shape their relationship.

In an important corrective, some authors working with the Tavistock model have attempted to redress this erasure of sexuality (e.g. Clulow, 2009; Hertzman, 2022; McCann, 2022). Some have specifically taken up the question at hand: Why do some long-term couples stop having sexual relations? Grier (2005, 2009), linking primal scene anxieties and Bion's concept of catastrophic change, suggested the "no-sex" couple is defending against an unconscious oedipal dynamic. Berg (2012) and Sehgal (2023) use the concepts of autistic–contiguous anxieties (Ogden, 1989) and the core complex (Glasser, 1979) to understand the problem.

Clulow (2009) edited an excellent collection of papers on the topic of attachment and sex in couple psychotherapy. However, in Fonagy's foreword to the book, the idea that attachment and erotic needs are at odds is proclaimed as fact: "The biology of sex and attachment, as well as their psychology, are incompatible" (Fonagy, 2009, p. xx). In contrast, Clulow framed the dilemma as a debate between biology and interpersonal processes, with Freudian theory posed as counterpoint to relational psychoanalysis.

> Relational narratives link biology and interpersonal processes in perpetual cycles of mutual influence. At its most minimal, sex in this context is a form of sociability, a medium of contact, a route to intimacy. Here, what might be attributed to body and instinct is understood as being shaped by social interactions. Both Freudian and relational perspectives recognise the significance of biology and environment in shaping sexuality; their differences are more in terms of whether psychological meaning derives from preformed forces, or, whether it is created and shaped through relationships.
>
> (Clulow, 2009, p. xxx)

Notwithstanding the false divide often posited in the literature, some explicitly consider the reciprocal relationship between attachment and sexuality. Caruso (2011), describing the dynamic interplay of the couple's object relations, attachment styles and sexual functioning, emphasized the importance of considering all these factors in couple psychotherapy. In a publication of papers presented at the 2004 John Bowlby Memorial Conference, the importance of the relationship between attachment and sexuality was explored, with particular emphasis on the link between emotional communication, the body and attachment (White, 2005). In an edited volume entitled *Attachment and Sexuality*, many contributors explored the convergence between these two systems, with the implication that they form a "bidirectional matrix" that beckons for an integrative approach (Diamond et al., 2007, p. 2).

The core concepts of psychoanalytic couple psychotherapy, especially those focusing on shared unconscious phantasy and projection identification, can be immensely useful in helping couples improve the quality of their relationships, and sometimes do result in a restoration of waning or inactive sexuality. But it has been my experience, along with other clinicians (Abse, 2009), that this sometimes results in couples who get along much better, yet have not resurrected their sex life and are left to question if they are still in love.

Working with the loss of sex in couples

If the diminishment of erotic love in couple relationships cannot be explained with a one-dimensional analysis positing attachment needs as the primary cause, how might we better conceptualize the problem? I propose that the diminishment or absence of sex in a previously fulfilling and sexually active relationship should be regarded as a symptom – one that is active in real time, functions communicatively and is rich with symbolic meaning. And, like all symptom presentations, this requires the therapist's receptivity to emotional communication, both conscious and unconscious, in the context of a consistent frame promoting reflection, understanding and thinking. Approaching couple dynamics within this framework provides the precondition for an understanding of the anxieties and defences that may underlie the problem at hand. Rather than reflexively assuming that the answer is in the tension between attachment needs and erotic desire, we may more open-mindedly examine an array of possible sources of difficulty.

Sexual problems may be disguised or revealed in interpersonal difficulties, and interpersonal problems may contaminate sex. All sexuality can be viewed as a form of "enactment": some enactments are playful, creative and generate metaphorical meaning; others are concrete, restrictive of metaphorical meaning and can result in rigid or compulsive sexual patterns. Colman (2009) advocates a two-way technical approach that explores interpersonal dynamics in terms of sexual metaphors, as well as the ways sexual activity (or its absence) may metaphorically reveal relational dynamics.

Working psychoanalytically with any type of sexual symptom must be approached non-moralistically and from the couple's point of view. It is their sex life, not ours. While they may generate powerful countertransferences, the specific sexual acts a couple does or does not do with one another (or with other people) may or may not be the focus of the work. Our role is to bring understanding, not to judge, denigrate or prescribe according to preconceived ideals or standards. This includes checking our biases that couples should want to be having sex together.

Much of sexual experience lives in non-verbal, bodily experience and is not easily represented in language. Talking about sex is difficult for many, if not most people. A feeling of safety is necessary for such conversations, and addressing what is threatening about the topic is essential before specific content can be discussed. Sexual fantasies and activities are often confined to the most private realms and are sometimes rife with insecurity and shame. Many people, including some clinicians, are not comfortable wading into this territory. Couples often have difficulty communicating with one another about their dislikes and desires, even within the confines of their own bedroom, let alone with a third person. In my experience, unless they are directly asked, it is not unusual for couples to avoid the topic completely. Nonetheless, some couples whose sex life has languished are aware of the sources of their difficulties and can, within the safe confines of the therapeutic setting, talk about them. However, many do not and the lack of sex in their relationship is experienced as a mystery, devoid of meaning – an impenetrable expanse filled with deadened desire, frustration and a longing for love.

Thinking beyond the false divide in the clinical setting

The loss of desire in relationships may rest upon a wide range of conscious and unconscious difficulties. Arguably, the immense scope of these potential problems mirrors the complexity and diversity of love and sexual experience itself. Nonetheless, I want to highlight some of the many factors that may contribute to problematic sexual relationships.

Breakdowns in communication can erode a feeling of connection at the emotional level that, over time, can impact sexual relations. The common, everyday interactions that arise out of different emotional states or needs can create dysregulating ruptures and failures in mutual recognition. Even small facial gestures, tones of voice or verbal references can be symbolically loaded with meaning and communicated via projective identification. A simple sigh or rolling of the eyes can be sufficient to begin a cycle of disruption. When the interaction is loaded with mutual anxiety, or when one or both partners have difficulty with emotional self-regulation, the conflictual interactions will tend to escalate and not easily be contained. In well-functioning relationships, when the partners possess depressive position capacities, failure of mutual recognition may be repaired, and the vitality of the emotional link may be strengthened. When this is not possible, the couple can be left to contend with rigid patterns of projective identification and splitting and are unable to reliably restore the loving connection between them.

Many couples suffer from a lack of psychic separation that can manifest in myriad problems including the end of sexual desire or activity. Healthy relationships rest on a psychic capacity for thirdness, the ability to hold onto one's own separateness, while at the same time being in relation to another person (Morgan, 2005; Nathans, 2021). In the absence of this capacity, regressive pulls for sameness or security may dominate, obscuring separateness and resulting in alienation or merger. Sometimes these types of relationships are characterized by excessive caregiving or parent–child dynamics that threaten the psychic security of adult sexual relations. In more extreme instances, the desire for merger rests alongside claustrophobic anxieties that infuse sexual activity with especially dangerous experience (Berg, 2012; Sehgal, 2023).

From an attachment perspective, a secure base provides freedom and psychological safety in both childhood and adulthood, making exploration possible and enhancing the pursuit of passion. Relationships between two securely attached people are more likely to have relational flexibility and boundaries that allow for satisfying separate and intimate forms of contact, including sex. These relationships tend to be stable and suffer less from the interpersonal turmoil that can threaten erotic connection and the feeling of love. By contrast, insecure patterns of attachment may recruit sexuality in the service of attachment needs: intimacy may be avoided to maintain a sense of control or anxiously maintained out of fear of abandonment (Clulow, 2009).

Difficulties in the non-sexual aspects of couple life can contaminate and spoil sexual relations. Disappointments, grudges and complaints, accrued over time, can dampen desire and assail the exciting and idealized aspects of the erotic link upon which the partnership was formed. While I have contested Mitchell's thesis as representing a universal truth, for some the risks and vulnerabilities inherent in mutually dependent sexual relations may be too frightening and can be obscured by the fictive mask of familiarity and comfort (Mitchell, 2002).

Alternatively, as Stein (2006) noted, counting sins and storing grudges may have a defensive function born out of superego anxieties based in oedipal guilt, inhibiting the couple from enjoying a satisfying sexual life and sustaining a feeling of love. In addition to guilt, other sources of unconscious oedipal conflict, such as shared catastrophic primal scene anxieties (Grier, 2005), may dominate in one or both partners and wreak havoc in the sexual sphere.

Healthy aggression is essential to love and its expression in sexual excitement. Unconscious conflicts about aggression can manifest in the sexual sphere, particularly when a relationship gets bogged down in excessive unconscious anxieties about destruction or when one or both partners possess insufficient empathy or concern about harm. A healthy integration of aggression and libido is necessary for sexual relations and the capacity to love (Kernberg, 1995). Eros may be destroyed by aggression and inhibition of aggression may ruin passion.

In relationships where one or both partners have a history of sexual abuse, sex may consciously or unconsciously resurrect the residue of trauma. This may manifest in a variety of problems with sexual performance or satisfaction, such as extreme inhibitions or compulsions, pain with penetration, erectile dysfunction or difficulties with orgasm – all of which may degrade the quality and frequency of sex. By its very nature, past trauma has the potential for causing dysregulated states, and when it is revived along with the potential deregulating aspects of sex, it can be overwhelming for the partners.

Conscious awareness of complaints specific to differences in sexual preferences may also be at play and can become ensconced in rigid dynamics that dull or destroy sexual desire and connection. In scenarios when one partner wants more sex than their partner, the struggle over psychic or bodily autonomy can engender an intractable power dynamic. If one person has a particular aversion to a sexual activity that the other partner desires, difficulties with boundary issues and maintaining the symmetry necessary for mutually satisfying consensual activity may blur the distinction between exciting surrender and frightening submission. In discussing the complexities of domination in relationships, Benjamin has pointed to a "breakdown of the necessary tension between self-assertion and mutual recognition that allows self and other to meet as sovereign equals" (Benjamin, 1988, p. 12). In my experience, these types of breakdowns and imbalances do not rest quietly. Rather, they emerge as repetitive, regressive, anti-developmental forces that exact their toll on many aspects of a relationship, but especially in the sexual realm.

With the passage of time, change is inevitable – and ageing bodies change. Older bodies do not function with youthful vigour, nor do they necessarily perform reliably in the bedroom. Libidinal desire may diminish due to hormonal shifts or illness. A couple's struggles with these losses may result from narcissistic vulnerabilities that interfere with accepting the realities of ageing, the return of earlier anxieties (Balfour, 2017), or long-standing difficulties in the capacity to mourn (Nathans, 2012). But despite the many challenges inherent in ageing, many couples can successfully navigate these losses and retain a lively erotic link to one another.

A vignette

I offer this vignette, composed of similar clinical presentations from several couples who have stopped having sex, to illustrate an approach to this symptom based on an exploration of unconscious anxieties and defences – a formulation that extends beyond the assumption that love and sexuality have been overtaken by the need for security and stability.

Alicia and Jonathan, a married couple with a two-year-old child, on the verge of divorce, came to therapy unsure if they were still in love. They reported having had an active, gratifying sexual connection for the first four years of their relationship, but after the birth of their child they've rarely had sex. Alicia said she was worried Jonathan wasn't attracted to her anymore because whenever she approached him, he rejected her. She said she felt she must attend to everyone else's needs and longed to be cared for. Jonathan said he was exhausted. He worked all day and then was obligated to share the childcare and domestic duties. Alicia countered that she, too, had a full-time job and Jonathan only imagined he was doing his fair share. She said he came home, ignored her, devoted his attention to their daughter, and left all the chores to her.

This is a common presentation in couple psychotherapy and it would have been easy to ascribe this couple's difficulties to the everyday strains of young, working parents, or to the reductive idea that the routine structure and needs of family life had created a sense of predictability or boredom, eroding their sexual connection and love for one another. But it quickly became evident that something more troubling was at play that would not be sufficiently addressed by encouraging them to create novelty or have more date nights. A full description of the clinical work is beyond the scope of this chapter, but I offer a brief description of their dynamics and a summary of my understanding of what lay at the root of their problems.

Alicia's parents divorced when she was five and her father died when she was a teenager. She never felt close to her mother, whom she described as a selfish person. She said she had never felt a strong desire for a child, had been unsure she would be a good mother, and worried about the impact on her career.

Jonathan said he always knew he wanted to be a father and had hoped to have more than one child but watching Alicia parent their daughter made him question if this would be possible. His parents also divorced when he was young, at the age of eight. He said he admired his father from afar and wished to spend more time with him. He described his mother as a highly anxious person whose chronic depression and judgemental critiques kept him wary and at bay.

Alicia had had a difficult pregnancy, a long and painful labour, and a complicated postpartum recovery. Jonathan felt he had to step up and take care of their baby in the first weeks after the birth. Rather than feeling that he was supporting her, Alicia experienced Jonathan as "crowding her out and taking over". She said, "he criticises me all the time; he thinks he is the better mother to our daughter". Jonathan claimed he was only trying to "show" Alicia how to be a better mother. For example, when she was nursing, he thought it was important for her to maintain eye contact and not get distracted by her phone. Additionally, he worried that Alicia's desire to sleep train their daughter could be emotionally harmful, so he started sleeping in the child's bedroom. Alicia said she feared he loved their child more than he loved her and she believed their daughter was more attached to him. As evidence, Alicia described feeling jealous and excluded when she came home from work, witnessing Jonathan and their daughter playing together.

My concerns in this case went well beyond the diminishment of this couple's sexual life, which I viewed as a symptom reflective of problematic unconscious dynamics. I worried that their daughter was being triangulated in a destructive dynamic that threatened the bond between Alicia and the daughter, the bond between Alicia and Jonathan, and the stability of the family. I speculated that the initial erotic link between Alicia and Jonathan was based on an unconscious wish for a dyadic union that offered the illusion of psychic repair to each of their internal divorced parental couple representations, as well as a phantasized reunion with a more perfectly attentive, caregiving parent. With this type of dyadic link, the couple could not easily integrate an actual third. The birth of their child revived the early attachment anxieties from each of their childhoods, resulting in a painful pattern of pursuit and rejection ensconced in a destructive projective identification process. Alicia, deeply insecure about her maternal capacities, had become a "bad mother" in both of their eyes, and this was projected onto their daughter who was viewed as insufficiently cared for by her. Jonathan, the putative "better mother", was unconsciously identified with his own judgemental mother and was critical of Alicia. This defensive stance allowed him to deny his own anxieties about parenting, as well as his critical superiority, which enabled him to distance himself from a "bad mother". While Jonathan consciously thought he was supporting Alicia and protecting their daughter, Alicia experienced this as a betrayal that excluded her. From within this field, they each projected an unavailable father onto one another, much like their own fathers who they felt had abandoned them in divorce or death.

The love between two partners in any relationship will undoubtedly contain elements of both dyadic and triadic excitement and anxiety but, in this case,

Alicia and Jonathan's love was swamped by triadic conflicts that their initial dyadic link could not bear. From an attachment perspective, the insecure attachments in each created an insecure couple attachment – a connection that was not secure enough to withstand the challenges inherent to parenting. Under the assault of these destructive splits and projections, replayed in real time in their day-to-day interactions, the love of their first years together could not flourish. Rather than the need for stability and security undoing their sexual life, insecurity was creating instability, undermining their erotic connection and love for one another.

Conclusion

In this article, I have made the case against the commonly held idea that attachment needs are necessarily in opposition to sexuality and that the need for security will inevitably create a sense of familiarity that dulls sexual excitement and its loving expression in long-term relationships. Although attachment and sexuality may be described as separate behavioural systems, they do not occur independently, and can be conceived as operating in a dialectical, mutually influencing relationship. Moreover, attachment and sexuality exist in a mutually influencing dialectic with the object relations fields of both partners in a couple. The integration of all these factors creates dynamics that impact the sexual and emotional life of the couple, all of which can be situated in the presence or absence of love.

One-person psychoanalytic models are inadequate to address the complexity of the myriad unconscious dynamics that create or degrade love, sexual desire and sexual connection in a relationship. Instead, I advocate a two-person, contemporary psychoanalytic approach to romantic love that is based on an integration of emotional experience, attachment needs and sexuality. This approach promotes consideration of a wide array of potential unconscious and conscious forces that may contribute to the extinguishing of sexual activity. I have emphasized that attachment, erotic experience and love originate in infancy, are rooted in both emotional and bodily experience, and develop in a relational context characterized by responsive, reciprocal communication between the infant and caregiver(s). The enigmatic erotic messages of maternal desire that Kristeva (2014) has theorized are transmitted in a relational context inseparable from the maternal care that also promotes security and lays the foundation for love in adulthood.

In adult relationships as well, attachment and erotic experiences emerge and are played out relationally. They are communicated, sorted, destroyed, negotiated and revived intrapsychically and interpersonally, through conscious and unconscious processes, in both the emotional and corporeal realms. The origin of the capacity for making love – the healthy surrender to one's own and one's partner's desires – does not reside exclusively in conscious experience. It is situated in the primordial history of comfort and security found in our earliest contact with another person's physical body. It resides there for lovers to re-find when embraced in the arms of one another, in the dynamic safety of secure erotic attachment. Ultimately, it might be attachment itself that keeps sex exciting, gratifying, and safe. By the logic of the theory that security needs to recruit familiarity in their contest against libido, novelty must be pursued to maintain necessary erotic tension, and sexuality is subsequently defined by its limitations. But if the source of libidinal desire rests in another arena – in the desire to re-find the erotic in the context of security – then love and sex may freely thrive and endure over time.

References

Abse, S. (2009). Sexual dread and the therapist's desire. In: C. Clulow (Ed.), *Sex, attachment and couple psychotherapy: Psychoanalytic perspectives.* Karnac Books, pp. 103–118.

Atlas, G. (2016). *The enigma of desire: Sex, longing, and belonging in psychoanalysis.* Routledge.

Balfour, A. (2017). Growing old together in mind and body. In: S. Nathans and M. Schaefer (eds), *Couples on the couch: Psychoanalytic couple therapy and the Tavistock Model.* Routledge.

Beebe, B. (2006). Co-constructing mother–infant distress in face-to-face inter-actions: Contributions of microanalysis. *Infant Observation*, 9 (2): 151–164.

Benjamin, J. (1988). *The bonds of love: Psychoanalysis, feminism, and the problem of domination.* Pantheon.

Ben-Ze'ev, A. (2022, May 10). Do lovers want change or familiarity? *Psychology Today.* https://www.psychologytoday.com/us/blog/in-the-name-love/202205/ do-lovers-want-change-or-familiarity. (Accessed 1 August 2025.)

Berg, J. (2012). "A bad moment with the light". No-sex couples: The role of autistic contiguous anxieties. *Couple and Family Psychoanalysis*, 2 (1): 33–48.

Bowlby, J. (1969) *Attachment and loss: Attachment.* Hogarth Press.

Bowlby, J., Miller, E., & Winnicott, D.W. (1939). Evacuation of small children. *British Medical Journal*, 2: 1202–1203. doi:10.1136/bmj.2.4119.1202-b

Caruso, N. (2011). The entangled nature of attachment and sexuality in the couple relationship. *Couple and Family Psychoanalysis*, 1 (1): 117–135.

Clulow, C. (ed.) (2009). *Sex, attachment and couple psychotherapy: Psychoanalytic perspectives.* Karnac Books.

Colman, W. (2009). What do we mean by "sex"? In: C. Clulow (ed.), *Sex, attachment and couple psychotherapy: Psychoanalytic perspectives.* Karnac Books, pp. 25–44.

Davies, J. (2005). The John Bowlby Memorial Lecture 2004. The times we sizzle, and the times we sigh; The multiple erotics of arousal, anticipation, and release. In: K. White (ed.), *Attachment and sexuality in clinical practice.* Karnac Books, pp. 57–80.

Diamond, D., Blatt, S., & Lichtenberg, J. (eds) (2007). *Attachment and sexuality.* Routledge.

Eagle, M. (2007). Attachment and sexuality. In: D. Diamond, S. Blatt and J. Lichtenberg (eds), *Attachment and sexuality.* Routledge, pp. 27–50.

Fonagy, P. (2009). Foreword. In: C. Clulow (ed.), *Sex, attachment and couple psychotherapy: Psychoanalytic perspectives.* Karnac Books, pp. xvii–xxiii.

Freud, S. (1905). *Three essays on the theory of sexuality.* In J. Strachey (ed. and trans.), *The standard edition of the complete psychological works of Sigmund Freud* (1953–74), Volume 7. Hogarth Press, pp. 123–246.

Friend, J. (2023). Love as creative illusion and its place in psychoanalytic couple psychotherapy. In: S. Nathans (ed.), *More about couples on the couch: Approaching psychoanalytic couple psychotherapy from an expanded perspective.* Routledge, pp. 33–46.

Glasser, M. (1979). Aggression and sadism in the perversions. In: I. Rosen (ed.), *Sexual deviation.* Oxford University Press, pp. 279–299.

Goldner, V. (2004). Attachment and eros: Opposed or synergistic? [Review]. *Psychoanalytic Dialogues,* 14: 381–396.

Goldner, V. (2006). "Let's do it again": Further reflections on eros and attachment. *Psychoanalytic Dialogues,* 16 (6): 619–637.

Green, A. (1995). Has sexuality anything to do with psychoanalysis? *International Journal of Psychoanalysis,* 76: 871–883.

Grier, F. (ed.) (2005) No sex couples, catastrophic change, and the primal scene. In: *Oedipus and the couple.* Karnac Books, pp. 201–220.

Grier, F. (2009). Lively and deathly intercourse. In: C. Clulow (ed.), *Sex, attachment and couple psychotherapy: Psychoanalytic perspectives.* Karnac Books, pp. 45–62.

Harlow, H.F. (1958). The nature of love. *American Psychologist,* 13: 673–685.

Hertzmann, L. (2022). Lesbian and gay couple relationships: When internalized homophobia gets in the way of couple creativity. In: S. Nathans (ed.), *More about couples on the couch: Approaching psychoanalytic couple psychotherapy from an expanded perspective.* Routledge, pp. 112–131.

Kahr, B. (2009). Psychoanalysis and sexpertise. In: C. Clulow (ed.), *Sex, attachment and couple psychotherapy: Psychoanalytic perspectives.* Karnac Books, pp. 2–33.

Kahr, B. (2015). Led astray by their half-baked pseudo-scientific rubbish: John Bowlby and the paradigm shift in child psychiatry. *Attachment: New Directions in Relational Psychoanalysis and Psychotherapy,* 9: 297–317.

Kernberg, O. (1995). *Love relations: Normality and pathology.* Yale University Press.

Kristeva, J. (2004). Some observations on female sexuality. *The Annual of Psychoanalysis,* 32: 59–68.

Kristeva, J. (2014). Reliance, or maternal eroticism. *Journal of the American Psychoanalytic Association,* 62 (1): 69–85.

Laplanche, J. (1989). *New Foundations for Psychoanalysis.* Blackwell.

McCann, D. (2022). *Same sex couples and other identities.* Routledge.

Mitchell, S. (2002). *Can love last: The fate of romance over time.* W.W. Norton.

Morgan, M. (2005). On being able to be a couple: The importance of a "creative couple" in psychic life. In: F. Grier (ed.), *Oedipus and the couple.* Karnac Books, pp. 9–30).

Nathans, S. (2012). Infidelity as manic defence. *Couple and Family Psychoanalysis,* 2: 165–180.

Nathans, S. (2021). Oedipus for everyone: Revitalizing the model for LBGTQ couples and single parent families. *Psychoanalytic Dialogues,* 31 (3): 312–328. doi:10.1080/10481885.2021.1898398.

Ogden, T. (1989). On the concept of an autistic–contiguous position. *International Journal of Psychoanalysis,* 70 (1): 127–140.

Perel, E. (2006). *Mating in captivity: Unlocking erotic intelligence.* Harper Collins.
Schwartz, J. (1999). *Cassandra's daughter: A history of psychoanalysis.* Viking Penguin Press.
Sehgal, A. (2023). Viewing the absence of sex from couple relationships through the "Core Complex" lens. In: S. Nathans (ed.), *More about couples on the couch: Approaching psychoanalytic couple psychotherapy from an expanded perspective.* Routledge, pp. 84–101.
Stein, R. (1998). Passion's friends, passion's enemies: Commentary on paper by Stephen A Mitchell. *Psychoanalytic Dialogues*, 8: 547–560.
Stein, R. (2006). Unforgetting and excess, the re-creation and re-finding of suppressed sexuality. *Psychoanalytic Dialogues*, 16: 763–778.
Stein, R. (2008). The otherness of sexuality: Excess. *Journal of the American Psychoanalytic Association*, 56: 43–71.
Stern, D. (1985). *The interpersonal world of the infant*. Routledge.
Van der Horst, F.C., Leroy, H.A. & van der Veer, R. (2008). When strangers meet: John Bowlby and Harry Harlow on attachment behavior. *Integrative Psychological and Behavioral Science*, 42(4): 370–388. https://pubmed.ncbi.nlm.nih.gov/18766423.
White, K. (ed.) (2005). *Attachment and sexuality in clinical practice.* Karnac Books.
Wilkinson, S.M. & Gabbard, G.O. (1995). On romantic space. *Psychoanalytic Psychology*, 12: 201–219.
Winnicott, D.W. (1964). *The child, the family, and the outside world.* Penguin.

Chapter 5

Love is where we start from

An examination of Winnicott's "use of an object" as it relates to mature love in the couple relationship

Ortal Kirson-Trilling

A most brilliant design feature of the human being is that in our state of utter dependence at birth, we are born "hardwired" for love. Even so, to love another is more difficult a task than one might imagine. Difficult, in part, because our hardwiring for love is but one building block in our capacity to truly love another. Psychoanalysts have long understood that our capacity to love another in adulthood follows in large part from the quality of psychic provisions offered in our earliest relationship(s). The presence and absence of essential elements of the early psychic environment are akin to uploaded "software" that shape our capacity to open-heartedly give and receive love as adults. Such "software" can also confuse, override, distort or outright block our inborn hardwired receptivity to love. Even so, love is arguably one of the greatest preoccupations of human beings. Because, more often than not, when we drill down to the heart of the matter, it is the *heart*, above all else, that *matters*. Love. To feel loved, beloved. This is what so many members of our couples long for in their relationships. Herein lies the ultimate challenge for couples; there is often a discrepancy between an experience of longing for love and an appreciation for the very need to grow and thus "*learn*" to love as Rilke wisely suggests:

> For one human being to love another: that is perhaps the most difficult of all our tasks, the ultimate, the last test and proof, the work for which all other work is but preparation. For this reason, young people, who are beginners in everything, cannot yet know love: they have to learn it. With their whole being, with all their forces, gathered close about their lonely, timid, upward-beating heart, they must learn to love.
>
> (Rilke, 2012, pp. 48–9)

Perhaps because we are hardwired for love we imagine love to be straightforward, easily accessible and naturally forthcoming in the couple relationship. When it is not, members of couples can feel frustrated and may begin to search for signs or evidence of their partner's love. Evidence in words or actions. But when the very same words and actions that once felt like love, no

DOI: 10.4324/9781003518129-5

longer feel like love, the very same words and actions no longer *represent* love. And this is not surprising because love cannot be pinned down or defined. Rather, love is an *experience*. We know love because we *feel* love. What is more is that one cannot demand love from another – it can only be "given" freely. It can be rather dizzying for couples to sort out why they or their partner may struggle with love in the couple, especially because the experience of longing for love can leave members of couples feeling pained and dejected.

Beyond the chemistry between two people, how do the same two people who felt a spark between them grow into a couple that supports feelings of love? While we may not be able to define love, as such, I believe we can identify conditions that foster the emergence of the experience and thus the feeling of love in a couple relationship. In this chapter I examine one essential, albeit complex, early psychic "provision", namely the destruction and survival of the object that I believe ushers in the capacity to love. I propose that psychic discovery of the other through a constant reshaping of our ideas about the other leads to psychic growth, to "learning" to love – from which the capacity for care, concern, respect, tenderness and generosity emerge to form mature love in the couple relationship.

In a letter to Jung in 1906, Freud wrote: "Psychoanalysis is, in essence, a cure through love" (Freud, 1974, pp. 8–9). Indeed, it is. Because we might say that, by examining the psychic environment of the earliest relationship, psychoanalysts have decoded or deconstructed the essential elements of a m/other's love that facilitate psychic development and translated them to the analytic setting. Fundamentally, psychoanalysts have long understood that love and psychic development go hand-in-hand. Love is both "where" we start from and "where" we grow from. Analytic work, whether with a couple or an individual, is the work of psychologically developing and growing through loving psychic provisions. We might imagine the sign of infinity with love and psychic development flowing into and from one another.

On the side of psychic development, we are aided in our task by an innate need to grow. Winnicott remarked, that in each baby is a vital spark "and this urge towards life and growth and development is a part of the baby, and … is carried forward in a way that we do not have to understand" (Winnicott, 1964, p. 27). Indeed, this impulse to develop is intrinsic to us all. Ogden (2022b) describes this urge to grow as "an intense, unrelenting force within us to hurl ourselves against the walls of internal and external constraints in our effort to achieve increasing depth and breadth of who we are and who we might become" (p. 1). But development, throughout the lifespan, just as in our earliest months and years of life, requires an ongoing psychic environment that supports psychic growth. Psychoanalytic therapy can provide this environment as can the couple relationship itself. We might say that, taken together, our inherited hardwiring for love along with our innate "urge towards life, growth and development" constitute two of the most central aspects of the human psyche that we, psychoanalytic couple therapists, rely on in our work with individuals and couples. Surely, this is a most obvious point. And yet it is this, our loving psychic provisions, (intimately linked to the m/other–infant experience) that aims to facilitate growth and development in the members of our couples.

To this aim, when thinking analytically about mature love in the couple, we begin with an understanding that, in order to love another, one must first allow them to *be* "an other". This is no easy or small feat. Tavistock Relationships theorists have long recognized that the capacity to experience the other as a true separate other is a critical developmental milestone for healthy couple relating. Why is this particular aspect of psychic life so crucial in the couple relationship? Because one cannot love another if the other is merely a psychic extension of oneself. While we necessarily build up conscious and unconscious "stories" in our minds about the other with whom we are coupled (and thus we are forever "creating" them in phantasy), an enduring feeling of love toward one's partner is predicated on the capacity to experience the other as truly separate. Because, if the built-up stories of the other remain fixed, immovable, the other – that is, one's partner – cannot be known, felt and experienced. The other, then, who is all the time in the process of "becoming", ceases to be known. When the channels to knowing the other are closed, so, too, are the channels to loving the other. They are, in essence, the same channels.

In order to truly encounter the other, we must be open to the "destruction" of our "built-up stories" of the other. Herein lies the potential for members of a couple to "do something with" the otherness of the other. In essence, to make genuine contact with the reality that is the other, as opposed to our ideas of them, we must be willing to supplant our "version" of the other with an updated version of them that incorporates an otherwise ignored aspect of the reality of them. This new version will be supplanted again at some point in the future because the other is never fully knowable. Still, each time we engage with this process we encounter the otherness of the other from a fresh place. This experience of registering the ways in which we were inevitably "erasing" the other fosters humility which ushers in important reflective inquiries (e.g., What else do I tell myself about you that is inaccurate?). "Learning" to love in the couple relationship is an active process. Psychic shifts born out of such realizations pave a path to discovery. As Mitchell wrote: "When we give ourselves over to loving somebody, it is not just them we are discovering and loving but who we will become when we are with them" (Mitchell, 2002, p. 83). It is the very act (I do believe something very active must occur here) of "seeing" the other, that is, supplanting our version and discovering ourselves and the other, that psychically creates the (ever discoverable) other anew. Only then can love emerge.

To my mind, the most helpful theory regarding the developmental leap into being able to experience the other as separate was put forth by Winnicott. His ideas about the development of the capacity to use the object is the very process by which we encounter the externality of the other. And yet, even Winnicott (1971) conveys how challenging it is to arrive at the capacity for object usage:

> In the sequence one can say that first there is object-relating, then in the end there is object-use; in between, however, is the most difficult thing, perhaps, in human development; or the most irksome of all the early failures that come for mending. The thing that there is in between relating and use is the subject's placing the object outside the area of the subject's *omnipotent control*; that is, the subject's perception of the object as an external phenomenon, not as a projective entity, in fact recognition of it as an entity in its own right.
>
> (Winnicott, 1971, p. 89)

Why does Winnicott suggest that this particular aspect of development is the most challenging? This certainly rings true and helps us understand why Tavistock Relationships theorists have written most extensively about the capacity to experience the other as "an entity in its own right".

Time and again, we encounter couples in our consulting rooms who are desperately attempting to "use" their partner, in the Winnicottian sense, only to be met with retaliation. Such "use" is simultaneously self-serving in the sense that it is meant to support the psychic development of one member of the couple while at the same time it is the very vehicle through which mature love can emerge. How I understand the "desire" to "use" the other is through our search for another who will facilitate our ongoing psychic growth.

Bollas (1987) suggests that the urge to grow is "baked in" as a powerful unconscious motivator to *seek* partnership. Bollas writes, "I think we have failed to take notice of the phenomenon in adult life of the wide-ranging collective search for an object that is identified with the metamorphosis of the self" (Bollas, 1987, pp. 15–16). Bollas thus posits that the pursuit of a love object is, simultaneously, a pursuit of a transformational object, an object that will usher in ontological transformations (here I mean to be pointing to our ongoing developmental striving to be more fully our real and true selves). For Bollas this search is driven by our earliest experience with the m/other as process, specifically, an ontogenic process – that is, a process in which the m/other facilitates our coming into being our unique self. He writes:

> I have termed the first object the transformational object … Before the mother is personalized to the infant as a whole object she has functioned as a source of transformation … the first object is identified with the alterations of the ego's state. This ego experience remains as an unconscious memory in the adult who relives it through his adamant quest for a transformational object.
>
> (Bollas, 1987, p 97)

That is to say, the quest, the yearning for an other to facilitate our development is a powerful aspect of our drive to be a couple. Indeed, throughout the lifespan, we seek personal transformation through contact with intimate others. Using the other, in the Winnicottian sense, carries one such powerful transformational experience.

I will briefly review Winnicott's theory of object usage. In the beginning, when the newborn infant is unaware of the care they receive, it is of utmost importance that they are not made aware of the demands they place on their m/other. In a good-enough environment, there is time for the infant to "place the object in the world". During this stage of development, the repeated uninhibited demand for adaptation from the m/other amounts to a continual destruction of the m/other. The ongoing "destruction" is not born of anger or hate. It is a natural and necessary part of the process (over time) of discovering the "externality of the object". Abram (2022) likens this type of destruction to destroying the food we eat in order to metabolize its value.

The m/other's sustained ability to tolerate endless (destructive) demands offers the infant a sense of continuity and reliability. From this offering of reliability and non-retaliation, made possible by primary maternal preoccupation, the m/other's identification with the infant's position of dependency and the father's holding of the nursing couple, the infant is able to move from absolute dependence to relative dependence with a gradual awareness of the environment that is the m/other. It is here that the baby begins to perceive the m/other as being a part of "Not-me". Abram writes,

> As the baby starts to see the same person in a different way so the previous imago of the mother is destroyed. The previous merger of the environment mother and the object mother that made the baby feel he had two different mothers due to such extremely different experiences of both, emanating from his stage of development, begins to change and he becomes aware of one mother.
>
> (Abram, 2022, pp. 40–1)

Winnicott (1965, pp. 267–8) explains that the baby puts one and one together and makes one. It is at this point that the infant can "use" the object. Winnicott (1971) writes:

> This is a position [the intermediate position between object-relating and object-use] that can be arrived at by the individual in early stages of emotional growth only through the actual survival of the cathected objects that are at the time in the process of becoming destroyed because real, becoming real because destroyed (being destructible and expendable).
>
> (Winnicott, 1971, p. 90)

Ogden asks important questions regarding the destruction of the object:

> Is Winnicott talking about the fantasy of destroying the object or the subject's really destroying the object as a separate entity? And what would it mean to actually destroy the external object? … And what does it mean for the object to survive if the destruction is the real destruction of the external object, not a fantasied destruction?
>
> (Ogden, 2022a, p. 78)

His questions bring to mind that Winnicott's theories, unlike Klein's or Freud's, are necessarily interpersonal – in every stage of development, Winnicott's theories of change/development are two-person phenomena – this is not exclusively intrapsychic but necessarily also "interpsychic". Something very real is happening to the mother who is "in [the] process of becoming destroyed because real, becoming real because destroyed". Ogden's (2022a) questions and analysis of Winnicott's ideas suggest an important distinction between a conception of the destruction of the "omnipotent internal object mother" and the actual, real m/other. In other words, what does it mean if it is not just the mother "in phantasy" (the imago, as Abram puts it) that is destroyed, (and survives), but that something very real is being *done to* the mother and that the mother *does something very real* in her survival, which is what ushers in "the real" as an experience of "placing the object outside of omnipotent control"?

In "becoming destroyed because real", the m/other can then become "real because destroyed". The lived experience of the m/other's destruction is a crucial aspect of the transition into the capacity for usage. While it is painful to experience the m/other's pain, the infant cannot turn away if they are to develop. Because it is here that they, the infant, discover and encounter otherness (for the first time) in their perception of the m/other's pain. Up until this point, in theory, the m/other has protected the infant from the experience of "noticing" the mother's pain. Ogden (2022a, p. 81) writes: "the mother's experience of herself (and the infant's experience of her) as a mother is *actually* destroyed in the course of the movement from object-relating to object-usage" (Ogden, 2022a, p. 81). What is being destroyed is the mother's very real sense of herself as a good-enough mother. Again, Ogden writes: "What mother has not had the very painful experience of feeling that she has utterly failed as a mother and what's more, she has ceased to be the person she was before she had the baby?" (Ogden, 2022a, p. 81). It is because the mother is truly feeling destroyed that the mother becomes real to the infant. This is not theoretical – it is a very real lived experience that is registered by the infant as the infant waits to "see" what the m/other will *do with* this experience of destruction?

Indeed, what does the m/other *do with* the experience? This, too, is crucial. If she is to facilitate her baby's transition from object-relating to object-use, she must draw on her sense of herself, her maturity, her conscious and unconscious capacities in order to survive. The point is that she does need to actively *do something with* her experience of destruction which is intrapsychic first before it can become "inter-psychic". The intrapsychic psychological work requires active engagement in the mother in order to survive and not collapse into the position of a destroyed mother.

The final step in this transition is the mother's communication that, having been destroyed "in reality", she has in fact survived, "in reality". The communication is offered in large part through her non-retaliation (registered by the infant who watches her closely) and through her ongoing love and aliveness in her care for the infant. It is here that the infant celebrates her survival and discovers the m/other as an other that can be used again and again for the infant's, child's and later adult's development. Having experienced "the externality of the other", it is easier for the infant, child and adult to continue to "use" objects throughout the lifespan to encounter the otherness of the other, again and again, because the stage has been set that otherness, not omnipotence, is what is *real*. Winnicott writes:

> The subject says to the object "I destroyed you," and the object is there to receive the communication. From now on the subject says: "Hullo object!" "I destroyed you." "I love you." "You have value for me because of your survival of my destruction of you." "While I am loving you I am all the time destroying you."
>
> (Winnicott, 1971, p. 90)

How is this relevant to the couple relationship and "learning" to love? Surely, one might point out that the couple relationship is not asymmetrical in the way that the m/other/infant relationship is. Actually, I believe that asymmetry *is* a universal aspect of the lived experience of the couple, alongside the experience of symmetry (i.e. being of the same generation). In reality, members of a couple often take turns in what might be thought of as "caring for" the other throughout the relationship. While imbalances can be problematic for some couples, my sense is that "taking turns" with caring for the other occurs organically based on the internal resources of each member of a couple at any given moment in time. Furthermore, when the care received and given *feels* good to members of a couple, this form of care supports the experience of love in the relationship.

I am reminded of the concept of "earned security" (Pearson et al., 1994) in couple attachment research. This term is used to refer to a once categorized "insecurely attached" member of a couple who married a person who is categorized as "securely attached" and has, as a result of the marriage with a securely attached individual, become recategorized as "earned secure". That is to say that being with a securely attached individual facilitated a transition from "insecurely attached" to "securely attached", thus newly categorized as earned secure. Without straying too far from the point I am trying to make, I imagine that the facilitation of this transition occurred through ongoing communication of "survival" on the part of the securely attached individual.

To illustrate these ideas, let's consider the following clinical vignette.

The flipped switch

In our initial phone contact, Sara's voice was pressured, her anxiety palpable. She explained that her partner of 23 years was pulling away from her. Sara was devastated. She hoped to save the relationship. We arranged to meet the following week. Sara called a few days later to inform me that Danny changed his mind and was no longer willing to meet for couple therapy. She then asked if I would call Danny to "convince him" to attend an initial session. I told her that while I could hear how painful this was for her and how much she wished we could meet, the decision was his to make. I also let her know that if he changed his mind, I would be happy to set up an initial appointment. A couple of weeks later, Sara called again and said that Danny was now willing to try couple therapy.

When they arrived for the initial session, I briefly summarized the phone contact with Sara and my understanding of her reasons for initiating couple therapy. Danny responded to my summary by saying, "that sounds about right". I asked Danny if he could share, from his perspective, how he hoped I might be of help to them. He said that he felt it was his "right to decide" whether or not he wanted to be in the relationship and added that he didn't "appreciate being dragged into couple therapy". Though his words sounded harsh, there was something about the way Danny said that he didn't "appreciate being dragged into couple therapy" that was unconvincing. Noting this internally though not speaking of it, I sensed that at least a part of him actually *did* appreciate Sara's insistence to meet, though clearly he was ambivalent given his cancellation of our first intended meeting. Danny went on to say that given his age, 65, he was no longer sure if Sara was the right partner for him. He needed space to sort out his feelings and Sara wouldn't give him space.

Exhibiting significant anxiety, Sara said: "It's like a switch flipped. I don't understand what happened." She spoke of the ways Danny withdrew love and affection. She described his pulling away as gradual, beginning about 7 months prior to our meeting. Sara's sense of security in the relationship was shattered. Danny no longer offered kindness. This pained her deeply. She explained that Danny complied with her requests to get together but "his heart wasn't in it". She had hoped the two of them would grow old together. Sara said that she loved him.

Though her anxiety about Danny withdrawing *his* love was unmistakable, when she spoke of *her* love for Danny, her voice changed. It had a quality of solidity. It was notable because it was the only time, in this initial meeting, that Sara's tone and cadence of speech slowed. But then, as though a switch flipped in her, in a pressured tone, she asked, "What did I do? Is there someone else?". Danny snapped back, irritated, and said, "No. There's no one else. I just need space to figure it out." Sara said that it didn't feel right to throw it all away without understanding what was going on. She added that if she let go, "there would be no relationship". She, alone, was doing the work of keeping them together. Danny shrugged and said, "Well, maybe it's not meant to be." Again, there was something unconvincing about Danny's comment. Taking a stance in defending his "right" to decide, I surmised, was perhaps the crux of the matter.

I gathered that they were caught in a dynamic in which Danny's "pulling away" created profound anxiety in Sara, which fed Danny's wish to pull away even further. When I shared this with them, Danny seemed to relax slightly in his chair while Sara nodded as if to indicate that she agreed with me. I added that it was clear they were having very different experiences and that perhaps it was difficult for each of them to feel as though there was room for their feelings. Danny looked surprised and interested in what I was saying. He said, "That's exactly right. I don't feel like I'm *allowed* to have my feelings." I asked Danny if he had a sense of when this feeling began and he said he wasn't sure. He added that Sara takes up a lot of room. He then repeated that he had a *right* to his feelings. At this point, I wondered out loud if it felt to him as though he needed to say this again and again because, *he too*, had a hard time believing this was true, that he had a right to his feelings. To this, Danny visibly relaxed in his chair. He softened his gaze for the first time in the session and there was a notable pause. He then said, "Yes, that's probably true." Sara quickly chimed in to say that she had feelings too, and she really needed to know why he was pulling away from her: "Is it something I've done?" She added that she felt she *deserved* an answer from him after 23 years. At this point, before I could say anything, Danny responded with a simple, "I don't really know". Danny appeared quite sincere in his response; perhaps even in pain himself about the dramatic shift in his feelings towards Sara, but, at the same time, he remained steadfast in resisting Sara's pressure. As the session continued, Danny's frustration with Sara's anxiety was apparent. He said: "It's just too much for me." As the session came to a close, Danny admitted that he was pleasantly surprised by his experience in the session and that he was open to continuing to meet. Sara was eager to continue meeting as well.

Over the next few months, I learned that Danny and Sara met soon after they had each divorced their first spouses. While they connected over their respective experiences, Sara's divorce was particularly contentious. A theme that emerged again and again was Sara's need for Danny to offer support in myriad ways. Danny consistently offered a sympathetic ear and was, in both of their accounts, immensely generous with Sara through consistently listening to, supporting, and comforting her as she contended with a contentious divorce.

An important historical event for the couple was that Danny hoped to merge his family with Sara's and raise their respective children under one roof early in the formation of the relationship. Sara insisted they not disrupt the children's lives further which was hard for Danny. The decision was made that they remain in their own homes, raising their children separately while sustaining a relationship from two separate homes. Sara recalled that Danny was hurt by her resolve to remain in their respective homes. Danny believed the children would have adjusted. Despite his feelings of rejection early in the relationship, Danny and Sara stayed together. In fact they both agreed that the relationship had felt largely satisfying to both of them, until Danny's "switch flipped".

Sara was the oldest of six children and very close with all the members of her family. She spoke to her ageing parents daily and was involved in her siblings' lives; she felt herself to be a vital resource to all members of her family and regularly counselled everyone. Her father was a maths professor, her mother a stay-at-home mum. Now in their 90s, both parents were nearing the end of their lives, which was profoundly anxiety producing for Sara as she couldn't imagine a world without them. Sara prided herself on her interest in psychology and ability to "read people". She also admitted that she suffered from anxiety, which she "managed" – admittedly at times unsuccessfully – by talking to Danny, her family and friends. She had never sought therapy before because the cost was more than she could afford financially (though I wondered if it also might be costly emotionally).

Danny, the youngest of five and the only boy in his household, lost his father at a young age. He said, "I had five mothers", explaining that his sisters took it upon themselves to "mother" him. Danny was compliant as a little boy. He recalls being cast in the role of "man of the house" when he was age six or seven. He took out the garbage, fixed electronics, raked leaves, etc. He felt a sense of pride at his capacity to attend to these matters. Even so, he felt smothered by the women in his household as a child. Ready to leave for college, he also remembers feeling considerable guilt about not being around to help his mother. She died when he was in his mid-40s. About a year prior to beginning therapy, Danny had retired from a successful career as an architect and was enjoying spending a good deal of time refurbishing his modest home. He felt pride in his abilities and competence in this realm of his life. He felt time was moving quickly and he longed to slow things down and just be. Pensive about mortality, Danny had become increasingly reflective and sought peace and calm.

Course of treatment

In the therapy and in their daily lives, as Sara anxiously pressed Danny, the two were caught in a dynamic of chase and escape. The more she pushed, the more he retreated from her. The more she pressured him, the more Danny dug his heels in. I often reflected on how painful it was for her not to know *why* Danny was pulling away and usually added something along the lines of what we *could* know was that it seemed clear that *how* she was engaging with him now was pushing him even further away. Sara was able to see this and in a relatively short period of time, she actively worked to allow for more space to consider these pressured feelings. As such, Sara began to feel curious about her lifelong struggle with anxiety, in particular because the one consistent message Danny *had* been giving her was that her anxiety was just "too much for him".

And so began our brief exploration. Sara described her mother's anxiety as overwhelming to her as a child and even now as an adult. Danny found this particularly interesting. Though at times defensive about her anxiety, Danny's interest and engagement was notable to Sara, which bolstered, supported and encouraged her further explorations into this most challenging aspect of her experience in life. In one memorable session, as Sara described in detail her experience with her mother, Danny nodded his head, conveying deep recognition of her experience. Sara was surprised by this, looked on at Danny and asked, "Is that what it's like for you?" Now Danny looked surprised, registering her genuine curiosity around *his* experience and answered unequivocally, "Yes, it's exactly like that". It was one of many pivotal moments in which Danny and Sara were "discovering one another". Though neither Sara nor Danny had been in therapy before, in a very short period of time both engaged rather seamlessly. As Danny was granted more space, he became curious about *his* feelings and made great efforts to describe his experience. As he did this, Sara relaxed considerably. Her interest in him registered with Danny, which had the effect of allowing him the space he so desperately longed for in their relationship.

There was an air of discovery coupled with profound pain (for both Danny and Sara) in learning about the ways in which Danny felt simultaneously smothered and left alone in the relationship with Sara. Though Sara became defensive at times, her genuine desire to hear more of his experience tempered her defensiveness. Over the next several months, we learned that Sara always had her phone turned on which left Danny feeling as though she could disappear at any moment. Sara regularly answered her phone, interrupting her time with Danny. Upon reflection, Danny said that it always felt as though she was waiting for "someone better" to come along and replace him. Both Danny and Sara were now starting to grasp why Danny had pulled away from the relationship. As he opened up, he talked about the impact of Sara's habit of going on and on analysing her friends' psychologies or sharing her anxiety about her children, parents or siblings. Danny had listened and been a support to her for too long. The relationship felt one-sided and he was tired of it. Ultimately, he felt there was little room for him and little room for the two of them to shut out the world and just be together. He had needs too, though he hadn't been able to articulate them without the help of therapy.

As Sara listened, she also presented her experience, which challenged some of Danny's perceptions of how one-sided the relationship truly was. She spoke of the ways she regularly cared for him too. Having the space to talk about his experience opened Danny up to Sara's expressions, in particular because she was no longer consumed by the anxiety of losing him. Danny was clearly open to hearing Sara's perspective and often agreed with her presentation of the ways she cared for him, reminding him of her genuine love for him. It was in these moments that Danny seemed to pause and truly contemplate and integrate Sara's thoughts and feelings regarding what was "good" about their relationship.

Danny and Sara used the couple therapy as a springboard for deeper conversations throughout the week. After eight months Danny spoke about how his feelings for Sara had begun to change again. Sara, too, noted the ways in which her anxiety had permeated much of how she related to Danny and began to pause for longer periods of time, allowing herself space to think through how she was essentially "employing" Danny to manage her anxiety for her. She found that her self-monitored "built-in" pauses led to a reduction of anxiety and, more exciting to her, she could sense Danny's movement towards her in acts of tenderness that were beginning to return. Furthermore, over the course of several months, he began expressing genuine loving feelings and missing Sara when they were apart.

However, at this point in the work, Sara struggled with an emergence of feelings of hurt along with a nagging worry that Danny's "switch" could "flip" again. Sara shared how terrifying it was to imagine her life without him when he "disappeared" on her. She expressed genuine concern that she might never be able to feel truly secure with him again. Sara was tearful and confused about Danny in this moment. Was she naïve to stay? Was he genuinely moving towards her? What if he changed his mind again and decided he didn't want to be with her? Danny listened to Sara. Over the course of several weeks, he increasingly exhibited tenderness toward her in sessions when she spoke of her experience when he was actively pulling away from her for the many months before they began therapy. Rather than only hear her anxious pleas to remain in the relationship, Danny was now able to register Sara's hurt at his pulling away and the legitimate worry that she had lost him forever. Danny's willingness to listen to Sara was comforting and reassuring to her. He did not argue with her. Danny eventually said to her that while he could not make any definitive promises about the future, he was now in touch with his love for her and felt hopeful that the two of them had learned how to listen to each other in ways that felt encouraging to him about the prospect of their future together. Over the next several weeks, both described a shift in their experience of their time together. Sara was experimenting with keeping her phone turned off when she and Danny were together. Their capacity to relax with one another had returned and there was talk of possibly moving in and building a shared home. It became increasingly obvious to all of us that they were ready to terminate the therapy though they both found comfort in knowing they could return if there was a need to do so.

Discussion

Recently retired, contemplating mortality and subsequent existential angst, Danny's assessment that he had, perhaps, "outgrown" the relationship, necessitated Sara's involvement and attention. In this way, *his* existential "crisis" became *their* existential crisis. Unconsciously bumping up against "walls of internal and external constraints", Danny registered feelings of unease that became increasingly hard to ignore. While his feelings of ambivalence and discontent signalled *something*, he was unable to decipher the meaning of the signal on his own, and Sara's anxiety further crowded out his thinking/reflections. Danny thus felt he had two choices. He could remain in a relationship that he now experienced as "too small" psychically, in which "a room/mind of his own" felt inaccessible, or he could leave Sara. He had essentially already left Sara, largely leaving the work of attending to his emotional upheaval and unrest to her. His initial refusal to engage in couple therapy, as well as his insistence that he had a "right to decide" was all he could muster in the face of his mounting dissatisfaction.

Consumed by anxiety, Sara was unable to think about the shift in Danny's feelings toward her. Sara anxiously reached for answers, pressing him time and again. Danny's inability to articulate *why* his loving feelings had disappeared was exacerbated by Sara's pressuring him. As such, the existential crisis was driven by two forces: Danny's "flipped switch" experience and Sara's unmanageable anxiety. In this way, both Danny and Sara could not truly encounter the other.

It might be said that Danny's withdrawal and dismissiveness had a ruthless quality. By withdrawing, he was, in fact, leaving the work of the relationship to Sara – destruction of her and the relationship be damned. The very real *damage* done to Sara and the relationship could not be registered in Danny (yet) though it was acutely registered in Sara. In this way, Sara's feelings for Danny – that is, her ability to sustain *positive* feelings despite his rejection – was a crucial and necessary aspect of the couple's capacity to engage in this time of crisis. In an important way, then, Sara was *surviving* the destruction (driven by maturational processes in Danny, his need to develop and grow), in her capacity to register and sustain access to what was "good" in the relationship – an aspect of the reality of the relationship. In this way, Sara was grounded in a mature perspective that incorporated elements of the relationship that Danny was actively psychically disavowing. If they were to grow as individuals and, possibly, as a couple, Sara first needed to survive his ruthless attack on the relationship and on her. She was, to my mind, exhibiting an aspect of psychological maturity in her capacity to hold onto the reality of what was good between them without knowing if Danny would ever come around and reclaim the relationship. However, Sara was only partially able to survive his ruthless attack on her and the relationship. Her anxiety was a form of non-survival that halted progress and made doing the work of sorting out their different feelings on their own impossible. Perhaps Danny unconsciously relied on Sara's sturdy feelings toward him and the relationship in order to *use* her. In this way, Danny's unconvincing comment in the first session, "I don't appreciate being dragged into couples therapy", revealed the opposite as I experienced him as quite amenable to the work. He needed help to be able to "do something with" his feelings of dissatisfaction, that is to register, metabolize and transform his experience through encountering the Sara who was in front of him rather than the version of her he carried in his mind. Until the therapy began, Danny's feelings of dissatisfaction, "the flipped switch", was a placeholder, a symptom that carried the potential to be a catalyst for change that could only come about through deeper authentic engagement with himself and with Sara. With the cycle of anxiety/withdrawal largely interrupted, both Danny and Sara were in a position to begin to encounter the other in new ways.

Concluding remarks

In order to truly love another, one has to be able to psychically "place" the other outside the sphere of omnipotence. This is achievable through an ongoing (lifelong) engagement with the other in which members of a couple necessarily destroy one another in real and psychic ways. It is the very real experience of being destroyed, that is, *feeling* destroyed, that offers the potential to usher in *the real other*. I'm reminded of what Maria Kodoma, Borges' wife, conveyed to Ogden during a morning he spent with her. She said: "The greatest gift we can give to those we love is what they do not know about us" (Ogden, personal communication, 2025). Like the infant who rejoices at the mother's survival because her survival leads to a most wonderful discovery of her, the real mother, couples are uniquely positioned to discover one another again and again in the intimate relationship that belongs only to them. The infant's exuberance, expressed with the playful "hullo object!" includes an exclamation because the discovery of another is truly magnificent. Moreover, it is the very discovery of the other that breeds feelings of love for one's partner. Nobel Laureate Olga Tokarczuk (2019) beautifully captures the experience of tenderness, a vital aspect of mature love in couples:

> *Tenderness is the most modest form of love. It is the kind of love that does not appear in the scriptures or the gospels, no one swears by it, no one cites it. It has no special emblems or symbols, nor does it lead to crime, or prompt envy. It appears wherever we take a close and careful look at another being, at something that is not our "self".*

Indeed.

References

Abram, J. (2022). *The surviving object: Psychoanalytic clinical essays on psychic survival-of-the-object*. Routledge.

Bollas, C. (1987) *The shadow of the object: Psychoanalysis of the unthought known*. Columbia University Press.

Freud, S. (1974) Letter from Sigmund Freud to C.G. Jung, 1906. In: W. McGuire (ed.), *The Freud/Jung letters: The correspondence between Sigmund Freud and C.G. Jung*. Princeton University Press.

Mitchell, S.A. (2002). *Can love last?*W.W. Norton & Co.

Ogden, T.H. (2022a). Destruction reconceived: On Winnicott's "The use of an object and relating through identifications". In: *Coming to life in the consulting room: Toward a new analytic sensibility*. Routledge, pp. 72–97. (Originally published 2016.)

Ogden, T. H. (2022b). Introduction: Notes on being and becoming. In: *Coming to life in the consulting room: Toward a new analytic sensibility*. Routledge.

Pearson, J.L., Cohn, D.A., Cowan, P.A. & Cowan, C.P. (1994). Earned- and continuous-security in adult attachment: Relation to depressive symptomatology and parenting style. *Development and Psychopathology*, 6 (2): 359–373.

Rilke, R.M. (2012). *Letters to a young poet*. Merchant Books.

Tokarczuk, O. (2019, December 7). Nobel Lecture: The tender narrator [Speech transcript]. NobelPrize.org. https://www.nobelprize.org/prizes/literature/2018/tokarczuk/lecture/.

Winnicott, D.W. (1964) The baby as a growing concern. In: *The child, the family, and the outside world*. Penguin Books. (Originally a BBC radio broadcast, 1949.)

Winnicott, D.W. (1965) The capacity to be alone. In: *The maturational processes and the facilitating environment*. International Universities Press, pp. 29–36. (Original article published 1958.)

Winnicott, D.W. (1971) The use of an object and relating through identifications. In: *Playing and Reality*. Routledge, pp. 115–127.

Chapter 6

You make me feel ...

The function of the transformational object in love relationships[1]

Karolina Pniewska

When I was a teenager, I covered one wall of my room with posters of Robert Smith, the lead singer of The Cure. His pale face, eerie hair, red lipstick, and the usually black background on which he was photographed created quite a depressing wallpaper. On the other wall, there was a poster of the Sex Pistols, with the words "*no future*" written in charcoal on it. In this punk-rock setting, I listened repeatedly to The Cure's album *Disintegration*. The fourth track on the album is "Lovesong", which reverberated through my teenage soul. In the context of my then-current heartaches, it didn't fill me with optimism; it expressed longing, unfulfilment and emptiness. At the time, I mounted a successful defence against the content of the lyrics and against accepting the fact that Robert Smith had written them at a time of his own romantic fulfilment – and, what was worse, as a wedding gift for his wife. In this room, clad with posters of my heart-throb vocalist, I of course fantasized that I would be the one he sang of, and that I would move from the suburbs of Warsaw to London – and everything would change.

Christopher Bollas links fantasies of this kind to the function of the transformational object. He writes that:

> As it is an identification that begins before the mother is cognized as an object, it is not an object relation that emerges from desire, but from a kind of proto-perceptual identification of the object with its active feature – the object as enviro-somatic transformer of the subject – and manifests itself in the person's search for an object (a person, place, event, ideology) that promises to transform the self.
>
> (Bollas, 1979, pp. 97–8)

Bollas relates this search to the first experiences of parental care, which was able to transform hunger and thirst into satiety, cold into warmth, and anxiety into calm – in short, care that transformed every discomfort into comfort, altering the whole world and the infant's sense of self. In essence, we are speaking here about the transformation of disintegration into integration, essential for survival at this stage of life. As adults, we look for objects that

DOI: 10.4324/9781003518129-6

we associate with a metamorphosis of the self, and which bring the hope of transforming our internal chaos into an integrated whole. Such an object can be a god, a new relationship, a change of job, or even the latest tech gadget. It can be anything or anyone causing a change to the external environment which we then associate with the promise of internal change. In his text, Bollas focuses on how the particularity of the analytic relationship is conducive to the search for the function of the transformational object in the person of the analyst. I want to apply Bollas's observations to romantic relationships because I am of the belief that, in adult life, most of us pin hopes of changing our fate on our entering into a love relationship, and that the melodies of our first relational experiences are to be heard particularly clearly here. I hear their echo in the lyrics of "Lovesong", when Robert Smith sings about his beloved as restoring a sense of wholeness.

During the second Warsaw Conference on "Working Psychoanalytically with Couples", Stanley Ruszczynski emphasized the fundamental importance of conscious and unconscious choice of partner (Ruszczynski, 2017). The line from "Lovesong" can be understood on these two levels of consciousness. The first level refers to the Platonic concept of halves, which, in my understanding, speaks of something conscious that we can recognize – something that couples often explicitly describe when asked what attracted them to each other. In these stories, we hear of how opposites attract, of the promise of fulfilling some sort of lack, and of the hope for achieving completeness together. These accounts might include statements like: "I'm so chaotic, he was so organized, I always needed that", or "I have a rational, logical mind, and my wife brought something emotional and expressive into my life". Here, we are in the realm of conscious choice.

The second level, which I will focus on in this chapter, refers to the unconscious and is closer to what Bollas has described – the operation of a transformational function of the relationship. We encounter this realm when, in response to the question about what brought them together, couples provide very brief answers, sometimes frustrating for those working with them, such as: "It just happened", or "Well, it just felt right … we liked each other, and that's it", "I felt we would be good together, and that everything would change, I felt it instantly, I don't know why", or even, indignantly: "Isn't it obvious from her looks?". I find myself moved by the absoluteness and intensity of these statements, expressed through words like "everything", "instantly", or "that was it". In working with couples, we can often get frustrated with this absolutist quality, the sense that a partner has unrealistic expectations, or that someone cannot really name what it is that they want, and that they seem unable to wait, tolerate something or think about things. We might say: "There's no thinking", "There's no reflection" and sometimes even "There's no couple".

What therapists struggle with here is primarily the nature of the emotional investment of the couples themselves. This difficulty is mainly related to the unconscious dynamics of a romantic relationship which can be analysed by adopting various theoretical perspectives. In this chapter, I aim to examine these love interactions through the lens of Winnicott's theory of development and Bollas's related concept of the transformational object. I believe that memories of the transformational object are intensely activated in the context of real, sensual and sexual contact with another adult. Furthermore, I suggest that (re-)finding and acknowledging the transformational function in the other person forms the foundation of falling in love, and of mature love in general. In this chapter, I would like to invite the reader into the world of these primal, unutterable experiences, related to the psychic drama of disintegration and magical integration. I will focus on how in my view, *love* sometimes *distorts in order to transform*, and I will aim to show how we can try to create an environment conducive to such transformation in the consulting room.

The promise of transformation: What is a transformational object?

It seems to me that the term "transformational object" is less familiar than "transitional object". We owe the latter term to Donald Winnicott, who described "the use of the first not-me possession" (Winnicott, 1971, p. 1). It is "something that is not me", something "between a thumb and a teddy bear" (Winnicott, 1971, p. 22). For Winnicott, the division into an internal and an external world was insufficient. He introduced the concept of a third "intermediate" area, which "lies in the middle" and is created by both internal and external reality (Winnicott, 1971, p. 2). Importantly, this area does not require differentiation of the two realities. It is a "resting-place for the individual engaged in the perpetual human task of keeping inner and outer reality separate yet inter-related" (Winnicott, 1971, p. 2). For Winnicott, the transitional object's appearance is when the child can move from the first oral relationship with the mother to a "real relationship with the object". The emergence of the transitional object creates a "bridge" between the internal and external world. Creating this bridge makes it possible to take some distance from a world of polarized oppositions: subjectivity and objectivity, unity and separateness, etc. (Phillips, 2007, p. 114). Bollas, whose thinking is deeply rooted in Winnicott's theory of development, focuses on the phase preceding the transitional phase and leads us to this black-and-white realm, where no intermediate solutions are possible, where there is no room for the subject's creativity, and where the key issue is simply to survive. For Bollas, the transformational object is the "first object", which, as I shall go on to elaborate, is available to infantile experience more as a process than as an object. *I believe that the life of a couple is tied to the constant movement between these two spaces: the space of the transformational object and the space of the transitional object.* I seek here only to point out this critical difference between the transformational object and the transitional object, and I will come back to it later when I describe the technical implications that emerge from the application of Bollas's concept to couples work.

At this point, a question might come up about the difference between the transformational function and *reverie* or containment, terms that we owe to the Kleinian tradition. I would venture to say that the transformational function refers to a narrower spectrum of phenomena, and that being contained is not always identified by the subject with a simultaneous metamorphosis of *the self* and the world around it. I decided on the concept of a transformational object because it is rooted in the Winnicottian perspective, which is close to my heart, and because my teaching experience with people working with couples shows that this concept seems to be intuitively understood and thus can be clinically helpful. Another important issue is what David Hewison highlights in his text "Re-visioning creativity in couple psychoanalysis – the importance of Winnicott and Bollas in clinical practice" (Hewison, 2022). Namely, that we should try to put the complicated, unconscious dynamics of the couple into words from various theoretical dictionaries and go beyond the dominant post-Kleinian narrative in the field of psychoanalytic couple therapy. I will now turn to a more detailed discussion of Bollas's text.

More of a function than an object

Bollas begins his text by defining the function that the mother fulfils for the child. He refers to the "supplementary ego" described by Paula Heimann and Winnicott's "facilitating environment". Winnicott emphasizes the function of the "environmental mother", who constitutes the whole world for the child at the earliest stage of life. The environmental mother ensures the continuity of the child's existence and creates the conditions for various interactions specific to this couple alone, related to the ordinary care that the infant receives. Bollas furthers his description with the observation that "the mother is less identifiable as an object than as a *process* that is identified with cumulative internal and external gratifications" (Bollas, 1979, p. 97, my emphasis). The child "gets to know" the mother through the repeated experience of being with her:

> As the mother integrates the infant's being (instinctual, cognitive, affective, environmental), the rhythms of this process, from unintegration(s) to integration(s), informs the nature of this "object" relation rather than the qualities of the object *qua* object.
>
> (Bollas, 1979)

The child does not recognize the mother as a separate individual, nor does it feel itself as a whole; it does not know where one ends and the other begins and it submits to her as a "transformational being" that provides an integrating metamorphosis of the *self*. Bollas argues that, in adult life, we do not so much desire to possess the object, as desire "to surrender to it as a process that alters the self" (Bollas, 1979). I believe that when a person who is single falls in love and begins to share their life with another human being, the loved one has an influence on them in all the dimensions mentioned by Bollas: instinctual (sexual desires are awakened and can finally be satisfied in a couple); cognitive (we start to see ourselves and the world around us differently); affective (the temperature of all the feelings we experience changes); and environmental (the world not only appears to us in different colours, it really becomes different because we are not alone in it, we are mirrored in the eyes of the world as a couple). Of course, we now see the other person more fully than how a newborn sees its mother, but it would perhaps not be possible to say that we see the other as an entirely separate individual at the stage of falling in love. Genuinely getting to know the other takes time and requires complex competencies, something described beautifully and in detail by Judith Pickering in her book, *Being in love: Therapeutic pathways through psychological obstacles to love* (Pickering, 2008). Pickering writes that "[t]rue love requires a marriage of altruism and alterity" (Pickering, 2008, p. 6). and these are undoubtedly the characteristics of mature love. In the present discussion, I want to focus on love's primal, greedy, aggressive and fearful incarnation, a face of love that may cause us to reduce our loved one to the function of satisfying our needs, but that also allows us to experience the pleasure and ecstasy of blurring the boundaries between ourselves and this loved one.

The promise of transformation: the mother and the loved one as a transformational process

Under favourable conditions, the infant repeatedly experiences the mother as a process of transformation. According to Bollas (1979), the mother assumes the function of a transformational object because she constantly changes the infant's environment to meet its needs and the infant's subjective perspective. The transformations she makes are real; we are not talking about some form of illusion here, but rather about the fact that the mother actually changes the world of the infant, of this there can be no doubt. At the same time, the infant's world is transformed by their emerging ego capacities. These achievements (the acquisition of language, the ability to differentiate objects, remember them, etc.) bring changes in the ego that transform the nature of the infant's inner world. The infant identifies these successes with the presence of the object. Can we transpose this phenomenon to the dynamics of adult relationships? Let us imagine how we might attempt to move heaven and earth for our loved one, especially at the stage of falling in love, and how being in love (the advent of a real change we experience in all the dimensions mentioned above) changes how we see ourselves, and this change is invariably connected with the presence of the loved one in our lives. We may also consider the less exciting but no less emotionally significant moments of crisis in life, and find stories of couples who changed their world in response to them. I often hear accounts of how a life crisis made the presence of another person invaluable. A person experiencing a crisis comes out of it stronger and has a basis on which to link the change in themselves with the presence of a loved one. As a result of such experiences, aside from developing mature feelings such as love and gratitude, we can also come to believe that the other person has the magical power to change the world outside us and inside us. Similarly, the person who has helped us in this way may become convinced of their own abilities in this regard. However, at another time, a moment comes when we require such transformation, but we do not experience it, or are unable to provide it, and then we can find ourselves in a painfully disappointing and sometimes unbearable place.

Psychosomatic sense of fusion

What follows is a crucial point in the couple's vital experience that we are occupied with here. It is worthy of note that in his entire text, Bollas (1979) refers only three times to a new person/new relationship as an example of an object that promises transformation. He seems to place a greater value on art, religion, ideology and psychoanalysis in this role than on a romantic relationship. In a clinical example, he describes a man who was cast in the role of transformational object by his mother during childhood and later sought a similar function in his analyst. Bollas recalls how the patient came to him after breaking up with his girlfriend, but he does not elaborate on this thread or ascribe any meaning to it. It may be hard to compare the transformation in an analytical relationship with that of a romantic one, but I am left curious as to why Bollas seems to avoid reference to love relationships quite so much. Even more intriguing is that in his discussion of how the psychosomatic sense of fusion comes from aesthetic experience, the issue of romantic relationships completely disappears from sight. Bollas writes about merging with a work of art or a beautiful landscape, while omitting the experience of a couple falling in love or experiencing orgasm. Are these not the moments when we most fully experience the "uncanny fusion with the object" (Bollas, 1979, p. 98), through feeling and touching another person? Are these not the moments that the vast majority of works of art to which Bollas assigns the function of transformational objects are precisely about?

Bollas emphasizes that these intense aesthetic experiences do not so much have a transformational function as evoke in us the memory of something "[...] never cognitively apprehended, but existentially known" (Bollas, 1979, p. 99). The aesthetic experience thus revives the memory of the transformational object. Susan Pacey's book (2024) integrates the "Sensate Focus" behavioural sex therapy technique with psychoanalytic thinking about the couple. She writes that "the complex, mysterious phenomenon of sex means that human beings have to grapple with the fact that no one is ever quite 'unchanging' or sexually 'ordered'" (Pacey, 2024, p. 100). In the transitional space of the bedroom, adults play with their bodies, touching not only what is physical but also what is emotional. This complexity of sexual life and the inability to be together in this transitional space is a frequent reason why couples end up in our consulting rooms. I would also dare to venture that this issue is often linked to the fact that sex has lost its function as a transformational object or that such hopes have even ceased to be associated with it. At the same time, when sex comes back into a couple's life, we sense it straight away. Linsey Blair, presenting some of her extraordinary work with couples, writes: "I knew when I went into the waiting room that the couple had had sex [...] A sex that allowed for something new to happen because they listened to each other's bodies, hearts and minds" (Blair, 2018). This is a familiar feeling to me, this impression when you open the door of the consulting room and it is immediately obvious that the couple has regained their sexual life. This dimension of a romantic couple's functioning fundamentally differentiates it from other relationships. On the one hand, this is obvious, but on the other hand, it is a topic that seems to be constantly avoided and silenced. I want to emphasize its importance here because I believe that the presence of sex is conducive to the appearance of memories related to the function of the transformational object.

Again, I would emphasize how these desires for transformation are rooted in real experience and the transformational function of sexual intimacy in the couple. Even if a couple uses sex defensively to reduce tension, the importance of this function cannot be ignored. The intensity of the sensations that sexual intimacy provides – both fulfilling and frustrating – takes us to a world where touch – and all bodily sensations, including even those that are very subtle – matter more than words. In my opinion, in such moments, we can clearly hear the echo of transformational experiences.

The transformational object and psychoanalytic couple therapy

In the literature on psychoanalytic couple therapy I found only one reference to the function of the transformational object in adult relationships. David Hewison, in his article "Projection, introjection, intrusive identification and adhesive identification", writes about it as follows:

> [...] We invest in it with excessive expectations because of how magical it was to us when we were too young to make sense of mother's role in this, and as a result are likely to feel betrayed that it does not have the same magical qualities we experienced as a vulnerable, dependent baby. (...) Unless we realize that it is ourselves we must invest in and look to for change potential, our hope in the object will turn to disappointment.

> Those who get into relationships with the idea that the partner will make them better are looking to love and sex as transformational objects, and they are bound to hit trouble. The longed-for thing outside cannot change us in the way that we hope – after all, we are no longer babies with mother.
>
> (Hewison, 2014, p. 162)

In this passage Hewison focuses on only one side of the love paradox: that indisputably "*we are no longer babies with mother*". However, I would like to add and emphasize the importance of the fact that sometimes we may still be such children, and that this is inevitable. Our primitive desires come alive in us in relation to our loved ones, and the distinctive environment of the couple relationship in particular lends itself to this. Sometimes we want to be a child, at other times, also omnipotently, we want to be the parent saving the other from some form of oppression. Some people are often frustrated that they don't get what they want; others are driven to despair by the inability to satisfy the other,[2] and these roles are of course not static or permanently assigned. To reduce love and sex solely to the function of a transformational object would definitely lead us into trouble, but, at the same time, to deprive them of this function would surely condemn us to a life devoid of amorous rapture, to some sort of sterile and boring vegetative state. Wouldn't we then find ourselves in an equally troubling situation? And what is the place of couple therapy in all this? Isn't this the moment when we arrive at Julie Friend's question: "Is it our aim for couples to be reasonably passionate?" (Friend, 2013, p. 7).

Creative sexual and loving exchange *really and truly* make us feel better and make us see the world in new colours. If we have had the experience that "this longed-for thing outside" changed us exactly as we wished in our adult relationship, why shouldn't we go on continuing to demand more of the same effect? These are not just childhood memories, they are also vivid recollections of transformations we have experienced in our adult relationships. We remember them, we can name them, and we long for their return. We may consider them to be irrational or immature moments of our adult life, but we can also see them as spontaneous gestures essential for the development of creative life within the couple.

Friend (2013) suggests that we listen to manifestations of love in two registers: the more mature register, and the less rational one, which traces back to our embodied experiences. The search for the function of a transformational object in the other and in ourselves undoubtedly takes us to this less rational world of embodied sensations. Bollas writes that "[…] it is folly for the therapist to deny that the culture of the analytic space does indeed facilitate such recollections" (Bollas, 1979, p. 102). I would add that it is equally unreasonable to deny that the culture of a romantic couple's space also facilitates such recollections. Moreover, due to the sexual and sensual nature of this relationship, these transformations are recalled with an even greater intensity when compared to that which occurs within the psychotherapeutic relationship. We now arrive at a point where we have a couple and the environment of their relationship, which foster the emergence of primal desires, all coming together in the therapeutic setting of the consulting room, which itself fosters regressive movements. Things are really heating up.

Anyone who works with couples will likely be well acquainted with those fraught moments when both partners are relentlessly demanding change in the other, convinced that if only the other person behaved differently, everything would take a turn for the better. In loud, sometimes harsh or even vulgar words, they demand this shift – a movement that, in line with Bollas's concept, promises to transform something unbearable into something enjoyable and satisfying. In couples where neither partner has had a good-enough experience of containment from their caregivers, these new love connections formed in the first period of falling in love are particularly important and vividly remembered, since they referred to primal states of blurred boundaries of the self. One partner in a couple I worked with once said: "You used to respond to my every sigh; but now when I yell at you, nothing, you don't even bat an eyelid!" Another couple described the first months of being together as a time of" "slowly dissolving and blending together", "like in paradise". They came to therapy because they were experiencing moments of severe disintegration, each of them feeling as if they had lost this magical connection that dissolves all the differences between them, and they felt as though they were expelled from the paradise and left alone in "a cold and dark dead end". They were suffering not only because the other person no longer ensured a magical transformation but also because they still longed for this experience of sensuous merger to return, even though their "reason" was telling them that it was time to let it go. Although those moments of miraculous transformations had become rare, their occasional return left the couple confused. What drove them to despair was the fact that, in many instances, they either couldn't – or, feeling hurt and resentful, wouldn't – offer each other this relief. One of them said: "I'm falling apart, and you do nothing! When you know you could do everything!"

In these conversations that dragged on for years, often like an unbearable cacophony, I too could despair. At times, I wanted to yell at them to finally grow up, start communicating with each other, or just break up and finally give each other – and me – some peace. Both of them wanted me to "do something" about it, while I had no idea what that "something" should be.

In calmer moments, I tried to use my own experiences to interpret the desires they directed towards me, but my words fell on deaf ears. I found myself drifting away from the couple. Hewison's otherwise valid point – that change should start with oneself – was utterly out of reach for either of them at that time. Confronted with both the couple's helplessness and my own, I often wondered whether continuing their therapy made any sense at all.

Hewison (2014) subsequently discusses how the space within a couple can become a place for both fulfilling our childhood desires and for enacting earlier conflicts. He sees this space as having the potential for working through the fact of being dependent on another, and that of being a person on whom another is dependent. Seeing couples over many years has taught me that this is indeed a key area of focus, especially in the case of those couples where partners were not provided with containment by their parents in a way that matched their needs or developmental capacities. The couple I mentioned above – who desperately sought to recapture their shared oceanic experience for a primal sense of boundless merger with another – clearly belonged to this group. I believe that the foundation for working through dependence is the recognition and acknowledgment of primal needs, within a good-enough environment in the therapy room for their containment. For this to occur, it is crucial that the longing for such a scenario can resonate and be recognized by all parties in the therapeutic triangle. I should emphasize that I am not suggesting that these desires actually be fulfilled, but rather that slowing down the pace of interaction within the couple can create enough space for the force of this desire to stop being perceived as a destructive attack and enable it to be understood as a profoundly important need. Of course, this is quite a challenging task in the context of the rapidly changing couple dynamics during a therapy session.

The power of the transference energy within a couple is immense and, in my view, difficult to compare with the strength of the transference and countertransference in the therapist–couple relationship. Therefore, when the couple described above did not respond to my countertransference interpretations, I decided to focus on their mutual desires and on the overwhelming disappointment brought about by their exile from a paradise. I also realized that in these moments of regressive functioning, the couple could not see me as an object, and that therefore formulating transferential interpretations would likely be counterproductive. I existed for the couple primarily in the capacity of a transformational function, not as a separate object.

I would like here to return to the notion of the transitional object and transitional space. One may wonder what this "paradise" constitutes for the couple described above. Is it a memory of the first object, the psychosomatic fusion related to the function of the transformational object as described by Bollas? Or is it a reference to a transitional object, a blanket that both hold onto and by which means they can differentiate between what is inside and outside, play together and remain in creative exchange? I believe that these experiences are inseparably linked, and that being in an adult couple creates the conditions for us to move back and forth between the phase of the transformational object and the phase of the transitional object. Perhaps being expelled from the paradise and left alone "in a cold and dark dead end" can be understood as a dramatic moment when transitional space disappears and there is return to the earliest phase of development, in which dependence on the other is simultaneously linked both with mortal danger and miraculous salvation. Adam Phillips writes that "the transitional space breaks down when either internal or external reality begins to dominate the scene, just as a conversation stops if one of the participants takes over" (Phillips, 2007, p. 119). If one or both partners cannot move freely within the transitional space, then there is a high probability that the couple will frequently revert to the earlier transformational phase – at once hoping for change and fearing it. After many weeks of discussing this topic, my couple surprised me with a creative act – they bought a new blanket for their bed and used it during moments of increased tension between them to feel "one step closer to our paradise". The couple created a shared transitional object and since then our conversations have been able to proceed on a much gentler course.

Bollas argues that:

> the search for a transformational object, in both narcissistic and schizoid personalities, is in fact an internal recognition of the need for ego repair and, as such, is a *somewhat manic search for health.* At the same time their idiom reflects a minimally transformative mother, a factor that becomes clear in the often meagre way they use the analyst in the transference.
>
> (Bollas, 1979, p. 101, emphasis added)

I propose that we view the acting out of an unbearable, unreflective exchange between a couple during the therapy session precisely as a manic attempt to return to something healthy. This is particularly evident in couples with narcissistic dynamics but, in my opinion, also occurs in most couples. If neither partner has had adequate transformation experiences, then it seems quite logical that such a couple would revert to the phase of seeking a transformational object. Subsequently, the couple may then move into a transitional space, and this will offer hope for the emergence of the true self.

In his recognition of the regressive level of a patient's functioning, Bollas responds to requests for "magical transformation", by proposing that we focus on "ordinary work of listening, clarifying and interpreting" (Bollas, 2018, p. 10). Mary Morgan, in her chapter on interpretation in *A Couple State of Mind*, a handbook on psychoanalytic work with couples, warns against formulating interpretations too quickly. In the same chapter, Morgan emphasizes the importance of tuning in to the current melody of the couple, learning their language, and allowing time for emotional experience (Morgan, 2019, pp. 152–75). This recommendation resonates deeply with me, especially when I think about those moments in the therapeutic process when we get in touch with memories of the transformational object. The intensity of unbearable emotions within the couple provokes an urge to formulate interpretations too quickly – it is natural to want to distance ourselves from the force of such experiences in an attempt to control the emerging chaos. In these moments, the couple do not perceive the therapist as a separate object, which is why a transference interpretation cannot fulfil its function. However, when I dared to risk a response in the simplest words possible and endeavoured to limit my interventions to listening and clarifying, it began to bring surprising results. One can attempt to draw on Bollas's concept by showing the couple the power of this first profound transformational experience – an experience that has come back to life in their relationship and lies behind not only their endless arguments and grievances but also (and perhaps even more so) their silent withdrawals from one other. How might we do this? I suggest doing it by the simplest means possible:

MAN: You haven't been able to sort this out for three months! What is going on here? You do nothing but wait for the world to give you everything. You wait for the world to change things for you; it doesn't make any sense. I don't even know how to talk to my wife anymore. Maybe you can bring her back to reason. It's like being with a child!

THERAPIST: What if that actually is what your wife wants right now – for the world to change for her?

MAN: And so I must react and make it happen. Are you saying that I have to fulfil her every desire?!

THERAPIST: That is not what I am saying. I'm suggesting that we slow down the conversation a bit and just try to think together about what lies behind this wish and how it becomes the case that you hear in it a desire that you feel expected to fulfil.

WOMAN: Exactly. I don't want you to do it for me, I just feel like I am falling apart when I must log into Booking and choose one vacation spot out of thousand.

MAN: And you think I don't fall apart when I must log in there? [to the therapist] I bet you probably lose it too …

This mundane exchange led us to a deeper conversation about their dependence on their omnipotent and controlling parents who, though well attuned to them in the earlier stages of life, later seemed to be preoccupied with other matters and to somewhat abandon their children. After years of therapeutic work, it became clear to me that the memory of these first magical transformations was still alive in them and that they desperately longed to regain this, while failing to notice how much they were already in reality providing for each other in their marital relationship. The couple were only able to regain the ability to reflect after an extended period of discussing what it was that they desired from each other, and what they believed the other expected from them. For another couple I worked with, the emphasis was placed on recognizing the significance of the transformational function assigned by one spouse to the other:

MAN: You proposed this outing, and I appreciate the gesture, but it's not something that I like to do; you know very well that this type of outing doesn't really do it for me. I would like you to surprise me with something I don't even know I like myself and for you to hit the bullseye with it. That's what I dream of.

WOMAN: Oh, of course! You want me to paint the world in technicolour for you! What kind of world are you living in?! How old are you?!

THERAPIST: Why do you think you can't paint your husband's world in this way?

MEN: Exactly! You can, you see.

WOMAN: Oh, come on! Maybe I want something for me? Maybe I would like you to paint my world for me?!

In both of these exchanges, I tried to help the couples move between the transitional space –where the use of an object is possible – and an earlier space, associated with seeking a transformational function in the other, using simple questions and comments.

Stephen Mitchell writes:

> Romanticism in relationships is like a sandcastle built by two people. It is a necessary condition for the emergence of passion, yet it is not a permanent sphere of expression. Due to the ever-changing nature of romantic relationships, sandcastles require constant reconstruction. Passionate intimacy demands complex bonds that do not fit into a simple, stable structure.
>
> (Mitchell, 2002, p. 200)

The self may be built from a more binding material than sand, yet this is never a material that guarantees it invulnerability. Like a sandcastle, our mature self can be seriously damaged or even collapse under the impact of a powerful wave coming from the outside, which triggers an equally intense internal response. In such moments – shattered, dependent, vulnerable and afraid – we become particularly sensitive to the reactions of our loved ones. Similarly, when we are in contact with someone close to us who is experiencing such a breakdown, we too become fragmented, dependent and frightened. One partner, hoping for reintegration, seeks in the other the function of a transformational object, while the other often tries to find this function within themselves. If this search immediately fails, the couple may spiral into despair, helplessness, or rage. It may also be the case that one partner, in an attempt to escape this state of hopelessness, turns to the other and says things along these lines:

MAN: We came here because there were storms raging between us – violent ones, razing everything to the ground. And now these storms have gone, they have faded, but from time to time, lightning strikes. My wife can't help me, and I can't stop myself from getting angry. How things are between us right now isn't representative – It seems like things have improved, but really, it's just an illusion. At the end of the day, nothing has fundamentally changed between us ...

WOMAN: I think everything has changed because, after these downpours, we don't separate from each other anymore. I experience it differently now, and I think you do too. Those horrible scenes don't happen anymore; they don't come back to haunt us as they used to.

MAN: I'm still afraid that they will. You could avoid these scenes, I could avoid them too, and yet we keep repeating them – why?

WOMAN: Because that's life.

This conversation comes from the second year of my work with a couple who were capable of both passionate and dramatic quarrels as well as deep, reflective conversations – both in therapy and outside of it. In this couple, the longing for the other to remove every discomfort, as well as the desire to be the one who protects the other from all difficulties, could be felt very deeply. They carried a heavy burden of their own traumatic experiences, as well as those inherited from previous generations. Has everything changed in this couple, or nothing at all? Does their love transform the painful experiences from their families of origin, or does it distort the "true picture" of life they took from their history? It seems to me that, although the ground of their new experience remains unstable, something fundamental has shifted – separations no longer feel life-threatening. The couple has begun to play with meanings, though they do not yet fully trust this change. On these shifting sands, both uncertainty and false certainty have their foothold, and each of the partners can attempt to find their footing in this new landscape.

Mitchell writes: "The ultimate form of self-understanding is not so much a precise comprehension, a correct interpretation, but rather a fully self-reflective experience that breaks the closed cycle of repetitive, self-destructive interpersonal relationships" (Mitchell, 2002, p. 254). In this couple, where one partner is the child of Holocaust survivors and the other the child of a passionately intimate couple who often excluded their children from their world, the longing to surrender to the other as a transformational being and to be miraculously saved is striking. Their life stories, and the way they narrate them, provide an abundance of material for brilliant interpretations and meaningful connections, but this couple have taught me not to make use of them. Instead, I began to focus on catching the longing glances of what Bollas (1979, p. 97) calls "the subject-as-supplicant", and to listen to the couple's less rational register. For weeks, we listened to the same emotional broken record: the couple kept each other in check, while I commented, "You really don't want to bring up this topic because it makes you feel like you're falling apart, while you [to the other partner] say you will fall apart if you don't talk about it. Each of you needs comfort and looks for it in the other." Last week, the couple broke out of this gridlock. They engaged in a conversation and took actions they had never been able to agree upon before. And they did it on their own – between sessions. The man said, "It's strange because lately, you haven't really done anything for us … and yet something has changed. Just like that."

Had I brought about no change at all, or had I changed everything? I would like to believe that my slow, careful attunement to their primal longings allowed them to soften their re-enactment of losing the *mother-environment* and to move towards a transitional space, where the decisions they took no longer felt life-threatening, where their movements became less constrained and where words lost their absolute meaning. Something unbearable was transformed into something tolerable, and the melody changed. The couple experienced the transformational function – not just in their relationship but within the therapeutic triangle itself.

Returning to Hewison's words about being too young to understand the significance of the mother in this magical transformation, I wanted to show that we can help partners in adult couples recognize their role in the daily transformation of life's chaos, allowing them to acknowledge it and see its constructive meaning. In my text, I have aimed to illustrate how this chaos of life can reflect an internal experience of a world without an object, where the other – whether a loved one or a therapist – can only be experienced as a function, not as a separate other. This is very delicate and unstable ground, upon which couples primarily need us to simply be with them, and in these moments, due to the intensity of their primal desires and fears, this is itself an incredibly demanding task. Psychoanalytic couple therapy, with its slow pace and diverse vocabularies attempting to describe these unbearable phenomena, as well as with the role of therapists who have years of analysis of their own desires behind them, seems to me to provide a good-enough environment for this kind of work.

Conclusion

Robert Smith continues to sing "Lovesong" to the same woman while the words "*no future*" have disappeared from my wall. I like to think that both Robert and I are using the transformational power of love – not as a sentimental ideal, but as an experience that alters the self from within. In one of The Cure's latest songs "Nothing is forever" from *Songs of a Lost World* album, one's ability to love appears as a transformational object: something that carries traces of the past and yet reshapes the present, offering continuity where loss once seemed inevitable.

Note

1 The first version of this paper was presented during the Warsaw Conference "Working Psychoanalytically with Couples" in 2025.
2 It seems that quite often people from these seemingly opposite ends pair up to help each other cope with their shared inability to acknowledge dependence and exchange in an adult relationship.

References

Blair, L. (2018). Mind and body: An integrated approach to working with sexual dysfunctions. Paper presented during the "Working Psychoanalytically with Couples" conference in Warsaw, Poland.

Bollas, Ch. (1979). Transformational object. *International Journal of Psychoanalysis*: 97–107.

Bollas, Ch. (2018). Transformational object. In: *The shadow of the object: Psychoanalysis of the unthought known*. Routledge.

Friend, J. (2013). Love as creative illusion and its place in psychoanalytic couple psychotherapy, *Journal of Couple and Family Psychoanalysis*: 3–14.

Hewison, D. (2014). Projection, introjection, intrusive identification, adhesive identification. In: D.E. Scharff and J.S. Scharff, *Psychoanalytic couple therapy. Foundations of theory and practice*. Routledge.

Hewison, D. (2022). Re-visioning creativity in couple psychoanalysis: The importance of Winnicott and Bollas in clinical practice. In: S. Nathans (ed.), *More about couples on the couch: Approaching psychoanalytic couple psychotherapy from an expanded perspective*. Routledge.

Mitchell, S.A. (2002). *Can love last? The fate of romance over time*, Norton Professional Books.

Morgan, M. (2019). *A couple state of mind: Psychoanalysis of couples and the Tavistock Relationships Model*. Routledge.

Pacey, S. (2024). *Sensate focus and the psyche: Integrating sense and sexuality in couple therapy*. Routledge.

Phillips, A. (2007). *Winnicott*. Penguin.

Pickering, J. (2008). *Being in love: Therapeutic pathways through psychological obstacles to love*. Routledge.

Ruszczynski, S. (2017). Why are we together? Understanding unconscious partner choice. Paper presented during the "Working Psychoanalytically with Couples" conference in Warsaw, Poland.

Winnicott, D.W. (1971) Transitional objects and transitional phenomena. In: *Playing and reality*. Routledge, pp. 1–34.

Chapter 7

Helping borderline couples find love

Philip Stokoe

Love for the borderline individual or couple

For the borderline couple or individual, merger is misperceived as love. Separateness is impossible to conceptualize and is experienced as catastrophic. The catastrophe requires instant repair, which is usually the return to a psychic retreat which Steiner has conceptualized as a safe place that protects the person from the perception of the absence of the ideal (Steiner 1993). Alternatively, separateness can be managed in a sado-masochistic arrangement. In this latter version, however, although the roles of sadist and masochist differ, the link between the two individuals is a shared view of relationship; thus, the apparent difference (given the roles) is transformed into total agreement. In this way we can see that merger and sado-masochism are merely two sides of the same coin.

Borderline couples usually come for help because there has been a loss of merger, which they take to be a loss of a loving link. This merger-confused-with-love is felt to be vital for the couple's identity. The work with a borderline couple is to help them to discover separateness, as it is only through accepting the "otherness of the other" that it is possible to love.

Literature

For the couple therapist, working with borderline couples can be very challenging and has been addressed by several writers. Abse, in two papers published in the same journal (2013a, 2013b), describes in the first paper the challenges presented and her reactions to them. The title, "When a Problem Shared is a Problem … Whose Illness is it Anyway", is evocative of the confusion one faces with the kind of presentation categorized as "borderline". Abse refers to Morgan's concept of the couple state of mind as a guiding framework that enables the therapist to become aware of being drawn into an idea, "that one partner is more to blame or more disturbed than the other" (Abse, 2013a, p. 164).

DOI: 10.4324/9781003518129-7

Abse asks: Is the guiding principle of shared pathology a useful concept with borderline couples? Do such couples need a different kind of therapeutic container and intervention from other couples?

In her second paper, Abse proposes a development of a technique for such work at Tavistock Relationships, a combination of psychoanalytic couple psychotherapy and mentalization-based therapy, as described by Nyberg & Hertzmann in two papers (2014, 2018). They comment,

> An important area of overlap between MBT [mentalization-based therapy] and psychoanalytic couple psychotherapy is the focus on the patient's mind in the context of a relationship with another person, whether with the therapist or an intimate partner. It is this inter-relational focus that we believe contributes to making the combination of these two models especially helpful with couples "on the borderline".
>
> (Nyberg & Hertzmann, 2018, p. 25)

This approach offers the borderline couple a view of the other as a separate mind with separate feelings, though it does not address the problem of the inconceivability of separateness itself.

However, their valuable point about the complex nature of borderline couples is also demonstrated very clearly in a compelling paper by Moran (2020) using the songs of Cole Porter as a form of clinical material. Moran (2020) describes a way in which two people, Mathilde and Yarda, who do not individually present as borderline, can nevertheless create a borderline couple. She makes what I consider to be a vitally important point:

> Each having internalised a destructive parental couple, they shared the unconscious phantasy that intimate relationships were dangerous. The atmosphere in the room, the way I would catch myself lecturing to them, confirmed the presence of unconscious beliefs – "unconscious phantasies that don't shift in response to an external reality that doesn't confirm them" (Morgan, 2018b, p. 67) [...] Mathilde and Yarda's unconscious beliefs were that they were in some way defective, and that allowing their relationship to flourish could only be catastrophic.
>
> (Moran, 2020, p. 65)

Later, I shall refer to a particular kind of shared unconscious belief that I understand to be crucial in understanding the borderline construction.

Bigda-Peyton (2019) also describes the same sort of coupling that manifests as a borderline couple: "In this case, a husband with a narcissistic character structure has formed an attachment to a borderline woman who periodically retreats into incapacitating depression" (p. 34). She continues,

> My countertransference can become unbearable. They can actually be a pleasure to be with – bright, interesting and engaging. They think well of me, too. But more prevalent are the countertransference experiences of dread, impotence, mindlessness, and hopelessness. I space out, or want to scream, to tell them what to do (though I know that will have no effect), or to end our hopeless treatment.
> (Bigda-Peyton, 2019, p. 35)

What these writers have in common is a recognition that borderline couples find the psychoanalytic approach used with other couples a big challenge and they offer different techniques.

Commentary

I feel very sympathetic to the descriptions of the difficulties in working with borderline couples, particularly regarding the emotional impact on the therapist. I've always felt the image of a borderline works rather well with the position of the therapist, precariously balanced on an edge: the edge between holding onto a therapeutic position and being caught up in the patient's material, the edge between maintaining a memory of the underlying problem and preferring to treat a neurotic problem, the edge between being able to love the patient and hating them.

There is general agreement, with which I concur, that the borderline phenomenon can be seen as a difficulty in accepting the otherness of the other. My response to this is to ask what it is about the human infant that leads to the development of the conscious, cognitive mind and, consequently, the discovery of this "otherness". Why is this happening at all? What is unique about the human infant that leads to such a complex development compared to other animals? My suggestion is that an understanding of this helps us to identify what has gone wrong in development that would lead to this borderline phenomenon. For instance, when Moran writes about her couple, she makes apparent each partner's different stage of development: "the way Mathilde's engrained sense of guilt and Yarda's deep sense of shame coloured their judgement."

In my understanding of development, shame is an emotion we are born with, guilt is something we acquire later as a process of mourning the loss of the ideal object, as described by Klein (Klein, 1935, 1940). I shall describe this in more detail below. The crucial thing that Moran is drawing attention to here is the vital role that a shared unconscious belief plays in enabling individuals at different stages of development to form a couple: "Mathilde and Yarda's unconscious beliefs were that they were in some way defective, and that allowing their relationship to flourish could only be catastrophic" (Moran, 2020, p. 65).

The capacity to feel guilt, I believe, depends upon working through the loss of the ideal and embracing what Freud called the reality principle (Freud, 1911; Stokoe, 2020). It suggests that Mathilde had worked through the depressive position and achieved the reality principle, however the shared unconscious belief holds her in thrall to an imagined ideal relationship. Their shared unconscious belief holds them together, but their fear of being two, separate people in a relationship turns their "couple" into a rigid psychic retreat. Interestingly, Moran suggests that it was only when she was able to free herself from the pressure to join in with their undifferentiated state and act as a separate person, that she could offer a different view, specifically that it was time for them to plan to end therapy, i.e. to separate from her. This enabled something to become freer in their relationship.

In what follows, I shall describe something of the early development of the conscious, cognitive, self-reflective mind showing how the breakdown of that process can provide an understanding of the prototype of borderline function. My experience is that the understanding of the beginning of a borderline state helps in understanding its expression in the consulting room.

I consider that the shared unconscious belief that establishes the creation of a borderline couple is that facing a particular piece of reality (most commonly, that there is no ideal other) would have a catastrophic impact.

Defining borderline – back to the beginning or a developmental perspective

The descriptions of borderline presentation that I've just been discussing are a view from the outside. My own approach to all psychoanalytic work starts from a different perspective, which we might call a developmental view from the inside. I work from the principle that human beings actually are quite well designed and, therefore, when we appear not to be operating well, it generates the question, "What's getting in the way of healthy function?". If we are to recognize those unconscious blocks to normal function, it must be helpful to have a good understanding of the process of normal development of the conscious mind. I'd like to share this approach in the context of working with borderline couples, who conflate love with merger.

I begin by describing "borderline" from the perspective of the work of Rosenfeld, Rey and Steiner. These authors share the concept of a defence as an attempt to manage a view of reality that is too threatening to be known about. From their perspectives, they are describing processes going on inside the mind, not behaviour, although these processes can be seen to result in the behaviours that others, such as Kernberg (1967) have observed. All three authors agree that the borderline state is a defensive organization, meaning something more complex than a primitive defence.

Rosenfeld (1971) described a psychological presentation that he called destructive narcissism:

> The destructive narcissism of these patients appears often highly organized ... The main aim seems to be to prevent the weakening of the organization and to control the members of the gang so that they will not desert the destructive organization and join the positive parts of the self.
>
> (Rosenfeld, 1971, p. 174)

In other words, he uses the analogy of a mafia-like gang attacking the loving self in order to suppress it completely because love is believed to make one vulnerable and at risk. It should be noted that these authors, as they develop a deeper understanding of a defensive organization, move from Rosenfeld's idea of destructive narcissism into a proposition that they are describing a borderline state.

Rey (1994) describes the massive dilemma these patients face. They cannot live separately from the other, but intimacy feels unbearably claustrophobic; he calls this the claustro-agoraphobic dilemma, to which Rey's idea of a complex organization offers a solution: "they live a most limited and abnormal emotional life which is neither neurotic nor psychotic, but a sort of frontier state" (Rey, 1994, p. 8).

It is important to note the reference to the impossibility of living separately. I would say that this is crucial to the borderline condition; they cannot even conceive of separateness, which is experienced as a catastrophe.

Steiner (1987) looked in more detail at the personality organization described by Rey and called it a pathological organization, writing that:

> the pathological organization functions as a defence, not only against fragmentation and confusion, but also against the mental pain and anxiety of the depressive position. It acts as a borderline area between the other two positions, where the patient believes he can retreat if either paranoid or depressive anxieties become unbearable.
>
> (Steiner, 1987, p. 71)

Later, he describes these pathological organizations as "psychic retreats" and indicates the difficulties the therapist faces in working with someone so well protected against any feeling of intimacy with a separate other.

In a similar vein, Rey writes, "They have an external shell or carapace, but no vertebral column. They live as parasites in the shell which they seem to have borrowed or stolen, and this creates a feeling of insecurity" (Rey, 1994, p. 13).

This is a very helpful conceptualization of the borderline condition. "Normal" development, I believe, provides us with an internal sense of ourselves as "loved by a loving couple", which we could call an "endoskeleton". Without something holding them up from inside, borderline personalities require something outside, a carapace, to support them. But herein lies the rub, for in clinging to the external skeleton, if this is another human being, they are subject to the claustro-agoraphobic dilemma.

In understanding the aetiology of this condition I draw heavily on these authors and on Bion, particularly his description of the innate (component) drives that account for how the human infant is able to turn to face reality. This is the consequence of an innate drive that he calls, K, meaning the urge to know, but I prefer to call it curiosity on the grounds that curiosity is the emotional experience of the activity of the K drive. This activity is something that Bion calls "alpha function" and I call "What's going on here?" (Stokoe, 2020).

Following Steiner I consider that there is a necessary precondition for the later development of the borderline situation. This occurs at a critical point in the "working through" of the depressive position, or, to use Freud's conceptualization, the move towards facing reality and thereby achieving the reality principle. In other words, it is very early in the child's development of a cognitive, conscious mind. The baby reaches a moment when they are struggling with the experience of the absence of their carer; they have been able to look at reality with sufficient clarity to recognize that their bad feeling (for example, hunger) was not caused by someone outside them, a hunger monster attacking them; it was caused by the absence of their carer. The first "explanation" to themself is that they are responsible for this by turning their fear and hatred against that other whom they believed to be this hunger monster. They project all their bad feelings onto their carer and believe them to be coming from the carer (projective identification). When the carer returns to their infant however, the baby is forced to find another explanation for the carer's absence. At this point in their development, the baby has only two rudimentary ideas of relationships, that with the hunger monster, which is retaliatory, and that with the carer who makes everything better. Either way, the only other explanation available to satiate their alpha function (the ongoing question, What's going on here?) is that, if the carer is not having yummy yummy with them, they must be having yummy yummy with someone else.

This is the point that can prove to be too much of a challenge to the embryonic borderline development. Although this is a necessary precursor for such a subsequent development, it does not mean that all babies who stall at this point go on to become borderline; there are many opportunities for repair during further development. The point is that the baby has a preconception (Bion, 1962b) of the impact of loss and a sense of not having the resources to deal with such an experience, so they withdraw in order to remain in a merger with the "Ideal", by which I mean the omnipotent good. Thus, they inhabit a world in which they have had no experience of separateness, which remains, in Bion's terms, a preconception. The choice to merge protects the baby from the process by which this preconception can turn into either a thought or a conception.

It is my understanding is that it is only the mourning process for the ideal "good object" that results in the acceptance of what Winnicott called the good-enough mother (1953). The baby discovers how much he depends upon this person and discovers the emotional link of concern, which is part of the component drive, Love. This step is essential for the baby to be able to take inside themself a sense of loving and being loved by a loving couple, which forms the first endoskeleton identity.

In contrast, the baby who retreats from this process remains in a paranoid-schizoid universe in which there are only two types of relationship: merger with the ideal or sado-masochistic – exactly the world inhabited by the borderline patient who retreats from that and from the requirement of mourning necessary to move into the reality-facing or depressive position, as described by Rosenfeld, Rey and Steiner. An understanding of the developmental process that leads to such a state proves to be very helpful to the clinician whose job is to try to understand how this has come to pass.

Having identified a particular crisis in the earliest development of the conscious, self-reflective, cognitive mind that is a necessary precursor to a subsequent borderline development, I need to go even further back in order to identify necessary processes that develop "conceptions" in Bion's terms, which become perverted in the service of most (if not all) emotional problems, but which have a unique meaning for the maintenance of a borderline state. To do this I must begin with Freud. What follows is necessarily schematic and may sound perfunctory.

In describing his drive theory, Freud commented that the unique change for the human infant was the moment when, instead of acting to alleviate the "pressure" of a drive, they "turn to face reality". At this stage of development all feelings are hugely intense, so much so that the infant is aroused to do something to get rid of this extreme discomfort, in other words to act. Freud called this the pleasure principle, meaning that pleasure was actually the cessation of overwhelming feelings.

Freud did not explain how the infant was able to choose to do something other than act in the face of such intensity at the point of turning to face reality (which is the beginning of the development of the conscious mind). Bion does (1962a). Bion proposes there is a third innate drive, which he called K (or curiosity), which operates through alpha function, or, in my terms, the question "What's going on here?".

The first answers to this question rely on the very few things that the baby already knows, which is why these answers can be found in all humans across the planet (this is so early in the baby's development that they have had no experience of anything outside themself other than a very limited experience of their carer). Klein called these "explanations" the primitive defences, and they are essential. Each of these creates psychic space in the form of a shift in the source of the emotion to outside the self, i.e. coming from the other. This is a rudimentary volume control for the emotions. It provides a way to reduce the overwhelming "pressure", allowing some space to move towards an alternative to action.

The next thing that is essential is the experience of container/contained. Here the baby has a direct experience of another who can do something to these powerful feelings, turning them into information from which comfort can derive. The carer provides the baby with a safe space in which they can share the baby's distress long enough to work out what's wrong. They are able to do this because of their own innate curiosity drive and their ability to love their infant. The baby's experience of a mother who is open to her own alpha function and is consequently able to address her baby's problem and restore contentment, is what Bion called "container/contained".[1]

The baby now has a mechanism for turning down the intensity of feelings, the primitive defences. This provides a rudimentary sense of space which might be thought of as a preconception (in Bion's terms) of a safe space. Thus, the experience of a safe space (container/contained) can be described as a preconception meeting with an actualization leading to a conception of such a space. This becomes the place in which the baby can play with thoughts, an activity that further reduces the need to act on the arrival of a feeling.

It's only the development of these two means to modify the intensity of feelings that make it possible for the baby to "turn to face reality" – which is the response to alpha function in this less intense environment.

The two perversions

As with so much of human development, mechanisms that allow for growth can also become the means to resist growth and change. In the case of these two crucial examples, i.e. the formation of primitive defences and the experience of container/contained, the former becomes the template for a different form of defence. Combinations of primitive defences can be utilized to protect us from knowing about the ways in which we have distorted reality. Such defences will always be found to protect an unconscious belief.

The second mechanism, the container/contained experience and the baby's learned ability to create such a space in their own mind, a safe space in which to play with a thought (the beginning of thinking), can also lead to a perversion of that space. Instead of being a safe space from which to look at reality, it can become a defence *against* contact with the outside world, a means to protect themself from reality (an immature version of a psychic retreat). We discover that the power of "playing with a thought" is that it can become a way to avoid a feeling altogether; not a place in which it can be thought about but one in which it can be triumphed over.

Thus, in adulthood, the "couple" created by two individuals can become rigidified into a similar escape from external reality. I propose that some arrangement of the couple relationship must serve this purpose for us to describe them as borderline, and that the presence of both the couple-as-retreat and the horror of separateness, are necessary symptoms for the designation "borderline".

This is a state in which the separate existence of the other is so intolerable that it has to be denied. Loving feelings have to be suppressed because there is an unconscious belief that love is dangerous. Curiosity, by definition, presumes difference; there is no need for curiosity when one "knows" the other – because the other and the self are the same. Thus, the combination of love and curiosity is always experienced as a dreadful threat by the borderline individual or couple. This is why many therapists feel they have to change the psychoanalytic approach in order to work with borderline phenomena.

The maintenance of the therapist's capacity to make this sort of enquiry is the ability to hold onto three-dimensional psychic space so that they can take up a third position. In couple therapy, this is central to Morgan's concept of "a couple state of mind" (Morgan, 2019)

Borderline couples

There are thus three central features of the internal world of the borderline patient, which can create borderline couple relating:

1 Terror of separateness.
2 Seeking and building a rigid container in which to protect against a dangerous world.
3 The presence of a very powerful but deeply held unconscious belief that distorts the view of themselves and the world they live in, which will always be some version of love being dangerous.

Along with Abse, I think it is important to consider the three types of borderline couple: one in which only one member of the couple is actually borderline, a second in which both individuals are borderline, and a third in which neither are borderline individually but, together, they create a borderline couple.

Any of those configurations could be the site of borderline function and it requires only one of the three qualities to create borderline couple. This is because the coming together of two individuals in an intimate relationship creates a "third" entity, the couple, often more unconscious than conscious (Morgan, 2019, 2025).

I consider the main feature of any one of the three types that we might describe as a borderline couple to be the shared unconscious belief that separateness is a catastrophic disaster, to be avoided at all cost, and that the formation of a couple offers this protection. It is helpful to bear in mind that love can only occur in a co-created relationship between two separate individuals.

Version 1: A couple in which there is only one actual borderline

The need for constant merger, the consequent reinforcement of the idea "we are the same" (our coupling proves this), and the deeply held but unconscious belief that distorts their view of reality, raises the reasonable question, what sort of person could not only enter, but maintain a relationship with a borderline individual?

If in doubt about such questions, my advice is to turn to Shakespeare. He has almost always got there first, and we can see this in one of his finest plays about coupling, *Antony and Cleopatra*. It describes the "fit" between a narcissist and a borderline.

Shakespeare's description of Cleopatra is one of the best descriptions of the borderline's way of relating, forming a merger. She does this through a combination of her sexuality and her skill at flattery, which is what the narcissist needs. Although they have not suppressed their loving capacity, the narcissist does not direct it towards any external person but towards themself. Cleopatra's flattery reinforces this. She says:

> I dreamt there was an emperor Antony.
> ...
> His legs bestrid the ocean; his reared arm
> Crested the world; his voice was propertied
> As all the tuned spheres, and that to friends;
> But when he meant to quail and shake the orb,
> He was as rattling thunder ...
>
> (Act 5.2, 81–5)[2]

The play illustrates the impact of the moments of separateness, which cannot be managed in a borderline couple. Antony has been drawn into a merger with Cleopatra in which she insists he must fight Octavius, who has decided Antony must be destroyed, at sea. Antony has demonstrated that he is unbeatable on land, but he has never fought at sea; to the despair of his generals, he agrees to this madness. But it requires Cleopatra to be at the head of her fleet, therefore separate from Antony. She reacts by taking her fleet and fleeing. This happens twice and it is after the second of these episodes that the couple come back together in the tragic scene in which both kill themselves, remaining united in death rather than facing the inevitable enforced separation that will be imposed by the victorious Octavius.

How does this help us to think about a therapeutic intervention for such a couple? I think the answer is to recognize that the very moment the couple feel in crisis about the reality of their separateness is the opportunity for engagement. The therapeutic container allows the therapist to notice subtle moments within the session in which each member of the couple responds to the therapist in very different ways. For example, Abse describes the pressure to agree that only one of the individuals is the real "patient" (Abse, 2013a) The intervention I have in mind addresses the different need each partner has of the therapist at this point; in crude terms, one requires the therapist to agree that the other one is the problem and the other requires the therapist to repudiate this. Noticing and describing these moments, particularly before they become warlike, provides each with an experience of how separateness can be held together in the same place by a loving environment.

Picking up these moments of separate expectations of the therapist at the earliest possible expression of it requires of the therapist a combination of an attitude of benign enquiry and an attitude of listening without memory or desire (Bion, 1970, p. 31). It is my experience that this works to reduce the incidents of angry assaults on each other and increases a gradual developing awareness of the benefits of accepting separateness.

By way of contrast, I wrote about my failure with such a couple in Chapter 2 of *The Invisible Matrix* (Stokoe, 2000) in which I agreed with the couple to see each of them separately and to have joint meetings once a month.

> I felt that it was a useful approach because the female partner was holding firmly to the line that the other was the patient and needed therapy; I thought that individual work would enable this idea to be explored in a more realistic way. What I hadn't done was formally to acknowledge that the task was different, that the individual sessions widened the scope of the therapy from the couple relationship to individual functioning. With this hindsight it seems to me reasonable that the woman, who believed the problem was lodged in the man, became very angry with me for making interpretations about her internal world and chose to break off the therapy.
>
> (Stokoe, 2000, p. 31)

The pressure to change the "frame" in work with borderline couples is very powerful.

Version 2: The couple created by two borderline individuals

What would be the necessary conditions that would enable two borderline patients to form a couple? Each seeks the illusion of love that arises from a merger. The thing that happens that destroys the belief of there being no difference between them is the sudden realization that the other has a different view to their own. This is not experienced as disappointing, irritating or sad – it is experienced as a catastrophe. Their external skeleton, the "carapace" suddenly dissolves. This is the main reason that working with a borderline patient is so different from working with other types of patient.

This means that for two borderline patients to form a couple, they have to be utterly committed to maintaining the illusion that they are the same and that this is love. This is most likely to be established if they share the same, or a complementary, central unconscious belief. Fortunately, the Tavistock Relationship model of shared unconscious beliefs provides a way for discovering unconscious beliefs in couples, including borderline couples, although the "catastrophe" problem will serve to make us cautious about how we use any discovery of these underlying beliefs. Finally, the shared concept of a defensive structure, the rigid perversion of the thinking space derived from the original container/contained experience, a place on the border between psychotic and neurotic, between paranoid-schizoid and depressive position, must become the required quality of the relationship.

I suggest that the attraction of creating a couple arises because the individuals have not yet developed a psychic retreat for themselves. Many years ago, the phenomenon of two borderline individuals creating a borderline couple often occurred in psychotherapy institutions like therapeutic communities. In lieu of a psychic retreat, they often developed another mechanism to hold themselves up in the absence of an internal skeleton: they held onto a grievance. Working with such individual patients is extremely challenging because, as I pointed out earlier, beliefs are always coins with another side and the other side of grievance is entitlement. This provides the ideal arrangement. One person's grievance is supported by the other's reassurance that they are entitled to whatever it is the grievance is about. This will work as long as there is an equal sharing of this arrangement.

It seems to me that sharing a grievance or having one's grievance supported creates a psychic retreat; this arrangement serves to keep reality well away. I don't know how many such couples actually come to couple therapy. My experience has been in the context of couples formed in residential communities or a group. In this case the purpose of the coupling is usually, if not inevitably, a resistance to the treatment process. Once this is understood, it becomes easier to work with them because the context of the group means that there are others who can comment on their own experience of being excluded by this "pairing". This sort of commentary will be experienced by the couple as an attack, usually an envious attack, on their relationship but this offers an opportunity for the therapist to provide a different view.

Vignette: Tom and Debbie

Tom and Debbie were just such a couple held together by a shared grievance that they were entitled to unconditional love. Both had mothers who had been unable to provide this experience for them as babies. The therapist in the group was able to understand that the absence of a possibility to provide love was lodged in the group. The group reacted to this by feeling that the couple were attacking the identity of the group. The therapist worked from the principle that a therapeutic community is based upon a shared agreement that patients and staff are engaged in a process of therapy for the members. This can be thought of as a boundary or contract and this was being "attacked" by the coupling. He was able to acknowledge both the group's experience of having their *raison d'être* attacked and the couple's belief that only by holding tightly to each other could they avoid the massive anxiety about trusting that the group was offering a loving, safe place.

By feeling confident in his sense of this process being alive in the group before it reached an expression of confrontation and, therefore commenting on it early enough, both the couple and the group were able to use the therapist's intervention make a benign exploration of the underlying anxieties on all sides.

Version 3: A couple that operates as a borderline entity even though neither of them are actually borderline

Once again, I shall approach this from the perspective of thinking about the necessary developmental trajectories that might lead two individuals to create a couple, a third, that has those borderline features that I've been describing.

Although neither of them might have developed a borderline identity, the fact that they can join together in a borderline relationship suggests that they share an early challenge in which the capacity, the internal resources, to work through the loss of the ideal were not developed.

Vignette: Jo and Jim

Jo and Jim are two such individuals, neither of them borderline but their relationship was a nightmare. Both came from what might be described as the professional class, households that knew the right way to behave and expected their children to accept this without question. Which they did. They both attended boarding schools, which excel in teaching how to suppress love (because of the hurt it causes) and instead substitute a way of behaving that masquerades as love but is actually based on the message: "I don't hate you". It provides an image of how an adult human being should be that brooks no deviation. Neither of them had had a successful relationship, but each had remained in disturbing and dysfunctional relationships much longer than most people would. They met and fell in love when Jim was moving towards divorce, and Jo was beginning to believe she'd never find "the right man".

It transpired that both had had very early traumatic experiences with their mothers. Jo's mother was a very successful businesswoman; however, she was never going to be able to manage mothering and I came to believe that the moment of her daughter's birth was likely to have been a devastating experience for her. Looking into her daughter's eyes for the first time felt like being fixed in a searchlight that showed what an abject failure she would be as a mother; I think she saw her own daughter as potentially able to do something that she could not; a trajectory that could lead to her daughter being able to love a baby. This evoked instant hatred, and the baby had to negotiate that view of herself as hated, unlovable and wrong.

Jim's experience was very similar; he was born to an alcoholic mother who found his existence profoundly disturbing. He was so frightened of her that he would stay away from home from an extremely young age, playing in the trees surrounding the family home until he was dragged back to the house to go to bed. Thus, although Jim was desperate to divorce his current wife, who had whittled away a huge amount of his inheritance, his sense that a proper gentleman should behave with stoicism and without malice meant that he could not claim a reasonable settlement because that required him to believe that his needs were not only reasonable but might outweigh hers.

This couple shared a deep unconscious belief that neither of them was "right" nor were they lovable. Much of their relationship was characterized by each individual perceiving the behaviour of the other as evidence of their own failure. The loving link that drew them together in the first place collapsed under the pressure to resume the beliefs about themselves and about the external world that had characterized their lives to date. I felt that the evidence was clear that the real problem was that the loving link that drew them together as a couple was not enough to survive their shared unconscious belief that "I am unlovable and not the right one", which organized their relationship. Thus, it became classically borderline and subject to a sense of catastrophe as soon as one or the other behaved in a way that indicated separateness. It was enormously helpful that each was in psychoanalytic therapy in which this shared unconscious belief could be brought into conscious awareness and could then be brought into the couple work as a mechanism to allow them to rediscover their loving feelings for each other.

Discovering love with borderline couples

To restate a basic principle, love is utterly suppressed in a borderline state for the very good reason that love is only possible between two *separate* individuals; it is their separateness and difference that provides the space for such a link. A baby only discovers their loving feelings when they have given up the merger with the ideal mother, which triggers the process of mourning. That is why the move to the reality-facing state was called by Melanie Klein the depressive position. As I described earlier, this developmental step is avoided by the potential borderline individual, who retains merger with the ideal as his way of relating and thus avoids the mourning process. This merged state is misperceived as love.

This is the point at which the psychoanalytic work with borderline individuals and couples is different from work with neurotic patients. The therapist's comments arise from their ability to observe themself in relation to the patients, a third position. This is not a problem for neurotic patients who arrive with the knowledge that relating happens between two separate individuals, but it will be terrifying for the borderline couple/individual. This clearly calls for a different way to *apply* the psychoanalytic understanding of what is going on in the consulting room. I think it is this challenge that causes some therapists to seek a different, non-psychoanalytic approach or technique. My suggestion is that, once we understand the patients' terror of the encounter with separateness, it enables us to "titrate" the analytic insight so that it is not experienced as an indication of separateness so much as a sense of being understood by the therapist.

For example, when I first understood the nature of the shared unconscious belief for Jo and Jim (that they were not the required one and could not be loved), I said that I felt that what they secretly expected from me, which was also what they most feared, was that I would take a position of judgement about them as a couple that would obscure how important their love for each other was. This comment did not provide them with a sudden, different and therefore separate view of the world, but is an example of the patients' experience of being understood.

Indeed, I would say that the process of gradually creating a space to be able to face separateness is entirely a process of tiny moments of feeling understood. Each of these moments arouses a background recognition, mostly unconscious, that, for me to understand this, particularly the point about me and the danger I represent, suggests that I was looking at all three of us from a separate position. This is the position Morgan calls the couple state of mind. It is painstaking work. It requires the therapist to wait for the "selected fact" (Britton & Steiner, 1994) to arrive in their mind but then to subject it to a process of thinking about the thought until it becomes clear how to express it in a way that does not confront the couple with the therapist's separateness so much as the therapist's understanding of them. This is why I call the analytic process a benign enquiry. The enquiry part requires patience and will be supplied by the emergence in the therapist's mind of the selected fact. The benign part draws upon one's loving link to the patients, which will guide the therapist towards an expression of that "fact" in a way that can actually be received by the couple. It is for this reason that I think it is a necessary element in the work that the therapist is able to feel a loving link; otherwise, this meticulous process might be given up in favour of something more confrontative.

The gradual dawning for the borderline couple that the feeling of a loving understanding *must* mean that I've been watching us all from a separate position can be a wonderful moment because it restores love to its proper place as intrinsic to each one's personality or identity. As a patient of mine said after making the discovery of separateness, when he arrived at the next session, "my whole world has changed, knowing that you are separate has allowed me to discover that I love you … I love you as a uniquely different person to me".

Notes

1 This is why Carpy (1989) and Brenman Pick's (1985) observations that it is the baby's awareness of the mother's struggle, rather than the outcome/interpretation itself that is transformative, are so important.

2 Shakespeare, 1993.

References

Abse, S. (2013a). When a problem shared is a problem … whose illness is it anyway? *Couple & Family Psychoanalysis*, 3 (2): 163–177.

Abse, S. (2013b). Further thoughts on When a problem shared is a problem … whose illness is it anyway? *Couple & Family Psychoanalysis*, 3 (2): 178–187.

Bigda-Peyton, F. (2019). can't live with you, can't live without you: Working with a primitive, hostile, dependent couple. *Modern Psychoanalysis*, 43 (2): 33–48.

Bion, W.R. (1962a). *Learning from experience*. William Heinemann. [Reprinted Karnac Books, 1984.]

Bion, W.R. (1962b). The psycho-analytic study of thinking. *International Journal of Public Administration*, 43: 306–310.

Bion, W.R. (1970). *Attention and interpretation*. Karnac Books, p. 31.

Brenman Pick, I. (1985). Working through in the countertransference. *International Journal of Psychoanalysis*, 66: 157–166.

Britton, R. & Steiner, J. (1994). Interpretation: Selected fact or overvalued idea? *International Journal of Psychoanalysis*, 75: 1069–1078.

Carpy, D.V. (1989). Tolerating the countertransference: A mutative process. *International Journal of Psychoanalysis*, 70: 287–294.

Freud, S. (1911). *Formulations on the two principles of mental functioning*. In: J. Strachey (ed. and trans.), *The standard edition of the complete psychological works of Sigmund Freud* (1953–74), Volume 12. Hogarth Press, pp. 213–226.

Kernberg, O. (1967). Borderline personality organization. *Journal of the American Psychoanalytical Association*, 15: 641–685.

Klein, M. (1935). A contribution to the psychogenesis of manic-depressive states. *International Journal of Psychoanalysis*, 16: 145–174.

Klein, M (1940). Mourning and its relation to manic-depressive states. *International Journal of Psychoanalysis*, 21: 125–153.

Moran, P. (2020). "I've got you under my skin": Borderline states in couple relationships. *Couple & Family Psychoanalysis*, 10 (1): 59–71.

Morgan, M. (2019). *A couple state of mind: Psychoanalysis of couples and the Tavistock Relationships model*. Routledge.

Morgan, M. (2025). *Couple relations: A contemporary introduction*. Routledge.

Nyberg, V. & Hertzmann, L. (2014). Developing a mentalization-based treatment (MBT) for therapeutic intervention with couples (MBT-CT). *Couple & Family Psychoanalysis*, 4 (2): 116–135.

Nyberg, V. & Hertzmann, L. (2018). A partnership of two therapeutic models: The development of mentalization based treatment-couple therapy (MBT-CT) within a psychoanalytic framework. *Couple & Family Psychoanalysis*, 8 (1): 23–37.

Rey, H. (1994). *Universals of psychoanalysis in the treatment of psychotic and borderline states*. Free Association Books.

Rosenfeld, H. (1971). *A clinical approach to the psychoanalytic theory of the life and death instincts: An investigation into the aggressive aspects of narcissism. International Journal of Psychoanalysis*, 52: 169–178.

Shakespeare, W. (1993) *Antony and Cleopatra*. Wordsworth Editions. (Originally published 1623.)

Steiner, J. (1987). The interplay between pathological organizations and the paranoid-schizoid and depressive positions. *International Journal of Psychoanalysis*, 68: 69–80.

Steiner, J. (1993). *Psychic retreats: Pathological organizations in psychotic, neurotic and borderline patients.* Routledge.

Stokoe, P. (2000). Holding the boundaries. In: S. Brookes and P. Hodson, *The Invisible Matrix*. Rebus Press.

Stokoe, P. (2020). *The curiosity drive: Our need for inquisitive thinking*. Phoenix Publishing House

Winnicott, D.W. (1953). Transitional objects and transitional phenomena. *International Journal of Psychoanalysis*, 34: 89–97.

Chapter 8

Primitive layers of love

The need or desire for the Other

Timothy Keogh

Introduction

Many couples we see in our consulting rooms have an impaired capacity to love, or their capacity to love has been impacted by a regression in their psychic functioning due to an emotional crisis. These couples often struggle to explain their difficulties with intimacy, which can at times be experienced as claustrophobic or engulfing. For the couple therapist it is the level of psychic functioning underpinning such experiences that determines the therapeutic focus of the work. In this chapter I wish to describe how some love relationships are characterized by a dominant mode of primitive psychic functioning wherein the other in the relationship is used to gain a sense of self-cohesion. I distinguish this from narcissistic relating which assumes a level of development that allows for the other to be an object capable of being projected into and for the self to be capable of introjection. It will thus focus on couples whose capacity to love and their associated sexuality are rooted in the more primitive layers of psychic development, that is, where the other is needed more as a means of psychic necessity rather than as a desired other. This represents a relatively new and often unacknowledged focus of couple functioning in couple psychotherapy.

The mode of relating to which I refer thus represents an immature form of relating more primitive than those dominated by narcissistic or paranoid-schizoid modes. These modes of psychic functioning, despite their capacity for introjection and projection, fall short of the achievement of a level of separation and individuation required for mature love. That is, they do not encompass what Britton (2004) has described as the capacity to be able to see oneself from the perspective of the other, a prerequisite of a capacity to love.

Our understanding about love relationships has emanated from a variety of disciplines and points to the fact that love relations result from a complex interplay between bio-psycho-social-cultural factors. Unlike psychoanalytic theories, however, many of these theories do not provide a useful, heuristic compass for assisting troubled couple relationships psychotherapeutically. Other theories have resulted in related interventions that focus on the

DOI: 10.4324/9781003518129-8

cognitive and behavioural aspects of troubled relationships rather than on unconscious or implicit processing of experience resulting from adverse developmental experiences.

Examples of prominent theories of love and love relations include the *Reward Theory of Attraction* (e.g. Myers, 2010), a psychological theory which proposes that people are attracted to others whose behaviours are rewarding to them and who provide positive and fulfilling interactions that require little reciprocation. Similarly, as a sociological theory concerning partner choice, "filter theory" (Janda & Klenke-Hamel, 1980) proposes that social structures and conventions limit the number of eligible candidates for a mate and mean that people frequently marry only those who are similar to themselves. Characteristics that are often taken into account are age, race, social status and religion. Theorists such as Rubin (1970) have also described and attempted to measure the elements of love relations. Rubin described three elements of a love relation: attachment (which encompasses needing to be cared for and to be with one's partner), caring (which involves valuing the other person's happiness and needs as much as your own) and intimacy (which involves sharing your private thoughts, feelings and desires with the other person).

Lee (1973) described love relations as representing either Eros, Ludos or Storge: Eros (which was seen to involve both emotional and physical passion), Ludos (as a playful form of love relation involving little capacity for commitment) and Storge (as the love that is involved in a friendship). Sternberg (1986), in his *Triangular Theory of Love,* further described love relations as comprising three components: intimacy, passion and commitment. In a similar vein Giles (1994) argued that romantic love is a complex of reciprocal desires for mutual vulnerability and care, suggesting both a desire to be vulnerable with someone in order to evoke care and vice versa. That is, he saw that being in love implies having sexual desire towards the other and a desire for a type of vulnerability and care.

These descriptive theories of love relations, although interesting, offer little in terms of implications for couple therapy. Moreover, based on four other main theoretical frameworks (cognitive-behavioural, humanistic, integrative and psychodynamic), a myriad of intervention models of couple therapy have developed. These include emotionally focused therapy (EFT), acceptance and commitment therapy (ACT), cognitive behavioural therapy (CBT), dialectical behaviour therapy (DBT), cognitive existential couple therapy, congruence couples therapy, structural and systemic-based interventions, attachment-based couple therapy and a number of author-specific approaches including the Gottman Method. All these therapeutic approaches, with the exception of attachment-based approaches, focus on learning skills to alter thoughts, feelings and behaviours that impede intimacy.

In contrast, attachment theory focused more on internal templates of relationships and their modification as the basis of couple interventions. This approach, which can be integrated with an object relations approach to couples therapy (Clulow, 2001), focuses much more on implicit psychic templates and unconscious processes.

Attachment theory contributions to understanding love relations

Attachment theory as a theory of love relations is based on Bowlby's original empirical findings about an infant's emotional experience when separated from its mother (primary attachment object). The theory argues that such reactions are linked to internal templates that lead to expectations about relationships based on one's implicit view about oneself and others. Based on Bowlby's original research findings, authors such as Hazan and Shaver (1987) have put forward the idea that romantic love can be conceptualized as an attachment process. Their theory of love relations argues that a person's attachment style is partially formed by the relationship that person had with his/her parents in childhood. Their research suggested that this is replicated in adulthood and becomes part of their expectations about romantic relationships.

Hazan and Shaver (1987) and Diamond et al. (2007) have also described how the sexual-behavioural system and the attachment system, although different, are connected, suggesting that individual differences in attachment-system functioning, which appear early in child development (in fact during the first year of life), do shape the functioning of the sexual system. That is, they note that although sexual and attachment behaviours are functionally different systems, they influence each other and contribute to relationship quality and relationship longevity, especially where there is secure attachment (Hazan and Shaver 1987; Diamond et al., 2007).

Attachment theory, which is empirically based, thus resonates with and supports psychoanalytic theories of love relations.

Psychoanalytical theories of love

In terms of theories that can inform therapeutic intervention with couples who struggle to establish and/or maintain a loving relationship, psychoanalytical theories have been among the most helpful. These theories have underlined that the capacity for mature love, exemplified by a capacity for empathy and a reciprocal relationship, is inextricably linked to the level of psychic development implicit in the couple relationship. These capacities facilitate the ability to think about the state of mind and feelings of another and attain what Morgan (2005, 2019) has termed a "couple state of mind". Linked to secure attachment status, these theories predict the ability to adaptively integrate what we now know to be the two separate systems of attachment and sexuality, which promote relationship longevity. When the optimal development of separation and individuation (achievement of depressive position functioning) that underpin such capacities does not occur, the ability to love is compromised and sexuality can be exploited in defensive ways.

Articulating the first psychoanalytic theory of love relations, Freud proposed "that the finding of the love object is in fact a re-finding" of the original love object (Freud, 1905, p. 222). He described romantic love as involving the linkage of sexuality and love, which, he argued, could be observed in an infantile form in the child breastfeeding. He argued that the child must master the developmental challenges associated with the psychosexual stages that he hypothesized (oral, anal and phallic [oedipal]), which entail a process where one becomes individuated from one's primary attachment figures in order (in adolescence) to be capable of what he described as "genital love". This, he argued, entails the ability to recombine the capacity for tender love with the re-emerging sexuality.

Interestingly neurobiological research supports this view. For example, Shih et al. (2022), in a meta-analytic review of neurobiological research concerning maternal and passionate love, argue that each shares a common evolutionary origin and neurobiological basis in the human brain. Their review of the research led them to conclude that it is the coordination of oxytocinergic and vasopressinergic pathways, coupled with the dopaminergic reward system, which contribute to the *formation and maintenance* of maternal and passionate love (Fisher et al., 2005).

They also found a greater involvement of cognitive-affective regulation in maternal attachment and a greater desire to combine liking and wanting in romantic love behaviours. This notion was supported by findings concerning the neurological structures involved in the different types of love responses. Specifically, the activation of the left ventral tegmental area (VTA), right thalamus, left substantia nigra and left putamen, was found in the case of maternal love, but for the passionate loving response the activation was in the bilateral VTA (Shih et al., 2022).

Freud developed his theory of love further after developing his theory of narcissism. It posited that we fall in love with people who are mirror images of our ideal self, and that love completes our deficient narcissist selves. He argued that when love is reciprocated, the tension between self and other is eliminated, and that there is a relief from the freedom from envy of the other person's qualities and abilities. This he argued produces a sense of reward and an associated idealization of the object of one's love.

Inherent in Freud's theory was also the role of ambivalence towards the love object in the early phases of development and during the oedipal phase towards the father.

Klein (1945) helpfully elaborated Freud's notion of ambivalence in a way that helps us to think about the ability to love and form loving relationships. She did not, however, depart from Freud's original and prescient remark that there is in adult romantic love relationships a desire to re-find, in a new way, the original love object. Her theory of psychic development argues that, as one develops from a split, unintegrated sense of self and other (a paranoid-schizoid psychic position), love and hate towards the object of attachment become integrated, allowing for a psychic state of separateness from the other and consequent ability to see the other as separate from oneself. Klein saw this leading to what she called the *depressive position* of psychic development. It is a position that is painfully achieved, never completely harnessed and always in a dialectal relationship with the paranoid-schizoid position. In clinical practice we find many couples who regress to the paranoid-schizoid position and, in doing so, lose their capacity for their love towards the object in order to contain the hate experienced towards them. Kernberg (1995) has argued that this capacity for love to contain hate is what gives the sexual component of the love relationship its exciting and stimulating edge or perhaps its *frisson.*

Moreover, in all psychoanalytic theories about love there is an emphasis on the importance of a capacity to see the other as separate from oneself or a capacity for intersubjectivity (Fairbairn, 1946; Balint, 1952; Bergmann, 1980; Kernberg, 1977; Benjamin, 2005).

From a more contemporary psychoanalytic vertex, a couple's ability to maintain an ongoing passionate loving relationship is thus seen to link to the couple's level of psychic functioning. In turn this provides an understanding of the anxieties and defences employed in their relationship that characterize their pathology and indicate the nature of therapeutic action needed to help them resolve their difficulties. For example, as noted, many couples who have previously reached a state of being able to have a mature love relationship present to us in a regressed state (representing the paranoid-schizoid position) where their capacity to love has diminished due to a loss of capacity to see the other as separate from themselves. As such they become invested in splitting off unresolved aspects of themselves and projecting them into the other, who then becomes experienced as a persecutor.

The relevance of primitive mental states in couple love relations

In more recent decades it has become apparent that for some couples the level of regression can encompass an even more primitive mode of psychic development, involving more intense and frightening emotional experience where the sense of self can feel threatened with annihilation.

Ogden (1988, 1989) has termed this primitive psychic mode of experience as the autistic-contiguous mode, which he saw as "having equal organizing significance to the paranoid-schizoid and depressive positions and as contributing equally powerfully to the dialectic constituting human experience" (Ogden, 1989, pp. 1/2). This state of primitive psychic organization represents an integral part of normal development through which a distinctive mode of experience is generated. Ogden notes that "this mode of organizing experience is characterized by specific types of defence, forms of object relatedness, quality of anxiety, and degree of subjectivity" (Ogden, 1989, p. 2).

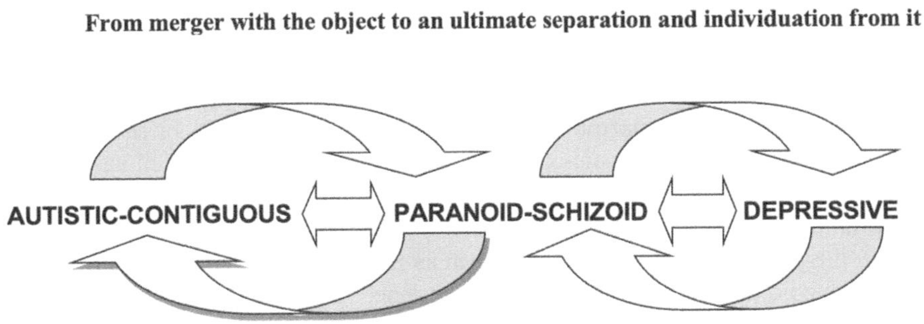

Figure 8.1 Dialectic of psychic modes of experience in couples (Keogh & Enfield, 2013; Keogh & Gregory-Roberts, 2018).

The term "primitive state of mind" thus describes a psychic mode of experience wherein the self is *experienced* as undifferentiated from its object(s). It is, however, a notion that has precipitated a certain amount of theoretical debate concerning the extent to which a baby, at birth, is already somewhat separate from its object, rather than in a necessary state of merger with it (Schellekes, 2021).

Primitive mental states of mind are those in which the capacity for symbolizing, fantasizing, dreaming and experiencing and finding meaning – that is, abilities requiring what Bion (1962) calls adequate *alpha functioning* or the ability to symbolically represent thoughts, are absent or extremely compromised in patients or couples experiencing the world and relationships through this primitive lens (Van Buren & Alahanti, 2010).

Bick (1968) importantly highlighted that such states involve an experience of an absence of what she referred to as a *psychic skin* of one's own. There is a need to use the skin of the other to create a sense of boundary, which, if all goes well, helps to develop a sense of what is "me" and what is "not-me".

Anzieu (1993), who had also written about a psychic skin or *moi peau*, suggests that there is:

> A stage of having a fantasy of an area of skin common to both mother and infant. The bodies of mother and infant are independent and located, as it were, respectively on each side of that area of skin. The bodies are also interdependent (the fantasy of "one skin for two" carries along the fantasy of "one thought for two") … and that … the baby goes through a stage of differentiation from the psychic apparatus of mother to disengage itself from the symbiosis with her.
>
> (Anzieu, 1993, p. 45)

Before such a differentiation takes place, the sense of self is precarious as it depends on this experience of shared skin. Any premature rupture to the sense of shared skin during this phase of development can create catastrophic anxieties. In adulthood there can be a regression to such anxieties in individuals or couples who experienced ruptures in their early development. The attendant anxieties can include fears of engulfment, fears of falling out of oneself and phobic type fears encompassing a sense "nameless dread" (Bion, 1988).

In couples this can result in a sense of catastrophic anxiety at the thought of separating and losing a partner which can result in panic attacks or phobic states. Ogden's concept of the autistic-contiguous mode of experience, which has attempted to capture many of these notions concerning primitive experiences, has been a helpful theoretical development in understanding such states in couples, especially when this mode of experience can be seen as part of a dialectic with Klein's paranoid-schizoid and depressive modes of experience (Keogh & Enfield, 2013).

When the poorly developed sense of self ruptures, there is a desperate need for an object to plug the sense of unintegration and provide a sense of bodily and psychic cohesion. In the couple relationship the Other is used to fulfil this function.

In terms of working with couples experiencing primitive mental states it is important to recognize that states of unintegration can lead to the experience of catastrophic types of anxieties that require extreme defensive manoeuvres in order to maintain a sense of equilibrium. This involves using the other or object as a means of achieving a sense of cohesiveness. This is a complex and double-edged device as, without a sense of boundary between self and other, too much closeness with an object can also lead to feelings of invasion and even annihilation by the other as there is a sense of losing oneself in the other. Bick suggested that the analyst needs to be available as an undifferentiated object. I feel with couples operating at this level the couple therapist needs to be available in the same way.

The identification of primitive mental states in couples thus entails a significant shift in our thinking about our intervention. In particular, it requires us to acknowledge that techniques based on the presumption of a capacity for projection and introjection are unhelpful with couples for whom the dominant mode of psychic experience entails primitive anxieties.

Related to the experience of fear and danger associated with such psychic states, Bleger (1967), who also agreed that a symbiosis with the object is a necessary stage of development, noted how some patients, such as psychotic patients who have difficulty maintaining stable differentiation from their object and a sense of the inside and the outside of themselves, deposit the most archaic aspects of themselves in the analytic setting. The analysis of the psychoanalytic frame itself can thus be an important tool in transforming these anxieties.

Lemma (2014), building on Bleger's work, has suggested that the analyst's body can function in this way as a depository, noting:

> "Embodied phantasies" not yet accessible to representation, may be communicated nonverbally to the analyst, leading to powerful somatic countertransference responses in the analyst. By this I mean a plethora of sensory and motoric experiences such as the analyst feeling discomfort in the body, alterations in breathing, feeling tired, sleepy or restless, feeling itchy or nauseous and so on.
>
> (Lemma, 2014, p. 228)

In couple therapy, we also speak about shared defences as a means of maintaining psychic equilibrium. In couples operating at a more developed level of psychic functioning this is usually achieved initially via projective and then via both projective and introjective processes. In couples with this more regressed functioning the key feature is merger and the employment of defences against separateness (Winnicott, 1949). There is an emphasis on a "we", that is, a merged unit rather than a true couple. The other is used as an autistic object, which helps to provide a sense of boundary for the other (Tustin, 1980). Any attempts at separateness are felt to be catastrophic and are resisted in the same way as they are in an individual therapy or analysis.

With such couples, small changes in the setting, such as changes in lighting and shadows in the room at different times of the day, can be disturbing. It means, however, that all these factors can be used to interpret and help transform primitive anxieties. This is what Bleger (1967) alludes to when he talks about the analysis of the psychoanalytic frame. This is because, as he notes, the frame acts "As an institution, as the receiver of the psychotic part of the personality, i.e. of the undifferentiated and non-solved part of the primitive symbiotic links" (Bleger, 1967, p. 517).

Bleger emphasizes the need for the frame to be analysed when it becomes prominent and links to the couple's repetition compulsion of the original symbiotic situation. The use of the frame in this way can manifest in couples noting that, for example, they only feel safe in the consulting room or how they feel calmed by the colours and texture of objects in the room. It speaks to their delicate psychic balance and ways of achieving this to which the couple resort. This notion is thus akin to that of *contextual holding* (Scharff & Scharff, 1991) in couples with developed levels of psychic functioning.

The development of metaphorization

Knowing that what we say is more likely to be used for its sensuous qualities (Maiello, 1995), such as its rhythm and tone, we discover why the voice can be such a helpful factor in terms of its containing effect. Linked to this, it is important that the couple is aware that they are in the presence of an object that is available for them to bind with, and that will ultimately help them make sense of their inchoate experience. This latter development occurs through the metaphorization of an otherwise threatening internal experience that allows a transition from beta elements to the beginnings of alpha functioning. As part of this approach, the analyst needs to tune into the unconscious aspects of the couple's material and allow for what Bion (1963) has referred to as a *selected fact* to emerge. This can be brought into the *liminal zone*, where the couple can begin to think with the therapist about their otherwise frightening and confusing experience that, until this point, they have had no alternative other than to evacuate.

In my clinical experience, inevitable ruptures to relationships underpinned by primitive mental states are often triggered by infidelity, which comes about as an escape from the build-up of claustrophobic anxieties that are part of the closeness–distance dilemma found in such relationships. Let us now consider these issues in the light of two such clinical cases.

Clinical case 1[1]

David and Judith were a childless Jewish couple in their mid-30s referred to me by their general practitioner (GP) after Judith had presented to her in an anxious state. The GP said this had been triggered by her discovery of secret text communications between her husband and a young woman who turned out to be a work colleague. She felt that the texts seemed intimate, and she wondered if they were having an affair. The GP had asked about their relationship and discovered that the couple had not been getting on well since Judith's mother had died one year prior. Judith had been very involved in her mother's care. Her mother's dementia had been worsening, and Judith's mother finally died of physical complications arising from the condition. I found out when they came to see me that Judith had an overly close relationship with her mother and was always guided by what her mother directed. After her mother's death it seemed that the dynamic Judith had with her husband, which was similar in nature, seemed to intensify.

David experienced his wife as increasingly needy and dependent, especially in terms of decision making. David was finding the relationship "very constrictive" and was increasingly looking to find reasons to stay longer at work and to go out on weekends on his own. This intensified her concern when she found the text messages that suggested that he might be having an affair.

Judith confronted him with her concerns and the fact that she had looked at his texts. He was furious and said that living with her felt like "I am in a prison". Ultimately, he admitted that he had been out with his young single colleague from work. He had shared with this young woman the tense situation at home that he felt he had to deal with. He had told her that he wanted "to separate from his wife", but he said that he felt she would not be able to cope on her own and that, despite the fact that he felt imprisoned in the relationship, he felt he could not leave her. This situation, where the one partner feels unable to leave the other for fear of the other not being able to cope, I find is a common experience in couples whose relationships regress to a more primitive level of functioning.

Apart from Judith feeling anxiously dependent and David feeling imprisoned in the relationship, they both said that when they were at home alone together, they could also both experience a sort of eery feeling. This could be relieved either by inviting people to stay with them or by arranging to stay with family or friends for the weekend. At times they could also retreat from one another, but this would have the effect of intensifying anxious feelings. This is a part of the dialectic of anxieties associated with closeness and distance found in such couples.

When they first came to see me as a couple they had a desperate clingy feeling about them, mostly given voice to by Judith. Strangely, as she put into words what their experience was, David would look at her anxiously, hang onto her words and then agree. This gave away that there were shared anxieties in the couple. During the session they commented on the feeling of solidness of my furniture and how comfortable and safe they found my room to be. My initial reaction to them, a somatic countertransference experience, was to feel overwhelmed and to experience a sense of breathlessness in response to their level of desperation and need.

Judith said that it was the discovery of the text messages that had really triggered her distress. David in contrast, pointed to the fact that things had really changed for them after her mother died. He said he found Judith increasingly clingy and needy and that it made him feel panicked, that he was not able to deal with her. He said that it was true that he had become quite drawn to a young woman at work who was supportive and reassuring. He said he knew that she too was needy and lonely. Although he said that he realized that there was a sexual attraction between them, he made it clear that the relationship had not gone any further than meeting together and talking. He said that he could see that it was moving to a point where it might become intimate, so he did draw the line, as he said he would never do that to Judith. She looked highly distressed as he discussed this possibility. It seemed that to her this was tantamount to an affair and that its effect felt irreparable.

When I asked her what she was in touch with, she said it was the thought of losing David and being alone and that this filled her with terror about how she would manage. I remember how, as Judith spoke anxiously, I found myself again becoming conscious of my breathing in a disturbing way, as if there was not enough air in the room.

In thinking about the fact that her mother's death had been a trigger to the developments in the relationships, it was tempting to approach the work with them with a focus on loss and failed mourning. However, I was struck with how the loss had triggered a regression to a primitive mode of psychic functioning and that this was temporarily relieved by relating to her husband in the same way she had related to her mother. In order to regain herself she had to use her husband as an object in a way that would help her regain a sense of self-coherence. I began to realize that it seemed the death of her mother had caused a regression in her, and in their relationship, to an autistic-contiguous mode of psychic experience. Judith acknowledged that the loss of her mother had led to a sense of rupture and a feeling that she was "falling apart". In such a state, it seemed that she needed to use her husband to plug this terrifying psychic experience.

What was less obvious was that her husband David had also been reliant on Judith in a similar way, but for him this had been more disguised. When the additional pressure in the relationship increased, he felt engulfed by her, which he experienced as being imprisoned. This relationship dynamic became more understandable as I explored their histories. David was the elder of two children. He had a younger sister who was frail and sickly. His father had died when he was six years old and, as he described it, he had to become "the man of the house after that". His mother had relied on her husband for everything and now she relied on him. They developed a very enmeshed relationship in which the loss of the father was never really mourned, robbing David of the opportunity to separate from his mother.

Judith, in contrast, was the youngest of three children and was born seven years after the middle sibling. For much of her childhood she had felt like an only child. Her mother developed intermittent multiple sclerosis, which meant she was seriously impaired for months at a time, especially when Judith was very young. She was sent to various relatives at these times as her father was unable to look after her because his work demanded that he travelled a great deal. When her mother was well, she had an overly close relationship with Judith, and it appears that she looked to Judith to compensate in some way for the absence of her husband. This was a further impediment to the development of Judith's sense of self which instead linked her further to her mother.

As she grew older, Judith said that she found it very hard to make decisions without her mother's help. When she married David, this dynamic also characterized their relationship. The death of Judith's mother therefore laid bare in both of them the failure of individuation and separation and the claustro-agoraphobic anxieties associated with a regression to an autistic-contiguous mode of psychic experience.

In terms of the therapeutic work and based on my experiences with other such couples I found that it was necessary to work with the primitive aspects of their couple functioning before interpretative work on their failed mourning could be achieved.

Clinical case 2[2]

Following an actual infidelity, Camile and Pascal, a French couple in their late 30s, sought help because, as Camile suggested, they needed "help in separating". The couple, who had been married for 16 years, were referred by Camile's therapist who felt the couple needed help because, despite an actual physical separation, they could not decide if they wanted to stay together or be apart. My initial countertransference to this couple was physically felt, urgent and disturbing.

Their relationship had been ruptured when Camile had discovered that Pascal had embarked on a sexual relationship with another woman after meeting her on a dating website. He said that he had started the affair in response to feeling he was "suffocating in the relationship", particularly about the need to see things in the way Camile did. Previously they seem to have agreed on everything and, as Camile put it, their relationship was "seamless".

Camile felt that the affair completely burst what she felt to have been this perfect connection between them. She was left feeling devastated by the infidelity and "as if I was going to pieces". She felt deeply hurt and considered the relationship to be irretrievable. She was also having trouble managing her work which involved looking after children with special needs.

The rupture of the relationship had caused a serious level of regression in the couple functioning. Camille felt phobic level anxieties and panic, while Pascal found himself depressed and in the grip of an obsessive relationship with the younger woman who texted him anxiously, much of the time leaving him again feeling hemmed in by this relationship as well.

When they attended for their first session there was a rawness evident in their emotional experience. Camille looked depleted and pale, almost as she had lost her energy source. Pascal was overweight and sluggish, as I was later to learn, a very different version of a previously more robust self.

With her eyes brimming with tears, Camile described her sense of shock and disbelief and the devastating impact the discovery of the affair had on her: "I felt like I dissolved into a state of panic; I felt I had come undone." She talked about their life previously as being "like two people who were part of the same organization". She went on to describe the extent of her distress and how anxious and upset she had become. She said she felt that it was "hard to know how to carry on".

Following this, Pascal talked about how before the affair it had felt unbearable at home for some time. He said that Camile had been complaining about him not being emotionally available. He said he felt she had become so needy. This coincided with the fact that their 12-year-old son had gone to boarding school.

Pascal also said, "I did not feel appreciated anymore and only felt wanted on her terms." He also said that these feelings about her had led to not having sexual feelings towards her. He noted that she was "difficult about sex anyway", noting that she had always seemed uncomfortable with sexual intimacy.

The couple said that they had met while working in the same company in their early 20s. Camile said that, for her, it was an instant attraction. She was so impressed by his confidence and she "just felt better as a person being with him". He said that he had felt intensely attracted to her physically and that he felt "more complete with her". There was a sense from his description that he was able to function better in the world with her, the opposite of how he had been since he had been apart from her.

As the couple work continued, I heard about the failed maternal containment and trauma in both their backgrounds. Camile had been brought up in a household where there was a child with special needs. She had become a parentified child who took on the role of a parent for a younger sibling who had a complex physical and emotional disability. This involved Camile having many frightening and overwhelming experiences with him that she was left to deal with by herself at a very young age, while her parents were very busy with their business. Her mother was described as having a psychosomatic illness involving being bedridden at times. There was also a history of marital infidelity, which had undoubtedly influenced a repetition in the relationship.

For Pascal there had apparently been an overly close relationship with his mother in the presence of a remote and emotionally distant father. This appears to have led to a failure to achieve the necessary psychological individuation for him to be able to be separate but together in the current relationship. He talked about his confidant-type relationship with his mother, who took refuge in the relationship with him from her critical husband.

This couple was ultimately able to come to understand that their problem in separating had deeper resonance and that it was in fact their early difficulties with separation and individuation that had drawn then together. This was the reason why they could not be a couple comprised of two separate individuals but rather one characterized by two people with an adhesive attachment where each served as an object that provided a sense of self-cohesion to the other. Gradually, they were able to see that the infidelity was a symptom of a more fundamental problem. The therapy enabled them to overcome the rupture and to eventually be a couple as differentiated individuals.

In working with couples such as the two I have described, I have noticed the importance and value of paying close attention to my moment-to-moment somatic countertransference reactions, sometimes shaped by the combination of the couple's responses to the clinical setting and the way the couple used me (the analyst) as an autistic object. To me, this vindicates what Bleger (1967) has pointed out about the setting being a re-creation of the symbiotic mother–baby relationship, a precursor to the development of a more differentiated ego.

Working with such couples also highlighted a paradigmatic shift in our understanding of the nature of the unconscious, that is, that it not only manifests in the intrapsychic, but also in the interpersonal and transpersonal realm (Keogh, 2020).

Implicit in the clinical case material provided I hope to have underlined the fact that central to transforming primitive states is not only generating a container-contained relationship, but relatedly, a gradual and titrated capacity to tolerate separation and to be alone. This requires an internalization of the container-contained relationship as a precursor to developing a mental apparatus capable of transforming proto-mental experiences. Moreover, this highlights the centrality of the developmental task of separation and individuation. In terms of the therapeutic relationship, it can often lead to a pressure to collude with patients through concordant and complementary countertransference type reactions.

Conclusion

In this chapter I have described the relevance of primitive mental states to couple presentations. Given that such states are often not acknowledged, it is necessary not only to be able to identify their presence, but also consider how to engage with and transform such states. This is particularly important when one considers that part of the dilemma of individuals and couples operating within such a mode of psychic functioning lies in their incapacity for introjection and projection. Unless one orients one's intervention to a style that does not presuppose such functioning, progress will be limited or stymied (Symington, 1985). In working with primitive mental states in couples the therapist must be able to make themselves available as a particular type of *undifferentiated object*.

The two couple cases were presented to illustrate a regression point involving primitive states of mind and a rupture to the sense of self as a result of an actual or perceived infidelity. In both cases it was a trauma that laid bare each partner's psychopathology as it contributed to the dynamics of the couple relationship. The rupture resulted from the precarious psychic equilibrium in their respective relationships that, disturbed by a crisis, caused their relationships to collapse into a state of primitive anxieties or into an autistic-contiguous mode of psychic functioning. It was argued that the dialectical model of developmental anxieties (Keogh & Enfield, 2013), which describes the typical anxieties associated with different levels of psychic functioning and countertransference responses to them, is a particularly useful heuristic device to monitor a couple's progression through the therapy with such cases.

Notes

1 *Confidentiality*: The clinical case material in this chapter has been redacted with personal and identificatory details disguised to protect the confidentiality of the couple.
2 *Confidentiality*: The clinical case material in this chapter has been redacted with personal and identificatory details disguised to protect the confidentiality of the couple.

References

Anzieu, D. (1993). Autistic phenomena and the skin ego. *Psychoanalytic Inquiry*, 13 (1): 42–48.
Balint, M. (1952). New beginning and the paranoid and the depressive syndromes. *The International Journal of Psychoanalysis*, 33: 214–224.
Benjamin, J. (2005). From many into one: Attention, energy and the containing of multitudes. *Psychoanalytic Dialogues*, 15: 185–201.
Bergmann, M.S. (1980). On the intrapsychic function of falling in love. *Psychoanalytic Quarterly*, 49: 56–77.
Bick, E. (1968). The experience of the skin in early object relations. *International Journal of Psychoanalysis*, 49: 484–486.

Bion, W.R. (1962). *Learning from experience.* Heineman; Basic Books.
Bion, W.R. (1963). *Elements of Psycho-Analysis.* Heinemann.
Bion, W.R. (1988). A theory of thinking. In: E.B. Spillius (ed.), *Melanie Klein today: Developments in theory and practice*, Volume 1. *Mainly theory.* Routledge, pp. 178–186.
Bleger, J. (1967). Psycho-analysis of the psycho-analytic frame. *International Journal of Psychoanalysis*, 48 (4): 511–519.
Britton, R. (2004). Subjectivity, objectivity, and triangular space. *The Psychoanalytic Quarterly*, 73 (1), 47–61.
Clulow, C. (ed.). (2001). *Adult attachment and couple psychotherapy: The "secure bas"' in practice and research.* Brunner-Routledge.
Diamond, D., Blatt, S.J. & Lichtenberg, D.J. (2007). *Attachment and sexuality.* Analytic Press.
Fairbairn, W.R.D. (1946). Object-relationships and dynamic structure. *The International Journal of Psychoanalysis*, 27: 30–37.
Fisher, H., Aron, A. & Brown, L.L. (2005). Romantic love: An fMRI study of a neural mechanism for mate choice. *The Journal of Comparative Neurology*, 493: 58–62. (Accessed from interwileyscience.wiley.com.)
Freud, S. (1905). *Three essays on the theory of sexuality.* In: J. Strachey (ed. and trans.), *The standard edition of the complete psychological works of Sigmund Freud* (1953–74), Volume 7. Hogarth Press, pp. 123–246.
Giles, J. (1994). A theory of love and sexual desire. *Journal for the Theory of Social Behaviour*, 24 (4): 339–357.
Hazan, C. & Shaver, P. (1987). Romantic love conceptualized as an attachment process. *Journal of Personality and Social Psychology*, 52 (3): 511–524. doi:10.1037/0022-3514.52.3.511.
Janda, L.H. & Klenke-Hamel, K.E. (1980). *Human sexuality.* Van Nostrand.
Keogh, T. (2020). Unconscious processes that inhabit us: A view from the Antipodes. *Australasian Journal of Psychotherapy*, 38 (1): 94–104.
Keogh, T. & Enfield, S. (2013). From regression to recovery: Tracking developmental anxieties in couple therapy. *Couple and Family Psychoanalysis*, 3 (1): 28–46.
Keogh, T. & Gregory-Roberts, C. (eds) (2018). *Psychoanalytic approaches to loss: Mourning, melancholia and couples.* Routledge.
Kernberg, O.F. (1977). Boundaries and structure in love relations. *Journal of the American Psychoanalytic Association*, 25 (1): 81–114.
Kernberg, O.F. (1995). *Love relations: Normality and pathology.* Yale University Press.
Klein, M. (1945). *Love, guilt and reparation.* Hogarth Press.
Lee, J.A. (1973). *The colors of love: An exploration of the ways of loving.* New Press.
Lemma, A. (2014). The body of the analyst and the analytic setting: Reflections on the embodied setting and the symbiotic transference. *International Journal of Psychoanalysis*, 95: 225–244.
Maiello, S. (1995). The sound-object: A hypothesis about prenatal auditory experience and memory. *Journal of Child Psychotherapy*, 21 (1): 23–41.
Morgan, M. (2005). On being able to be a couple: The importance of a "creative couple" in psychic life. In: F. Grier (ed.), *Oedipus and the couple.* Karnac Books, pp. 9–30.
Morgan, M. (2019). *A couple state of mind: Psychoanalysis of couples and the Tavistock Relationships model.* Routledge.
Myers, D.G. (2010). Relationship rewards. In: *Social psychology* (10th edition). McGraw-Hill, pp. 418–420.

Ogden, T.H. (1988). On the dialectical structure of experience: Some clinical and theoretical implications. *Contemporary Psychoanalysis*, 24: 17–45.
Ogden, T.H. (1989). On the concept of an autistic–contiguous position. *International Journal of Psychoanalysis*, 70 (1): 127–140.
Rubin, Z. (1970). Measurement of romantic love. *Journal of Personality and Social Psychology*, 16 (2), 265–273. doi:10.1037/h0029841.
Scharff, D.E. & Palacios, E. (2017). *Family and couple psychoanalysis: A global perspective.* Karnac Books.
Scharff, D.E. & Scharff, J.S. (1991). *Object relations couple therapy.* Jason Aronson.
Schellekes, A. (2021). Early emotional development and primitive mental states: A brief perspective. *British Journal of Psychotherapy*, 37: 594–605.
Shih, H.C., Kuo, M.E., Wu, C.W., Chao, Y.P., Huang, H.W. & Huang, C.M. (2022). The neurobiological basis of love: A meta-analysis of human functional neuroimaging studies of maternal and passionate love. *Brain Science*, 12 (7): 830.
Sternberg, R.J. (1986). A triangular theory of love. *Psychological Review*, 93 (2): 119–135. doi:10.1037/0033-295X.93.2.119.
Symington, J. (1985) The survival function of primitive omnipotence. *International Journal of Psychoanalysis*, 66: 481–487.
Tustin, F. (1980). Autistic objects. *International Review of Psychoanalysis*, 7: 27–40.
Van Buren, J. & Alahanti, S. (2009). *Primitive mental states: A psychoanalytic exploration of the origins of meaning*. Routledge.
Winnicott, D.W. (1949). Mind and its relation to psyche-soma. In: *through paediatrics to psychoanalysis.* Karnac Books (published in 1992).

Chapter 9

On love, loss and longing in lesbian couple relationships

Rachel Cooke

Introduction

The most auspicious beginning of a couple relationship includes a mysterious and magical feeling of attraction that leads to what we collectively call "falling in love". After the exciting, often mutually idealizing beginning, the potentially lifelong "established" phase of a couple's life together ensues and, in order to establish a strong foundation, each individual has to manage the loss of that heady early stage and grapple with the reality of their differences. It can be challenging to navigate the transition from the "beginning", with its illusion of permanent gratification, to the "middle", with all its reality laden disappointments. Just like the necessary loss of the infant-mother connection, the beginning phase of the couple must be relinquished in order for the relationship to mature. This is of course the case for all couples regardless of how they are gendered: all couples have to navigate the exchange of novelty and instability for a more lasting structure. I will attempt to describe here what might be stimulated unconsciously at this juncture for lesbian[1] couples, which I believe involves an unconscious return to the mother of early life, or "primary maternal object", and why this transition is suffused with particular complexities, especially for women who suffered loss or trauma early in life.

In my more than 20 years in clinical practice I have been struck by how many lesbian couples speak about their longing to be "seen", and how acute the pain of feeling "unseen" can be. This longing for attunement is felt very strongly to be an aspect of love. The better attuned their partner is, the more fully they feel "seen", and the more accurately seen, the more they feel loved. Conversely, the pain of being unseen is synonymous with feeling unloved. This longing to be seen, loved, understood and accepted has an intense cast to it: we all want to be loved, but this feeling is distinguished by its enduring, often unconscious, unrelenting quality, even in women who are ordinarily quite comfortable with their separate sense of self. I will attempt to link this longing for attunement to an origin early in life: under conditions of novel, adult, intimate connection, lesbian women often seem to pursue an unconscious return to the primary maternal experience with an attuned mother.

DOI: 10.4324/9781003518129-9

There is a high level of dependency and need for attunement, and the perceived shortfall in the partner's ability to meet these needs can feel very painful.

The physical and emotional intimacy of two people in a couple naturally evokes echoes of the earliest aspects of the mother-infant bond. If all goes well, infants are born into an environment of maternal provision in which they have their first sensory experiences and begin their slow emergence into separate existence. When Winnicott famously said "There is no such thing as an infant", he implied that it is impossible to speak of a baby without also considering the mother and her provision of care (Winnicott, 1965). The mother's love creates the facilitating environment in which the baby's earliest psychic, bodily and sensual experience of love is formed, and the mother is the baby's first love object. The roots of all couple attachments are buried deep down in this formative sequence of exchange.

It makes sense, then, that the couple relationship reactivates early aspects of the mother–infant connection, as well as the desire for an attuned and good-enough mother. The search for a deep and reparative emotional connection has strong unconscious reverberations from the infant–mother bond – especially for certain lesbian women, in the experience of a sensual-sexual return to the woman's body. Where the mother has not been "good enough", or there have been significant failures in provision, the longing may intensify. If a woman's personal history includes emotional abuse or neglect or significant early loss or trauma, there is likely to be a larger cavern of unmet longing. A felt history of not being seen may thus lead to a compensatory need in adulthood for attuned "seeing", which can strain the capacity to sustain love: having unrealistic expectations or making unrealistic demands invariably gets in the way of the couple achieving the closeness they wish. Part of a reality based or mature loving connection includes the ability to weather inevitable ordinary misattunements and disappointments that arise in the course of daily life. However, the early, mutually idealizing phase confusingly holds out the possibility of fulfilling those archaic desires, which stimulates needy and dependent feelings that militate against everyday adult states of self-reliance and independence. And in those women who are unconsciously looking to re-find the depth of that early lost connection, the phantasy[2] of gratification is very persistent and strong.

We might describe this kind of love as a longing to *be* loved, and the need to be seen, tenderly and lovingly, as the expression of need for a kind of maternal care. When this desire persists as a demand, conscious or unconscious, however, there is no way for the partner, who is not and cannot be the mother, to satisfy it. The phantasy is that the mother who "sees" her infant will care for her infant's every need, and this phantasy can be set in motion in the process of falling in love. There are moments in my clinical practice when I see partners interacting with each other, unconsciously, as mother and baby, offering or signalling a need for care. Roles can reverse or swap in an instant and are not rigidly held but rather oscillate in a way that demonstrates a shared unconscious phantasy. This is not solely a lesbian couple phenomenon, but I am raising it here as an aspect of how love may be represented by the provision of and a longing for highly attuned care.

The experience of being seen accurately, as one sees oneself, is an affirmation of the right to exist. For lesbian women, especially women over the age of 50, or from less accepting sociocultural backgrounds, the wish to be seen may also be intensified by a history of invisibility. Many LGBTQ+[3] people grow up invisible to their parents and even to themselves. This layer of not being seen leads not just to the later yearning for visibility but also to the *expectation* of not being seen. In this chapter, I explore the longing for maternal attunement and the unconscious pressure to restore something akin to the blissful connection that was lost. In what follows, I make use of several papers that reconceive the oedipal situation in order to shed light on the difficulty some lesbian couples have moving from the beginning to the established phase of relationship. Instead of a couple that offers both stability *and* an ongoing sexual connection, I have found that lesbian couples who get stuck at this transition often diverge into one of two directions: either there continues to be a lively sexual connection, although in a context of relational instability, or else the opposite unfolds, in which there is a stable relationship that has lost its exciting aspect, leading to the well-known phenomenon of LBD (lesbian bed death). I conclude with brief, composite vignettes drawn from lesbian couples I have seen in my practice and a discussion of the movement between dyadic- and triadic-relating.

The Trump administration, since taking office in January 2025, has acted with catastrophic effect to intimidate and disempower all marginalized populations, among which, in the current misogynistic climate, I include the entire category of women. Over the last 50 or 60 years, queer activists have notched up many successes in the fight for equal rights and gained greater acceptance by the heterosexual mainstream. Over the last two decades, there has been a significant shift in contemporary psychoanalytic writing about LGBTQ+ individuals and couples: psychoanalysis has taken strides to outgrow its longstanding bias towards heteronormativity. However, we do not have to go far back in US history to observe systemic injustice. Until 1973, the American Psychiatric Association classified homosexuality as "deviant behavior" (APA, 1973) and did not remove this as a category until 1987. In 1993, under President Clinton, lesbians and gays were finally granted protection against discrimination in every workplace. As recently as 2015, the Supreme Court affirmed the right of same-sex couples to marry in all 50 states. This law gives married same-sex couples important rights and protections that had previously been denied at the federal level. These include the right for one spouse to visit the other in hospital, the right to own property together and the right to inherit, all of which had previously been the sole province of heterosexual couples. History does not rest: MAGA ("Make America Great Again") Republicans and the Heritage Foundation's retrograde Project 2025 are pushing frighteningly hard to turn back the clock on civil rights.

This sociocultural, historical context of LGBTQ+ people is integral to my discussion of invisibility and the longing to be seen. The historical backdrop to growing up queer in the United States and Europe ("coming out" is still largely forbidden in many parts of the world) is one that requires each individual to make the journey from ignorance of their own sexuality to an emerging self-awareness, through unbidden but very real same-sex thoughts and fantasies, usually beginning in adolescence. Heterosexual adolescents also emerge into nascent adult sexuality, but they grow up in a world that reflects and approves of their experience at every turn. By contrast, each queer individual must travel an alternate path of often isolated self-awareness in order to "come out" to self and others. Almost every LGBTQ+ person has a coming-out story. For some, there has always been a sense of being "different". For others, an unexpected sexual identification arrives with a shock: "The hetero life I expected for myself is one I no longer want". Everyone who grows up with "non-normative" thoughts and sexual fantasies has had to go through this passage away from the mainstream, which often involves suffering and isolation. Many people came of age at a time or place when they were offered models for alternative sexualities that were frightening distortions created to dissuade young people from inhabiting those parts of themselves, or where there were no models at all. Many grew up feeling bad or guilty about same-sex desires, and, in all but the most accepting of families, they were often shunned and rejected or remained hidden. One member of a couple in my practice described coming-out to her mother, who told her on the spot and for several years thereafter: "You're confused. You'll regret it. Life will be much harder for you if you don't marry a man", and so on. The resultant internalized homophobia has a distorting effect on a person's view of their own sexual orientation and self-worth, making it a challenge to achieve a layered sense of self respect. LGBTQ+ activists have worked with resilience and determination for decades to get the outside world to reflect back a set of positive images rather than rejecting, disparaging ones.

One core element of being lesbian or gay, therefore, is a history of invisibility and an ambivalent relationship to it, beginning with invisibility to oneself, then to others, and often the concurrent fear of being seen. Being visible is complicated when being seen (by homophobic parents, for instance, or in the wrong part of town) can lead to rejection or physical assault. Even so, coming of age at the margins of the heteronormative world can result in profound compensatory needs for visibility and authenticity, represented in LGBTQ+ phrases such as "coming out of the closet", and "We're here, we're queer. Get used to it". It is hard to imagine being lesbian or gay without having a complex relationship to visibility in the world. One couple considering retirement in a European country argued over whether they would feel safe living openly as a couple or whether they would have to present themselves as "close friends". There are also profound implications for the "internal" world. In lesbian couples with an early history of trauma, the experience of *not* being seen and the *longing to be* seen are thus intensified by the possibility that it is *dangerous* to be seen. This can manifest in high stakes emotional situations in which the need to be seen is juxtaposed uncomfortably with the impulse to stay hidden. The sociocultural backdrop of having had to "come out" thus sets the stage for a more conflictual relationship to being seen and at the same time, a stronger desire to retrieve the original loving presence of an idealized and all accepting mother. The less there has been access early in life to a "good enough" mother, the more intense the desire and the more idealized she is likely to be.

Psychosexual development: desire and loss

I now turn to some contemporary revisions of Freudian oedipal theory in order to consider the possible impact of the oedipal transition on lesbian couple relating. Contemporary contributors have continued to maintain the important organizing role of oedipal psychic structures across psychological development, but the old paradigms of Oedipus complex and oedipal situation have at last had their heteronormativity laid bare, such that nowadays, we have a revitalized Oedipus "for everyone" (Nathans, 2021). Oedipal theory is increasingly described along triangular lines in which the emphasis is on dyadic and triadic relating and has moved on from outdated normative constraints of "mother" and "father". From this new perspective, the "resolution of the Oedipus" is no longer viewed in gendered terms but is charted instead in terms of the achievement of important developmental capacities: the ability to accept exclusion from the parental couple, which allows the child to develop their own separate sense of self and, later, to form a new, generationally appropriate, loving and romantic connection. Also crucial is the recognition that "thirdness" allows for the development of thought. Oedipal theory is thus no longer a constraining, awkward attempt to shoehorn female psychosexual development into a fundamentally male design. All individuals must grapple with relinquishing early dyadic experience in order to develop the capacity for mature relating. Nathans writes,

> Since the oedipal situation requires a gradual relinquishment of the phantasy of exclusive possession of the desired parent, as well as acceptance of the reality of being excluded from the parental couple, this promotes a capacity to tolerate loss and results in an increased capacity for mourning.
>
> (Nathans, 2021, p. 318)

Note that she writes, "the desired parent", which is deliberately inclusive and open to all forms of parent and family structure: the heteronormative mother and father, LGBTQ+ families, single-parent families, blended families and so on. This nomenclature itself demonstrates the movement away from the pathologizing tendency of the past towards greater inclusiveness and an everyday language that is much easier to understand.

A century ago, Freud tied himself in knots trying to explain female sexual development. In *The primary maternal oedipal situation and female homoerotic desire* (Elise, 2020/2002; reprinted in Hertzmann and Newbigin, 2020), psychoanalyst and gender scholar Dianne Elise argues that Freud's self-acknowledged "circuitous" ideas about female heterosexual development in fact reveal a much more straightforward route towards lesbian object choice. In Freud's formulation, the little boy is said to unconsciously desire the mother, for which he is threatened by the father with "castration" and therefore must defer to the father's authority in order to secure his place in the family. Aside from honouring age-old incest taboos and generational distinctions, as Elise points out, Freud's theory of *male* heterosexual object choice hangs together much better than his theory of the evolving sexuality of little girls. The threat of castration has always been understood as symbolic of the boy having to give up his first love, his mother, in order to continue his psychological development. Contemporary theorists have jettisoned the move from "mother" to "father" in favour of the shift from dyadic- to triadic-relating. A boy's trajectory at three or four years of age is surely more straightforward than a girl's: he must separate from his mother but gets to identify with his father in a fully compensatory way, and they get to be "boys" together. The girl, by contrast, is obliged to lose her exclusive relationship with the mother. She must separate from her mother yet at the same time remain identified with her, which is both more complex psychologically and also complicates the loss. A possible corollary of this developmental exigency is that girls develop greater empathy early in life, having had to suffer the loss of the mother as primary yet stay emotionally connected with her at the same time.[4]

Consequently, despite Freud's attempt to explain as normative the development of heterosexual object choice, given the depth and tenderness of the female infant's connection with her mother, Elise asks, "Why would the girl let go of this first object of desire and reroute to the father?" (Elise, 2020/2002, p. 106). Back in the 1980s, lesbian poet and essayist Adrienne Rich similarly stated that the assumption of innate heterosexual preference in women was only achieved via the most convoluted and strained of arguments. Rich wrote with frustration about feminist scholars who are "stuck … trying to reform a man-made institution – compulsory heterosexuality – as if … there is a mystical/biological heterosexual inclination, a preference or choice which draws women towards men" (Rich, 1986/1980, p. 34). Furthermore, Rich objected to how *this* preference does not require explanation – "unless through the tortuous theory of the female Oedipus complex or the necessity of female reproduction" (p. 34). What the mainstream *does* appear to require is an explanation of lesbian sexuality. This mystified and angered Rich, who challenged her feminist colleagues to investigate "whether the search for love and tenderness in both sexes does not originally lead toward women; why in fact women would ever redirect that search?" (p. 35). Rich and Elise align with many other feminist and queer scholars who conceptualize psychic bisexuality and desire for the mother as a primal experience for women *and* men, asserting the primacy of each infant's embodied, sensual connection with the mother.

Freud's notion of the girl's "negative" oedipal denotes a same-sex orientation of the girl to her mother which he considers misplaced and in need of "straightening" out. Elise replaces it with the primary maternal oedipal situation, thereby restoring the primacy of the mother's position. Looking at the psychosexual theory of desire, she points out that in contrast to the boy's desire for the mother, which sets in motion his Oedipal phase, the girl's desire for her mother is not discussed. Although Freud acknowledged that the baby girl's first desire is for her mother, this desire is not recognized in an erotic way. Instead, the girl's desire is omitted from the sequence of her psychological development. Elise contends that an unrecognized or disallowed homoerotic charge between the mother and baby girl constitutes a central point of origin for the future loss or absence of desire in adult women; the original tenderness between mother and daughter is now supposed to be re-found with the replacement of the father.

Elise's reading of Freud suggests the unconscious communication early in life of a position of inferiority. The "gradual relinquishment" Nathans writes of is likely the preferred route towards psychological maturity. Still, there is a meaningful distinction to be made between a relinquishment that is necessary for development, and an imposed distortion of their emotional experience with which proto-lesbian girls have had to comply, reducing their sense of their own value and desirability. A return to the blissful connection with the primary-maternal mother promises to heal that wound and restore the value that the mother confers on her infant girl by attuning to her with full acceptance. In the psyche, it does not matter whether this is a ph/fantasied mother or an actual mother. What matters is the reinstatement of love and acceptance, and it is this powerful experience that lesbian women often encounter unconsciously when first falling in love. No wonder that some women, especially those with a history of early trauma, do not want to let go of this deeply integrative experience, once they feel it has been recovered. The difficulty, of course, is that the experience of absolute acceptance and attunement is transitory. No one can offer absolute acceptance, and the mother who is sought is part real, part phantasy and part archaic object. The arc of temporal development requires that the early mother is lost and, phantasy notwithstanding, never re-found.

This is the exact terrain Leezah Hertzmann takes up in her paper, "Losing the internal oedipal mother and loss of sexual desire" (Hertzmann, 2020/2018), in which she suggests that lesbians are often unconsciously seeking a state of harmonious connection with the mother. For the lesbian couple, the beginning of the relationship brings with it, unconsciously, a sense of having re-found that primal, sensual, perfectly attuned mother. Falling in love offers the illusory promise of dyadic bliss that may have a tenacious grip on the mind of a woman who is unconsciously still searching for a mother who is receptive to her erotic longings. Letting go of that desire can become an intensely fraught process, and Hertzmann's main interest is in tracing the fault lines of the loss of the longed for mother and its repercussions.

In a similar vein as Elise's "primary maternal" oedipal situation, Hertzmann's "internal oedipal" mother alludes to the girl's emergence from dyadic experience towards awareness of not having the exclusive attention of her mother, which is the beginning of the development of thirdness. Her phrase calls to mind both the original dyadic, sensual connection between baby and mother as well as the unavailability of the mother in an absolute way: the attuned, devoted mother is there but also has an eye elsewhere, perhaps on the father/other parent, or on a newborn sibling. I think she is trying to capture experience at the cusp of triadic relating, to invoke a set of moments which look back at dyadic bliss, and toward triadic loss and the ensuing ambivalent experience of desire. The "internal oedipal mother" is both dyadic *and* triadic in nature, which captures some of why she is the object of such longing.

Hertzmann remarks that the loss of the beginning phase of the couple is psychologically distressing in different ways from the experience of the loss of the internal oedipal mother during toddlerhood, with its limited capacities for self-awareness and nuanced language. As much as the toddler may suffer and insist she "wants Mummy", the adult's self-awareness and complexity of thought add different dimensions to the loss. In her words, the "early oedipal experiences of merger and simultaneous loss … are reawakened and now have to be managed in adulthood, but this time with all the 'undone' boundaries, conscious and unconscious vulnerabilities, and investment that adult sexual relating involves" (Hertzmann, 2020/2018, p. 89). The loss of the recently recovered, longed-for primary maternal mother may be as wrenching as the original loss, particularly for women like the couple in her clinical example, both of whom had experienced early childhood trauma. That couple were unable to solidify their relationship without the diminishment of their sexual intimacy, which became a source of significant sadness to them both. The couple therapy revealed that one of them had jumped into an affair as an attempt to ward off her sadness, while the other became ruefully convinced that she was being abandoned, at times experiencing the couple therapist as the encroaching other lover. We can hear the triadic themes of loss, exclusion and betrayal as well as the dyadic anxieties of being abandoned and destroyed. Hertzmann notes with the couple that the sadness they had been feeling after their sexual encounters was likely to have been an indicator of the loss of the illusion that they could possess the oedipal mother and sustain that phase of relating.

This brings me to my central point, which is that lesbian couples are in the unfortunate position of having to suffer and manage *additional* psychic losses both in infancy/early childhood and in the course of establishing an adult couple relationship. These losses can give rise to an experience of love that appears to restore the lost primary-maternal love object, only to insist on the repeat of that loss. Love can thus be tinged with the kind of longing that comes from *not* having the illusory, imagined, archaic, erotic maternal connection that was glimpsed and then lost again. Every adult couple, straight and gay, having experienced the mutually idealizing beginning of their relationship, is obliged to navigate the loss of the beginning in order to make a full entry into the more mature and established phase of the relationship, but for lesbians there can be these additional *unconscious* losses to manage.[5]

The additional psychosexual loss which Elise posits occurs in early childhood. It consists of the lack of recognition by the mother of the girl's homoerotic desire and the pushing her off to her father. Unless she has the good fortune to be mothered by a woman comfortable enough with her own bisexual fluidity, the girl suffers a kind of rejection. Proto-lesbian girls whose mothers are able to sustain a mutually enlivening homoerotic experience may grow up to be adults who have an easier time building a firm foundation in their couples, while those whose mothers leave them wanting may be the ones who have a harder time. The loss of a certain quality of maternal attention has implications throughout life which may diminish the lesbian woman's access to her own (agentic) desire and sense of value. It almost certainly leads to a revival later in life of "wanting and not getting the mother – never getting the mother" (Elise, 2020/2002, p. 115). This results in the quality of longing, sometimes uttered as demand, which some of the lesbian couples in my practice give voice to. The mother's lack of recognition of her daughter's desire likely also sets in motion the earliest experience of being invisible, long before the emergence of conscious sexuality brings with it an awareness of not being seen, or of not being the heterosexual daughter who parents and society expected.

For Hertzmann, the additional loss occurs at the end of the beginning phase of the adult lesbian couple relationship. The initial phase arouses unconscious infantile longings and stimulates unguarded, unregulated, primitive emotions. In this undifferentiated early phase, there awakens in the unconscious the sense of having re-found the primary mother and, at the same time, the unconscious knowledge of her loss. The experience of being in love therefore stimulates the repeat of the loss of this early, blissful state. In Hertzmann's words, "The unconscious knowledge that the oedipal mother has been lost before and symbolically will be again is then related to as if it is happening in the here and now" (Hertzmann, 2020/2018, p. 97).

This knowledge increases the likelihood that one or both partners, (especially where there has been childhood trauma or rejection by the family of origin), will unconsciously expect that being in love brings with it a further experience of loss, which turns being in love into a state of anxious trepidation. In a way similar to Winnicott's observation in "Fear of breakdown" (Winnicott, 1974), I am describing an unconscious fear of a loss that has already been experienced. A childhood experience can be so overwhelming or disruptive that the child cannot experience it, which renders it, in Ogden's word, "unlived" (2024, p. 286). Certainly, the child has no capacity to mentalize or verbalize this experience. Psychotherapy in adulthood can help provide integration and meaning, but the couple on their own are likely to be destabilized when this seismic early experience gets repeated in the unconscious in adulthood, exactly when they are at their most vulnerable.

It follows, then, that out of an unconscious wish to avert repeated loss, couples sometimes resort to defensive manoeuvres or even place the new relationship in jeopardy. They may enact a kind of manic defence in order to avoid the felt repetition of the early loss, such as one person having an affair or abruptly ending the relationship. Or they may collusively establish a kind of relationship stasis, in which the relationship continues but the liveliness dries up. This stasis contrasts with the speed with which lesbian couples often hasten the pace of their union. Most lesbians know the oft-told joke about what a lesbian brings on her second date (a U-haul moving truck). However, perhaps the frozen quality of such couples is a consequence of how the relationship began, in that the rush to the "established phase" of the relationship can later be understood as an unconscious effort to stave off the significant loss that takes place over the course of this transition.

It is important to understand why it can be so difficult for certain lesbian couples to establish their relationship fully, and why one or both partners are likely to feel destabilized as their relationship reaches the cusp of the transition to a more mature state. Unconscious fear of the repeat of an archaic loss is the fissure along which some lesbian couple relationships either fall apart or freeze, because the unconscious impact of the repeat of this early loss is so very difficult to bear.

Clinical examples and discussion

I first noticed the phenomenon of an overlap between love and longing, and a kind of "deathly stasis" in particular, in my work with lesbian couples who happened to have lost their mothers – in reality, to mental illness, prolonged physical illness or death – early in life. The attempt to ward off the repetition of that loss, unconsciously, was met in each couple by creating a mostly friendly and safe couple space but one devoid of sexual intimacy. In such couples, a protracted state of dissatisfaction is felt to be inevitable. Although not conscious, there are signs of longing for a mother who will never return that show up in unmet desires that do not feel worth pursuing. One couple complained that life seemed boring, repetitive and lacklustre, and said they longed for a change, but neither had any impetus to do anything about it. Each spent years in solipsistic acts of self-absorption: one obsessively organized generations of family photographs, and the other sank herself into an overly demanding legal career. Both avoided self-reflection and intimate engagement with each other.

Over the years I have had other lesbian couples who formed, without intending to, a long-term pattern that keeps things static between them as much as possible. On one side of this dynamic is the woman responsible for making the other one wait – for sex, usually. On the other side is the one who carries the frustrated desire for sexual intimacy. The one desiring intimacy is in thrall to a desperate longing, while the other remains largely depressed and shut down. In and of itself, this is not a wholly unfamiliar dynamic in straight couples, but I have found the length of time the wait continues and the shared investment in the status quo to be a lesbian phenomenon, which I now understand as part of an unconscious effort to ward off intimacy in order to avoid unconsciously reawakening the calamitous experience of maternal loss.

The timeless, static quality of the relationship is similar to what Morgan has named "projective gridlock" (1995). As part of the pattern of static relating, attempts to ward off loss can lead to a persistent experience of "wanting and not getting", or of avoiding desire altogether. There can be all kinds of demands, which are frequently unmet. Sometimes the stasis is an attempt to avoid coming into contact with the painful awakening of primary-maternal desire, or the possibility of claiming more agency in the couple. At other times, the longing is a demand to be seen, mixed in, as I have suggested, with an expectation of remaining invisible. For example, an older couple came to therapy to address the years-long wait for physical intimacy that one had imposed but the other had also yielded to, albeit with increasing resentment and confusion. They considered each other "best friends" but one wanted a kind of intimacy that the other was afraid to acknowledge she did not. This had a "cat-and-mouse" quality, with the sexually reluctant member of the couple looking like a "tease", although she adamantly denied wanting to deprive her partner. The therapy helped galvanize and validate the frustration of the partner who was waiting, and the arrangement seemed to serve the woman who was not available for sexual intimacy but who did not want to lose her partner's deep and abiding emotional care. Both women tried for a long time to get something lastingly accepting and loving from the other in conditions which made it impossible to get their needs met.

I have occasionally had lesbian couples in my office still in the "hungry" phase of love, where their sexual energy is electric and excessive. In this climate, disruptions of their coupling run just as hot. Fully establishing the couple is precarious and one such couple came to therapy in tumult. They had moved in together after only three months. As long as they wanted the same thing and felt the same way, things were relatively easy, but if one of them forgot for a moment about the other or said something the other found offensively unlike her stored image of the other, a fight quickly ensued. Although they had developed the shared expectation that each would provide for the other a kind of maternally preoccupied level of care, the realities of adult life got in the way of maintaining this level of attention and generosity towards each other. It took several weeks before I could identify the unconscious pact they had made, by which each was now finding herself so constrained. They seemed to have made the unconscious agreement to put each other first, *always*. Maintaining the illusion of this arrangement required each of them to obfuscate the reality of what each could and could not provide, and they had agonized, confusing dialogues in front of me. When one of them had an independent need that imposed some limit on their availability to the other, it required a fight or an intense negotiation. I said I thought they had secretly vowed to be each other's everything, and that although this had felt blissful at the start, it was beginning to have them both in a choke-hold, and it had certainly had the paradoxical effect of making them invisible to each other. Things exploded irrecoverably when one of them was discovered to have been putting her own needs first at the other's expense and lying about it. This blew the lid off the shared belief that they could be each other's "everything", and the relationship fell apart. The relentless demand to put the other first was an effort to provide a compensatory level of maternal care, and also an unsustainable attempt to triumph over and refuse the primary maternal loss.

Another new couple who struggled to establish themselves securely kept having difficulty managing anxieties about the destruction of their relationship by one or another kind of "third". At times they believed their ex-spouses represented a threat to the couple. To each of them, the *other's* fear seemed absurd, but they both demanded loyalty and couldn't tolerate any expression of loyalty to the ex. They also both brought a child to their blended family, and each would sometimes feel not only painfully excluded but at times abandoned by the other's closeness to her own child. In one instance, during a fight about travel plans, and with a young child upset by the argument, one partner chose to sleep in her child's bedroom. The other partner went ballistic at this and issued all manner of threats and ultimatums. She did not realize it until a couple therapy session made the link, but she had been feeling rejected by her family of origin, such that in that moment she had felt utterly cast out. Later, she could rationally acknowledge a child's need for care and a mother's need to care for her child, as well as her own overreaction. In the heat of the moment, however, *she* felt like the child in need of maternal care. In couples with a trauma history, any closeness of one partner to a different family member has the potential to unleash abandonment anxiety. Lesbians without trauma histories who blend families also feel these exclusions deeply but navigate them more securely. This sort of incident constellates what I have been describing: an intense though mostly unconscious conflation of love with maternal care, and a demand or need for that desire for care to be seen and accommodated. When unmet, there is likely a starkly painful reaction due to the person feeling unseen and unloved.

Another couple unwittingly created a stasis that was intermittently punctured by heartbreak. This couple, who had been together many years, described having been "wonderfully in love" for the first years of their relationship, a state they thought would last forever. These women embodied opposing ways of attempting to deny the loss of the primary maternal connection. Darla was a teeming mass of feelings, forever overflowing in all directions. Unconsciously she held tenaciously to the belief that dyadic attunement between them was always present, until, in an instant, evidence pointed to the contrary and she would explode in angry, wounded demands for care. Marj, by contrast, was largely tuned out to Darla until an explosion occurred. She had little awareness of her own feelings and told me early on that Darla was an "ocean" but that she, Marj, lived "at the surface". Unconsciously Marj lived in the "deathly stasis" arena, warding off desire and emotional experience and apparently impervious to much of her wife's pain. Both of their childhoods were traumatic: Darla grew up with a violent grandfather who terrorized the household, and from whom there was no escape. Marj lived in the shadow of her mother's chronic illness and her father's inattention, so she coped with being invisible by tuning out from herself too. At their best, both Darla and Marj did have the desire and capacity to offer each other care, but their successes were compromised by the deafness and misattunement of one to the other when it came to understanding their historical relationships to emotional states. At the outset Darla had brought to therapy such an agonized and angry longing to be seen and cared for that this frightened Marj, who felt entirely inadequate to the task. This perpetuated the pattern of Darla feeling let down by Marj and Marj feeling walled off and afraid. They brought many examples to therapy in which Darla described how, from her vantage point, she would be crying out in pain, but Marj seemed unable to hear or see her, which exacerbated Darla's suffering. Hobbling along in a status quo of "one feels, the other doesn't", they repeated this decades-old pattern until couple therapy began to open up their vision to each other in new ways. Darla awoke to the realization that Marj was not *deliberately* blind to her but living in a very attenuated, frightened world. Marj became aware of Darla's pain outside of the accusation that it was all her fault, and began to show considerable empathy, which was all the more remarkable given how many years she had spent being emotionally closed down. Marj also began asking Darla to speak to her more kindly, and Darla faced for the first time the ways her angry outbursts impacted Marj. All this was a great relief to them both and led to their having greater access to loving care for each other. When Darla could say she "had an ouchie", and Marj could hear and see her and offer some soothing words, the inflamed arguments settled down considerably. Although they had been emotionally invisible to each other for years, their love survived the long stasis and they began to make real effort to see and get to know each other anew.

Concluding thoughts

In her discussion of Nathans' (2021) "Oedipus for everyone" paper, Morgan (2021) asks, "Could the difficulty in establishing 'healthy triadic relating' stimulate the wish to return to the lost dyadic space?" (p. 347). I think this is the precise pattern that plays out in some of my lesbian couples in the process of establishing their couple more firmly. These couples sometimes approach the threshold of triadic relating only to trip up on it, falling back into states of reciprocal blame and accusation. As discussed, when the mother does not see or accept her daughter's early homoerotic desire, this constitutes a rejection of a vital component of the most foundational loving connection. When the early experience – "You don't see (or want) me" – becomes the unconscious expectation, a part of adult relating is likely to consist of desperate demands to be attended to and results, for example, in the hours-long, mostly fruitless conversations that keep some lesbian couples up half the night, in which both women insist they do not feel seen or understood.

Is it possible that an early experience of invisibility sets in motion the wish to return to the lost primary maternal object for a kind of psychosexual "do-over"? If this is so, in a context of unreliable triadic-relating, the lesbian couple may revert to the phantasy that they can or should be able to experience "dyadic bliss" again. When this project fails, they encounter their own and each other's persecutory responses to repeated experiences of the loss of maternal attunement. It is as if the unconscious holds out continuous hope for the intact dyad and maintains the illusion that this has been reached, only to be shockingly, perturbingly disabused of that notion over and over again. This unconscious pattern represents an ill fated attempt to secure a loving connection that is not available and refuses the losses described. Listening for and noticing this pattern helps couples become conscious of their wishes for attuned connection and mourn what is not available. Then they can move on to a more mature form of loving and caring for each other.

Morgan answers her question thus: "This movement, backwards and forwards, might be part of the process of creating more secure triangular space" (Morgan, 2021, p. 347). In my work with lesbian couples, this process is particularly clear. In the course of repeatedly coming up against the impossibility of restoring dyadic experience, lesbian couples paradoxically have the recurring opportunity to begin to accept its loss. Accepting this loss is very much in the service of creating more space for thought, for reality and for a more mature kind of love. It has often struck me as interesting that almost as soon as toddlers first start to grasp language, they master the concepts and words for opposites: hot and cold, up and down, near and far. Adults have often not developed any further: take a look at our frighteningly polarized world. Many adults still need to develop the capacity to step back from these opposing pairs in order to create a "shaded", triangular, more reality-based view and identify some places in between. When fantasy insists that it can or should be reality, things do not go well. We can entertain fantasies (and there will always be unconscious phantasies), but the reality of human interaction consists of movements towards and away from each other in a continual oscillation. Sometimes there are spontaneous experiences of joy and connection and at other times there are disappointment and loss. This back and forth is where we live. We can pretend otherwise, but the costs of privileging the belief that the fantasy *must be* the reality, both to the psyche and to the world, are severe.

In the course of making a life together, lesbian couples, like all couples, come up against the inevitable challenge of seeing and accepting each other's differences, and loving each other across that divide. The alternative – insisting on the present-day fulfilment of an archaic ph/fantasy of absolute attunement – squanders time and energy in a fruitless pursuit. An adult experience of love can be reparative of early losses but only by accepting that we cannot go back in time, though we can make something of lasting value by valuing each other.

Notes

1 In this chapter, I use the word "lesbian" rather than queer or bisexual, because the women in my practice, who I refer to here, are cis-gendered women who use she/her pronouns and identify as lesbians. They may also identify as part of the wider "queer" world, but their primary identification is lesbian.
2 I am using the term "phantasy" to describe an unconscious fantasy, as opposed to "fantasy", which is a conscious process.
3 LGBTQ+: lesbian, gay, bisexual, transgender, queer and other gender-fluid and non-binary sexual identities.
4 Shelley Nathans, personal communication.
5 We could argue that for straight men there's a return to the mother by way of the female partner's body, and that for straight women there's the acceptance of the love of the father, now symbolized by the desire of the male partner. However, this description is too binary and does not take into account the fluctuating gender identifications people experience both consciously and unconsciously. I agree with Hertzmann that it can be crucial for couples to come to "understand and acknowledge a wide range of identifications with, and desire for, both genders" (2020/2018, p. 102).

References

American Psychiatric Association, Board of Trustees. (15 December, 1973). Resolution removing homosexuality from the Diagnostic and Statistical Manual of Mental Disorders.

Elise, D. (2020/2002). The primary maternal oedipal situation and female homoerotic desire. Reprinted in L. Hertzmann and J. Newbigin (eds), *Sexuality and Gender Now.* Routledge.

Hertzmann, L. (2020/2018). Losing the internal oedipal mother and loss of sexual desire. In L. Hertzmann and J. Newbigin (eds), *Sexuality and gender now.* Routledge.

Nathans, S. (2021). Oedipus for everyone: Revitalizing the model for LGBTQ couples and single parent families. *Psychoanalytic Dialogues*, 31 (3): 312–328.

Morgan, M. (1995). The Projective Gridlock: a form of projective identification in couple relationships. In: S. Ruszczynski and J. Fisher (eds), *Intrusiveness and intimacy in the couple.* Karnac Books.

Morgan, M. (2021). Triangular dynamics and triangular space: A response to Shelley Nathans' "Oedipus for everyone: Revitalizing the model for LGBTQ couples and single parent families", *Psychoanalytic Dialogues*, 31 (3): 340–348.

Ogden, T.H. (2024). Rethinking the concepts of the unconscious and analytic time. *International Journal of Psychoanalysis*, 105 (3): 279–291.

Rich, A. (1986/1980). Compulsory heterosexuality and lesbian existence. In A. Rich, *Blood, bread and poetry. Selected prose 1979–1986*. W.W. Norton & Co.

Winnicott, D.W. (1965). *Maturational processes and the facilitating environment*. Karnac Books.

Winnicott, D.W. (1974). Fear of breakdown. *International Review of Psychoanalysis*, 1: 103–107.

Chapter 10

Obstacles to love in gay male coupling

Gary Grossman

As one of the few openly gay psychoanalytic psychotherapists practising in San Francisco in the early/mid-1980s, most of the people I have seen in therapy have been gay[1] men, including the couples I have worked with. With over 40 years of clinical experience, I have had the honour of accompanying hundreds of gay men, from late teens and early adulthood to old age, in their pursuits of securing, maintaining and ending loving relationships.

Identification as a gay man only captures a portion of an individual's identity. Gay men are as diverse as humans are generally. Although I do not think it is possible to generalize to all gay men from the sample I have seen in individual therapy, psychoanalysis and couple therapy, I hope to offer some insights that may be useful to individual and couple psychotherapists working with gay men.

One commonality shared by all gay men, regardless of culture and place, is the experience of growing up in a society that values other-sex eroticism and relationships and devalues same-sex eroticism and relationships. Every adult gay man has lived a childhood encompassing a time of life prior to his awareness of same-sex desires and the subsequent discovery of his erotic interest in other males. Each gay man discovered his erotic life in the context of a familial and cultural milieu that could not explicitly recognize or celebrate his desires. Although much has changed in society's attitudes towards homosexuality, with greater recognition, acceptance and equity within countries of the West, persecution continues in other parts of the world. In the contemporary United States, a backlash against LGBTQ individuals and communities has proliferated in Republican-led states, creating increased stigma for LGBTQ youth and adults.

Every gay man has also travelled his own unique pathway of discovering and expressing his homoerotic desires, experiencing varying degrees of acceptance, rejection and conflict as he incorporates sexuality within his identity. His relationships with parents, siblings, extended family, community and peers will significantly impact how he experiences, perceives and understands his same-sex attractions. The role that feelings of love play along his pathway into adult erotic and intimate relationships will be influenced by

DOI: 10.4324/9781003518129-10

these relationships, both prior to and after his conscious awareness of same-sex desire and identification as gay. To understand the challenges in finding and maintaining love in gay male couples, it is important to recognize the developmental antecedents to adult romantic love in a boy who grows up to identify as gay.

In this chapter, I describe my understanding of the developmental precursors to mature romantic love, during the child's oedipal phase. I will highlight the experience of the boy whose erotic interests and romantic fantasies are contrary to expectations of his parents and culture, and the internal object-relational world that is created in response to these formative relationships. Recognizing the influence of both internal self and object representations and the concurrent defence mechanisms, I draw specific attention to a tenacious strategy many proto-gay[2] boys employ to cope with the injuries they have suffered in the discord with their parents. I elaborate the omnipotent fantasies, ordinarily so active in early childhood, that serve to protect the child from the profound helplessness and humiliation he experiences in the face of environmental failures and their future impingement on the development of satisfying romantic relationships in adolescence and adulthood.

Romantic love: Its development and expression

I first encountered psychoanalytic perspectives on romantic love in 1992 at a weekend conference sponsored by the American Psychoanalytic Association, "How Men and Women Love", featuring presentations by Ethel Person, Jessica Benjamin, Nancy Chodorow and Otto Kernberg. Although the presenters did not address the specificity of same-sex relationships, they each described models of development for the experience and expression of romantic love. The presentations by Person and Kernberg stood out and have stayed with me all these years, and each have published a major contribution on the topic. Person elaborated her model of love in her 1988 book, *Dreams of love and fateful encounters: The power of romantic passion* (Person, 1988). Kernberg, best known for his work on borderline and narcissistic personality disorders, focused his attention on love, passion and sex in *Love relations: Normality and pathology* (Kernberg, 1995).

Kernberg's account of the antecedents to adult love relationships includes the recognition of the emergence of sexual excitement in the infant's earliest relationship to the mother. His developmental trajectory recognizes the potential differences in the mother's relationship with a boy or girl, suggesting failures in her erotic attunement with her daughter. Kernberg presumes the heterosexuality of mother and daughter in his theorizing of the earliest seeds of romantic love.

Rufus Wainwright's song, "Imaginary love", poignantly captures the experience of early romantic love, highlighting romantic love as always being initially a form of imaginary love. This song immediately resonated with my understanding of unconscious fantasy; it captures the way our earliest internal object relationships shape the timing, nature and objects of our desire.

Person (1988) elaborates on the subjective experience of falling in love, emphasizing the idealization of the beloved. Although the individual believes that the object of their affections possesses unique characteristics that are the exclusive source of their attraction, Person highlights the flaws in this conviction.

> The lover thinks his love is aroused solely by the virtues of the loved one. It will not help to tell him that this is an illusion, that it is he who has endowed the beloved with so much value. Outsiders say that beauty is in the eye of the beholder, that love is a projection, but the lover feels enthralled by what he believes to be the actual attributes of the beloved. The lover … invariably attributes his love to the loved one's specialness, not to the creative powers of his imagination.
>
> (Person, 1988, p. 42)

The reverse may also be at play. The lover believes that it is solely their attributes that have aroused the love in their beloved. Within this construction is also the belief that loss of love is solely due to their attributes and/or the lack thereof.

Dating is risky business. If we are attracted to and interested in someone, we must face the uncertainty about whether our desires will be reciprocated. Each of us must discover our own means of managing the anxieties that are activated in our pursuit of love. Our unique histories and the internal object-relational world we live in, along with the strategies we have employed to manage emotional pain in our earliest relationships, informs our experience of contemporary relationships.

There has been an abundance of psychoanalytic literature that attempts to account for the emergence and developmental trajectory of erotic desire in individuals who grow up to identify as heterosexual, beginning with Freud's (1905) *Three essays on a theory of sexuality*. Notable contributions include Fonagy (2008), Laplanche & Pontalis (1968) and Stein (1988). Although efforts have been made to explore differences based on gender, fewer contributions have focused on the unique experiences impacted by sexual object choice.[3] Although our understanding of the determinants of sexual object preferences in childhood remains quite limited, we must recognize that every adult gay man has early life experiences that informed his adolescent and adult sexual and romantic interests.

If we accept that sexuality emerges in the context of the infant's earliest relationship with their primary caregiver, the trajectory of the child's erotic life will be idiosyncratic depending on their experiences in relation with significant others. A chance encounter with my neighbour, a couple years after the APsA 1992 "Love" conference, highlighted for me the importance of the oedipal stage in the development of adolescent and adult romantic love.

My neighbour was excited to share with me an experience he had with his 4-year-old daughter earlier that day when his wife was at the grocery store. His daughter said to him, "Daddy, wouldn't it be great if mommy didn't come home and then it could be just you and me, and we could get married!" He responded to his daughter saying, "Honey, that is so sweet. I love you to pieces! I think you are the most beautiful little girl in the world. But we love mommy too", and she said, "Yeah …" He continued, "And we don't want mommy not to come home, do we?" "No", she said with a pained look on her face. "How about this," he continued, "from now on, every Saturday afternoon you and I will do something special, just the two of us." He described his daughter's response as beaming. The delight was so evident in my neighbour's animated voice, I had no doubt that not only was he fully engaged in his daughter's fantasy but was thoroughly enjoying it. He seemed empathically engaged with her imagination and was, at the same time, helping her to find a satisfactory solution to her wish to have him all to herself. He did not reject her overtures, nor did he shame or scold her for killing off her mother. He recognized her ambivalent feelings towards her mother, the rival for her father's affection.

As I listened and shared in my neighbour's excitement, I thought how lucky his little girl was to have a daddy who could so readily participate in her romantic play and assist her in managing her internal conflicts. And to myself I thought, that is definitely not the experience gay boys have with their daddies.

The oedipal stage, and the unique compromises each child forms in their effort to manage the varied conflicts that emerge, plays a pivotal role in subsequent development, particularly regarding adult romantic relationships. For the young child who is deeply immersed in romantic fantasies about their parent, the oedipal experience serves as a dress rehearsal for later romantic relationships. The degree to which parents recognize and empathically respond to their child's fantasies will have a profound effect on the developing child's internal image of themselves as lover and beloved, and their internalized object as desiring and loving.

Although we have achieved a much greater level of recognition and acceptance of same-sex relationships in contemporary Western society, it is likely that most parents expect to participate, whether consciously or unconsciously, in a fantasized romance with their child of the other sex. What then is the impact on the oedipal-age child whose primary romance fantasy involves the same-sex parent? The child who grows up to identify as gay is immersed in an oedipal drama involving empathic failures that may result in a lack of recognition at best to humiliating rejection and hostility at worst. Lynch (2002) describes the segregation of love and sex in many of the gay men he has seen in treatment. Published well before the advent of dating and hook-up apps, Lynch strives to understand his gay patients' preoccupation with cruising for sex independent of love. Drawing on Freud's "On the universal tendency to debasement in the sphere of love" (1912), Lynch cites the impact of such empathic failures, "when the environment withholds approval of an individual's sensual desires, the mind finds a way to maintain a separation between love and sex" (Lynch, 2002, p. 178). As our cultures evolve and the prohibitions against, and anxieties about, same-sex eroticism lessen, I expect more children with same-sex erotic fantasies will have experiences more like those of my neighbour and his daughter. Currently, it is likely that the adult gay men we see in couples and as individuals in our consulting rooms will have emerged from discordant oedipal experiences.

When Freud (1900) first described the Oedipus complex, his narrative focused on the boy's wishes, impulses, and fantasies about his parents, and his psychological strategies for managing conflicts and discrepancies between internal and external reality. In this family drama, the boy strives to cope with his desire for his mother and rivalry with his father. And although this oedipal story was considered a universal phenomenon by subsequent analysts, Freud (1923) made it clear that this account represented only a simplified version of the Oedipus complex, and that "one gets an impression that the simple Oedipus complex is by no means its commonest form" (p. 33). Freud adds,

> Closer study usually discloses the more complete Oedipus complex, which is twofold, positive and negative … a boy has not merely an ambivalent attitude towards his father and an affectionate object-choice towards his mother, but at the same time he also behaves like a girl and displays an affectionate feminine attitude to his father and a corresponding jealousy and hostility towards his mother.
>
> (Freud, 1923, p. 33)

Although Freud recognizes the presence of homoeroticism in the oedipal fantasies, his cultural bias constrains his imagination. He is unable to conceptualize same-sex desire and affection outside of a heterocentric viewpoint: for the boy to desire his father, Freud asserts that the boy must first adopt a feminine identity.

Also missing in Freud's narrative of the oedipal drama (and most of the subsequent accounts by other psychoanalysts prior to 1987) is the participation of the child's parents. One exception was Kohut's (1971) self-psychology, which placed a greater emphasis on the role of parental empathy and responsiveness on the development of an independent self in the child:

> it would be misleading to consider the child's oedipal experiences in isolation … the child's experiences during the oedipal phase become understandable only when they are considered within the matrix of the empathic, partially empathic, or unempathic responses from the side of the self-object aspects of his environment …
>
> (p. 230)

For Kohut, the parents' empathic responsiveness to their child's oedipal strivings is crucial for the child's developing self. From an object-relations perspective, the child–parent interactions during the oedipal phase are internalized and form unconscious self and object representations. Emerging through the oedipal phase with parents who have been empathically responsive fosters the development of internal self-representations as loved, desired and treasured, including the roles of lover and beloved. Concurrently, object representations as excited, loving, desiring and accepting are internalized. These early object-relations units will then play a pivotal role when the child reaches adulthood and pursues romantic relationships. I could readily imagine the formation of such an internal object relational world for my young neighbour.

Richard Isay (1987) was the first to write, from a non-pathological perspective, about oedipal dynamics in the boy who grows up to identify as gay. Challenging earlier theories (Bieber et al., 1962) suggesting that overly involved mothers and distant critical fathers fostered homosexuality in boys, Isay (1987) argued that it was the father's discomfort with his young son's erotic attachment that precipitated his withdrawal and critical attitude. Isay's narrative, however, failed to address the oedipal boy's conflicted relationship with his mother. Goldsmith (1995, 2001) broadened the oedipal story in his descriptions of the proto-gay boy's struggles with both parents. Highlighting the role of parental involvement in the child's oedipal drama, Goldsmith's insightful account describes the emotional consequences of the mismatch between child and parents' expectations and fantasies.

As the child enters the oedipal phase, parents anticipate, consciously and unconsciously, a special romance with their other-sex child and rivalry with their same-sex child. However, when the child's erotic and aggressive strivings are discordant with parental expectations, as is the case when the child's attachment is to the same-sex parent and rivalry is with the other-sex parent, an empathic breach occurs with significant consequences for the child's developing sense of self.

From the boy's perspective, the father has become his primary love object and the mother his rival. The boy must then contend with both the libidinal and aggressive components of his oedipal conflict, his love for his father and jealous hostility towards his mother. Keeping in mind the existence of the complete Oedipus complex, the boy must also manage his continued attachment to and dependence on his mother, the wish to have her to himself, and his jealousy towards his father.[4] The boy's experience of this romantic drama and the compromise formations[5] (Brenner, 2002) he develops to cope with his conflicts will be greatly affected by the response of each parent.

For this contribution on love, I am focusing on the boy's relationship with his father. The father, who consciously or unconsciously is expecting to be the son's rival for the mother's affection, is not anticipating being the object of his son's desire. Under such circumstances, the boy's early romantic overtures will likely be missed, and an empathic break occurs. The father's subsequent responses to his son's erotic attachment, as Isay (1987, 1989) has suggested, will colour the quality of the internalized object relationship and influence the form of the boy's compromise formations. If a father is conflicted about his own erotic feelings towards his son and uncomfortable with his son's erotic attachment to him, he is likely to respond with some form of rejection and withdrawal. The level of a father's discomfort with the erotic strivings of his son will influence the severity of his reaction. For some fathers, this may be in the form of quiet withdrawal, distancing and loss of interest in their son. For others, where the conflict and discomfort are greater, the father's response could take the form of angry, harsh criticisms, hostile rejections and violence.

The rebuff of his affections, particularly if there are hostility and anxiety in the father's response, can leave the boy feeling foolish and humiliated. The boy's reaction to his father's rejection will depend on multiple factors, including the degree to which he has achieved earlier developmental milestones. In my clinical experience, a common reaction is the boy's defensive turning away from his father. Converting passive into active, he rejects his father in kind, thereby defending against feelings of hurt, loss and humiliation.

> Early in his therapy, Alex reported a distant relationship with his father. He described his father as a harsh, critical and punitive man who he had hated as a child and teenager, gradually softening to indifference as an adult. Alex adamantly denied that he had ever felt love for his father. Initially, Alex treated me with indifference, or, not infrequently, with rage and resentment. In the third year of treatment, after a period of more conscious awareness of loving feelings and erotic longings toward me, Alex recalled a highly pleasurable early memory of playing in a swimming pool with his father and older brother, and remembered feeling an intense attraction for his father, clad only in a bathing suit. He and his father actually had a close relationship, he recalled, that was both intimate and affectionate. All that changed around kindergarten, when his father became distant and critical of him and more engaged with his athletic brother. Alex remembered feeling hurt and rejected by his father, as well as humiliated for having expressed his unrequited love. He protected himself by becoming angry and rejecting toward his father, warding off the hurt and helplessness, as well as his frustrated loving feelings. As Alex grew older, his father would occasionally make overtures for greater involvement with his increasingly distant son. Alex responded with disinterest or disdain. Eventually, his father stopped trying and their relationship evolved into the hostile distance that Alex described at the onset of therapy.

And because of the predominately narcissistic view of a young child, that child is prone to feel responsible for his father's disinterest or contempt, forming the belief that there is something essentially wrong with him. The internal self-representation that may form is one of being faulty, lacking, disgusting, unlovable, bad.

A vivid portrayal of a father's aggressive reaction to his young son's expression of romantic interest is captured in the 2015 pilot episode of the television drama, *Empire*, starring Terrence Howard as the patriarch, Lucious Lyon, and Jussie Smollett as his adult gay son, Jamal. In a flashback scene, we see Jamal, looking to be about three or four years old, dressed in a woman's scarf and high heels, prancing playfully in front of his father and a living room full of family friends. Lucious, upon turning around and seeing his son, jumps up from his chair, grabs Jamal and throws him into a garbage bin outside the kitchen. The flashback scene is interspersed with adult Jamal, a professional musician, singing an autobiographical song that adds meaning to the memory we are witnessing. In the lyrics, Jamal sings of his desire for his father to look at him and see that he is good enough and, therefore, worthy of his father's love.

The lyrics provide credence to the inference that Jamal's dress up and prancing were an effort to attract his father's attention and love. They also offer insight into the character's understanding of his father's rejection: Jamal believed he was not good enough or worthy of his father's love. That he is singing this song as an adult also reflects the persistence of an internal self-representation as unlovable, unworthy, not enough.

The intensity of the father's aggressive reaction suggests that Lucious feels threatened by his son's erotic overtures. The self-representation that forms within a father–son experience such as the violent one depicted in *Empire* may additionally include a self that is dangerous.

The discordance between a boy's romantic fantasies and those of his parents, especially his father's, becomes the unconscious template for adult romantic relationships and, I believe, accounts for many of the challenges our gay male patients encounter in their pursuit of love. As painful as the experience is of feeling defective and holding the belief that something is bad or wrong about oneself, these beliefs may take on a secondary defensive function. A key component of a young boy's experience in the empathic disruption with and rejection by his father is that of powerlessness. The belief that the reasons for the rejection and hostility resides within the boy fosters the fantasy that receiving or losing their object's love is fully up to him. Drawing on Jamal's lyrics, we can infer the belief, "If I was good enough, you would love me". Such a belief reflects an internal self-representation as "bad" and serves as an omnipotent defence against helplessness and humiliation. All the power to determine being loved resides in the self and the object is stripped of subjectivity and agency. The multideterminism (Boesky, 2007; Waelder, 1936) in the construction of this belief fuels its tenacity across the lifespan. To recognize the autonomy of the object's desire and affection is to confront one's helplessness in the pursuit of love. For some, the suffering of a degraded self is more bearable than the pain of powerless loss at the hands of another, in part because it reifies the omnipotent fantasy that the agony of loss could be prevented.

Oedipal rejection, internalized homophobia and pursuit of love

The following narrative is my effort to capture the childhood experiences of the adult gay men we are currently seeing in our consulting rooms.

As the proto-gay boy struggles with his oedipal strivings and frustrations he is also growing up in a culture that devalues same-sex love. I believe that for the boy who has experienced the kind of oedipal rejection that I am describing, the anti-LGBTQ attitudes of our culture will resonate with his internal world, further reinforcing his conviction that something is terribly wrong with him.

Broadly speaking, the term homophobia refers to a fear of homosexuality. More typically, homophobia is understood as anti-gay attitudes and beliefs or hostility towards gay people. Homophobia can be conscious and/or unconscious. Internalized homophobia refers to anti-gay attitudes, feelings and beliefs in a person who is gay. Homophobia is internalized through processes of identification. Negative attitudes about homosexuality are accepted as one's own and endorsed as correct. Internalized homophobia can also be conscious and unconscious.

The sexual, competitive and aggressive dramas of the oedipal period are quieted as the boy enters latency. Erotic longings and romantic fantasies are repressed, and the child has no conscious memory of his frustrated desires, nor is he able to appreciate the meanings of his parents' empathic failures. Although he is not yet aware of his sexual orientation and may have limited understanding of what homosexuality is or what it means to be gay, he will continually be exposed to anti-gay attitudes in the surrounding world. As he approaches puberty, the boy gradually becomes aware of his sexual attraction towards other boys and men. He may fall in love with a best friend or develop a crush on a favourite male teacher. Ashamed and fearing rejection, fuelled by his early childhood experiences and his awareness of society's hostility towards gay people, he, unlike his heterosexual peers, must keep his feelings and fantasies a secret. Once he has become aware of his homoerotic desires and fantasies, the adolescent knows that the contempt towards gay people he has witnessed is also directed towards him. His success at keeping his secret, along with the degree of his gender typicality, will determine the extent to which he will be the direct recipient of homophobic hostility from his peers. The gender-atypical gay teen is especially vulnerable to harassment, ostracism, rejection and violence from other boys.

Because adolescence is often a recapitulation of oedipal conflicts, rejection and hostility from peers will resonate with the boy's unconscious internal world. To defend against hurt and humiliation, he is likely to identify with his persecutors, internalizing their hostile attitudes towards his gayness, resonating with and reinforcing his existing self and object representations. Whereas earlier in his life he may have consciously felt like something was wrong with him, without understanding what it was, he now attributes his sense of defect to his same-sex desires. From this point on, reckoning with his sexuality becomes a conscious endeavour and each boy's path will be a unique one.

"Coming out", a term used to describe the process of recognizing and accepting same-sex desires and disclosing it to others, is a significant life experience that has no counterpart in heterosexual development. The point at which a boy becomes aware of his same-sex attractions and then identifies himself as gay will vary, as will the label he chooses. He may think of himself as a faggot, queer, sissy, freak, pervert, sinner or possibly something more benign such as homosexual, gay or the more recently reclaimed "queer" with a positive valence. The degree of denigration in his self-labelling will likely impact the length of time before he begins to reveal his sexuality to the important people in his life.

We tend to assume that the more comfortable a person is with their same-sex desires, the more openly gay they will be, and that people who are openly gay are comfortable with and accepting of their sexuality. From a conscious perspective, I believe that these assumptions are reasonable. However, such resolve and self-acceptance may also serve to keep hidden unresolved feelings of degradation and shame associated with oedipal rejection and empathic dissonance from parents. That these early traumas associated with oedipal development continue to impact the lives of gay men is especially evident among those men who come to us for therapy.

Clinical implications

A significant portion of my gay male patients have sought therapy primarily because of disappointments, and/or difficulties, in finding and forming a love relationship. For some, this has been years of short-term love affairs and casual sexual hook-ups. For others, a series of longer-term, serious relationships that have ended. One of the most common complaints I hear is that the patient is interested in men who do not reciprocate and/or the patient is not interested in the men who are pursuing him. For some, the unavailability of the object of desire, resonating with their earlier oedipal longings, seems to heighten the attraction.

Alex's experiences in romantic relationships as an adult mirrored his childhood experiences with his father. He was drawn to men who were notably different from him: older, more traditionally masculine, taller and more muscular. He enjoyed having sex with these men and would become quickly infatuated and they would begin dating seriously. He described these boyfriends as self-involved, aloof and highly critical of him. He became preoccupied with working out, trying to become bigger and more masculine. When the boyfriend ended the relationship, Alex felt terrible. He was overwhelmed with self-hatred, blaming himself for the problems in the relationship, certain that he was deficient. Had he not been so deficient, the relationship would have survived.

Alex also had a couple of boyfriends he described as "boyish". They were slightly younger, closer to his slight physique, more emotionally expressive and playful in the way they engaged with him. He enjoyed the sex but lamented that it was not as exciting as with large muscular men. These boyfriends seemed to idolize Alex, and he luxuriated in their love and attention – initially. Gradually, Alex would find fault with his boyfriend and became increasingly disturbed by their presence. Little things annoyed him: they chewed too loudly, stomped when they walked, were too feminine, too sensitive and too needy. Eventually, Alex would end the relationship.

With the older men, Alex was reliving his early experience with his father. He was again in the position of trying to win the love and attention of a critical and distant man, feeling small, insufficient and defective. He felt bad about himself, convinced he was not worth loving. With the younger men, Alex initially felt loved and admired. However, when the relationship became more serious and Alex became more aware of his boyfriend's attachment and dependence, his anxieties about losing his autonomy intensified. In this dyad, the small vulnerable boy-Alex, longing for love, was split off and projected onto his boyfriend. Alex, immersed in a defensive identification with his father, became the strong, self-sufficient, critical and rejecting man.

In recounting his history and, over the course of therapy and living out similar scenarios with different men, Alex became immersed in self-reproach, harshly attacking himself for his relationship failures. His lack of a satisfying relationship was evidence that something was wrong with him. He was too critical, too rigid, too self-centred to be loved. Or he was too small, too weak, too needy, too lacking.

These same dynamics came alive in Alex's relationship with me. Initially, Alex experienced me as distant and lacking empathy for him. I was aloof and critical, and he frequently felt defensive in response to my observations. Concurrently, Alex was highly critical of me. He critiqued how I dressed, the décor in my office, the sound of my voice and my choice of words. Although I found sessions with Alex to be engaging and alive, I would also feel dread before greeting him in the waiting room, wondering how I would be scrutinized that day. Alex frequently felt frustrated and angry with me and was never shy about expressing his annoyance. He was indifferent or gleeful in response to my absences. I was left feeling small, ineffective and insignificant. Approximately 3 years into this 10-year therapy, and after surviving his attacks without too much defensiveness or retaliation on my part, Alex began to acknowledge his attachment to and affection for me. It was during this period that he shared erotic fantasies about me, became more openly curious about my life and recalled his earlier experience of a close relationship with his father.

Alex had been in several previous therapies, though never for longer than six months. Those treatments ended when Alex became too frustrated with the therapist's fallibilities, and he became convinced of their ineptitude. He wondered what was different in his work with me and why he continued even though he had a lot of criticisms about how I worked with him. My ability to tolerate his experience of me as an unloving and rejecting object while remaining engaged, interested and welcoming helped to modify his internal self and object representations. At the same time, Alex was convinced that if he was a different kind of patient, one who was more open and grateful, who paid more and had more frequent sessions, I would become more like who he wanted me to be. I would tell him more about myself, my experiences in relationships, my family, my personal preferences, and I would directly express my love for and admiration of him.

Daniel and Evan, both in their late 20s, had been together for three years. They sought therapy to address the discordance in their interest in opening their relationship. Prior to meeting Evan, Daniel, who came out in his late teens, had been in two shorter term relationships and had enjoyed various casual sexual encounters. This was Evan's first relationship. He came out towards the end of college and dated sporadically prior to meeting Daniel. Although he enjoyed sex with the men he dated, he did not seek out casual hook-ups. Both men expressed feelings of love, connection and commitment to their relationship, however, Daniel believed that opening their relationship to sex with other men would bring more excitement to their life as a couple and would deepen their sexual connection with each other. Evan had no interest in sex outside the couple and felt confused and threatened by Daniel's interest in other men. Although he expressed openness to talking about and exploring the option of non-monogamy, Evan felt threatened by an open relationship.

Evan experienced Daniel's desire to have sex with other men as a reflection on him. He had trouble understanding how their relationship was not enough for Daniel as it was and worried that it meant there was something essential that he lacked. If he was lovable and desirable, Daniel would be satisfied with monogamy. Daniel's desire for an open relationship meant to Evan that something was wrong with him. Efforts to talk about and explore opening the relationship in the therapy evoked feelings of deficiency and shame in Evan, often leading to impasses in their struggles in finding a path forward.

Evan grew up in a religiously conservative family with parents in traditional gendered roles. He experienced his father as remote, with high expectations of his son and as harshly critical of Evan's interests in art, music and reading. He grew up with the belief that he was not the "right" kind of boy to interest his father. He felt awkward in his body and embarrassed by his slim build. He was shy with his peers as a youth and was slow to begin dating after he came out. Daniel's parents divorced when he was very young, and he grew up primarily with his mother and sister, having little contact with his father. Athletic and involved in sports, Daniel felt at ease in his body and experienced a sense of power and excitement in his first sexual encounters with other boys. As a classically attractive young man, Daniel had rarely experienced rejection in his pursuit of casual sex and dating. He felt confident in his desirability, craved the attention of men, and felt like something vital was missing if he was not sexually active.

Over the course of the therapy, I gained a window into each man's internal world and their views of themselves and the objects of their affection. I could gradually appreciate how each partner had developed their specific preferences for a romantic relationship. For Daniel, the option of having sex with other men felt exciting and expansive and did not seem to disrupt his feelings of love and connection with Evan. Evan, however, experienced Daniel's desire for other men as a reflection of his deficiencies. His anxieties about loss and rejection, along with feelings of humiliation, made it very difficult for Evan to consider changing the framework of their relationship. The course of the couple therapy would entail helping each partner recognize the underlying meanings of their desires and anxieties and the preconditions for feeling lovable and loved, before they could equitably engage in exploring an open relationship.

Conclusion

To understand the unique desires for love and loving in our adult patients, we need to recognize the impact of their first experiences with romantic play that occur during the oedipal period of childhood development. If we accept the psychoanalytic premise that erotic life begins at birth and is actively engaged in the infant's attachment to caregivers, then we can appreciate, as the capacity for language develops, the emergence of the child's oedipal romance fantasies. This romantic play becomes a dress rehearsal for later adolescent and adult relationships. The immersion in oedipal romance fantasy and play populates the child's unconscious inner world with self and object representations that form as a response to these relational experiences. The unique array of the child's self and object representations will inform their erotic attractions and preferences and will come alive within their mature romantic relationships.

When parents can empathically recognize and participate in their child's oedipal romance fantasy and play, they facilitate the child's development of lovable self and loving object representations and shield the child from experiences of shame for their desires. The adult gay men that we see in our consulting rooms have more likely experienced a mismatch between their oedipal fantasies, in which the father has become the primary object of their erotic attachment and mother the object of rivalry, contrary to their parents' conscious, or more likely unconscious, expectations. In addition to forming unlovable, defective self and hateful, rejecting object representations, they are also inclined to develop omnipotent defensive strategies to manage the humiliation, helplessness and loss in response to their unrequited love. Such a defensive strategy serves to protect and maintain a "good" paternal object while also protecting against humiliating powerlessness through creating a fantasy that by becoming someone better (stronger, bigger, smarter, attractive, etc.) they will be able to win the love of the one they desire.

Alex was locked into a pattern of frustrating romantic relationships. He was either in the position of desiring and pining for an unavailable man or becoming annoyed and disinterested in a man who expressed attachment and dependence on him. In both scenarios Alex became immersed in an internal world of self-attack, blaming himself for the failed relationship and bemoaning what he lacked. As painful as this self-hatred was, it also served to maintain a fantasy that obtaining love from his desired object was all up to him, warding off feelings of powerlessness and vulnerability. The pain of self-reproach and blame was more bearable because it originated from within and served to defend against the potential humiliation and hurt he could be subjected to if he depended on another. Over the course of therapy, as Alex began to feel loved by me and could risk experiencing and expressing love and desire for me, he began taking more risks in his dating life. He developed greater tolerance for uncertainty, and could experiment with feeling small, desiring and dependent, without completely losing touch with his sense of autonomy. He could experience lack without a complete collapse of his self-esteem.

The couple therapy with Daniel and Evan served to foster their capacities to explore their desires and anxieties more openly. As Evan became more aware of his beliefs about himself and doubts about his lovability, including previously unrecognized persistent conflicts about being gay, he was more able to listen to and understand Daniel's sexual interest in other men. Although he was more aware of how vulnerable he felt in his relationship with Daniel, he was less defensive and able to consider his partner's desires as independent and not a reflection of his own desirability or worth. Daniel was initially flummoxed by Evan's assumption that his interest in other men reflected a loss of desire or love for Evan. The therapy helped Daniel to see their relationship from Evan's perspective and he, Daniel, was then more able to draw from his empathy in their continued explorations of their relationship's framework.

Psychoanalysis has vividly demonstrated the imprint of the past on the present. Each of us forms an internal world populated with self and object representations, created in response to our earliest relationships with caregivers, that inform who and how we desire. Growing up in a world that privileges heterosexuality provides continuity and resonance for the child who grows up desiring someone of the other sex. For the proto-gay child, the discordance of his desires with parental and cultural expectations creates disruptions with lifelong consequences. By expanding their understanding of the developmental experiences of proto-gay boys, particularly during the oedipal period, psychotherapists can better empathize with their adult gay male patients and the challenges they face when seeking romantic partners.

Recognizing the obstacles to love both in individual therapy, especially within the transference to the therapist, and in couple therapy through interactions between partners, will facilitate the therapist's sensitivity and specificity in their approach to treatment.

Notes

1 I use the term "gay" to refer to men who have a primary erotic attraction to and desire a relationship with other men. Some of the men I work with prefer "queer" and some eschew labels all together.
2 A term I use to refer to an adult gay man's childhood, prior to his awareness of sexuality and same-sex desires.
3 Lynch (2002) is one of the earlier psychoanalytic contributions to the understanding of erotic desire in gay men, specifically exploring the separation of sex and love.
4 I believe that this conflict is distinctly different than for the boy who grows up to be heterosexual and whose primary libidinal object is the mother and rival is the father. Although the proto-hetero boy must contend with both aggressive and libidinal impulses towards his father, the father is not the object of primary dependence, whereas for the proto-gay boy, the rivalrous object, his mother, is still the object he depends on.
5 Compromise formations are unique solutions to the tensions between desires, anxieties and defence mechanisms. The defensive strategy that the child employs to manage these tensions, in my experience, plays a significant role in adolescent and adult romance.

References

Bieber, I., Dain, H., & Dince, P., et al. (1962). *Homosexuality: A psychoanalytic study.* Jason Aronson.

Boesky, D. (2007). "The principle of multiple function": Revisiting a classic seventy-five years later. *Psychoanalytic Quarterly*, 76 (1), 93–117.

Brenner, C. (2002). Reflections on psychoanalysis. *Journal of Clinical Psychoanalysis*, 11 (1), 7–37.

Fonagy, P. (2008). A genuinely developmental theory of sexual enjoyment and its implications for psychoanalytic technique. *Journal of the American Psychoanalytic Association*, 56, 11–36.

Freud, S. (1900). *The interpretation of dreams.* In: J. Strachey (ed. and trans.), *The standard edition of the complete psychological works of Sigmund Freud* (1953–74), Volume 4. Hogarth Press, pp. ix–627.

Freud, S. (1905). Three essays on the theory of sexuality. In: J. Strachey (ed. and trans.), *The standard edition of the complete psychological works of Sigmund Freud* (1953–74), Volume 7. Hogarth Press, pp. 123–2460.

Freud, S. (1912). On the universal tendency to debasement in the sphere of love (Contributions to the psychology of love: II). In: J. Strachey (ed. and trans.), *The standard edition of the complete psychological works of Sigmund Freud* (1953–74), Volume 11. Hogarth Press, pp. 177–190.

Freud, S. (1923). The ego and the id. In: J. Strachey (ed. and trans.), *The standard edition of the complete psychological works of Sigmund Freud* (1953–74), Volume 19. Hogarth Press, pp. 3–66.

Goldsmith, S. (1995). Oedipus or Orestes? Aspects of gender identity development in homosexual men. *Psychoanalytic Inquiry*, 15, 112–124.

Goldsmith, S. (2001). Oedipus or Orestes? Homosexual men, their mothers and other women revisited. *Journal of the American Psychoanalytic Association*, 49 (4), 1269–1288.

Isay, R. (1987). Fathers and their homosexually inclined sons in childhood. *Psychoanalytic Study of the Child*, 42, 275–294.

Isay, R. (1989). *Being homosexual: Gay men and their development*. Farrar, Straus, & Giroux.

Kernberg, O. (1995). *Love relations: Normality and pathology.* Yale University Press.

Kohut, H. (1971). *The analysis of the self. A systematic approach to the psychoanalytic treatment of narcissistic personality disorders.* International University Press.

Laplanche, J. & Pontails, J.B. (1968). Fantasy and the origins of sexuality. *International Journal of Psychoanalysis*, 49 (1), 1–19.

Lynch, P. (2002). Yearning for love and cruising for sex. *Annual of Psychoanalysis*, 30, 175–189.

Person, E.S. (1988). *Dreams of love and fateful encounters: The power of romantic passion*. W.W. Norton & Co.

Stein, R. (1998). The enigmatic dimension of sexual experience: The "otherness" of sexuality and primal seduction. *Psychoanalytic Quarterly*, 67, 594–625.

Waelder, R. (1936). The principles of multiple function. *Psychoanalytic Quarterly*, 5, 45–62.

Chapter 11

All you need is love?

Monica Vorchheimer

Introduction

Several questions underlie my everyday practice almost since the very beginning when I started seeing couples in a psychoanalytic setting. Why do people consider being a couple as a way of substantiating love? Why, if we know that couples' lives are generally turbulent, do people still believe in this form of linkage? Is love enough? And, more interestingly, what promotes the togetherness that we call a couple?

This last question has been answered from different theoretical perspectives, and I will return to it. Meanwhile, I will address the first three questions.

The couple as conceived of today has not always been in its present form. What is known as the modern couple, described by Rougemont (1983), has only emerged as a relatively generalized form of coupling after the First World War in the urban West. Unlike couples whose marriage was arranged by their families of origin, still found in certain religious communities and Eastern cultures, the modern couple is one that is freely constituted by those who institute it and are part of the bond. It is a choice of the lovers. Moreover, what creates this modern couple is the assumption of reciprocal love. It is interesting to recall that in his excellent book, Rougemont has stressed that this modern couple is an invention of Western cultures and this idea of love as an invention will be my focus.

There have been, and still are, various attempts to question this modern couple or to invent new forms of couples. The new open couples, such as polyamorous or "free love", as acclaimed in the 1960s and 1970s, have not created significant new versions of coupledom. At least for now. Divorces are more common, yet our society holds to the ideal of romantic love. This is so powerful that a single or unmarried person can be seen as someone miserable, or very neurotic, or as someone who has seriously failed in life. The ideal of romantic love is still the norm, and the expectations of coupledom are even more demanding. This romantic ideal is supposed to sustain love, sexual passion and communication between the two members of the couple without them having to renounce individual freedom, projects, friendships, jobs and so

DOI: 10.4324/9781003518129-11

on. Although many couples fail to achieve these ideals, this does not challenge the prevailing model of modern couples. It is not uncommon today to think that young people fall in love quickly, only to become just as easily disappointed in their marriages. This view suggests a fragile capacity to sustain love – one that reflects a more narcissistic way of being in the world, oriented towards the self rather than towards the other, and lacking the object-related capacity to truly love. Even the openness implied by the recognition of same-sex couples has not challenged the modern couple model; on the contrary, diverse couples have often claimed the right, in their political struggle, to constitute themselves in the same way and following the same models as heterosexual couples.

If things have changed so much since the establishment of the so-called modern couples' format, why do people still hold on to this "old" model? What does this kind of couple provide in terms of psychic economy? How does this reciprocal love provide the experience of togetherness? And, last but not least, I would like to consider if the title of the famous song by the Beatles, "All you need is love", is any more than wishful thinking?

The link model

In order to address these questions about love and the modern Western couple, I turn to the link model which I will introduce briefly.

Link is a word used in ordinary conversation as well as in general psychoanalytic theory; it refers to a relationship in general, to that which ties together, puts in contact, and in some way unites two or more entities.

It is my impression that the need to understand and assess couples in a psychoanalytic setting requires a specific metapsychological concept that goes beyond the established theory developed for individual analysis. Since couples are approached from different social and human sciences such as sociology, anthropology, law and others, there has been a need to differentiate a psychoanalytic understanding from those disciplines. Moreover, insofar as the psychoanalysis of groups, institutions, families or couples has been viewed as a second-class practice, as a mere application of concepts, there is an increasing necessity to demonstrate how the field is able to stand on its own feet, having its own weight and based on its own metapsychology, though without departing from the analytic core concepts. In addition, many traditional analysts claimed that multiple person treatments detract from the intimacy needed for any psychoanalytic process to be possible, as if treating couples is conceived of as two individual treatments being held, simultaneously violating confidentiality and intimacy.

Practitioners were aware early on that the couple relationship could be described as two egos linked together, and that the result was more than the sum of two individuals. This was initially understood as the effect of reciprocal projective identifications, described by Henry Dicks as a "joint marital personality" (Dicks, 1967).

The concept of a shared unconscious phantasy is a theoretical tool to convey the emotional web that holds two psychic minds and hence two people who are linked and related in a steady, ongoing relationship. It has become a synonym of the unconscious life of couples, the lens through which couples experience their partners and play out stories together, and which serve to connect their individual selves. It is worthwhile noticing, however, that the concept of shared unconscious phantasy, however overarching, did not require substantial modifications to the formulations of the unconscious. The couple's relationship is understood as the result of an interplay of unconscious projections and introjections, a point of intersection, an unconscious complementarity or coincidence of internal objects that might or might not coalesce, through a phantasy which is both shared and unconscious.

As we know, concepts that have been incorporated by a scientific community are so powerful that frequently, after a certain time, they may lose their abstract dimension. They may become reified as if they are not a convention accepted by a group of peers to grasp a piece of reality, but as being the reality itself, an ontological being. I believe that such a phenomenon may risk concepts becoming something with which we "fall in love", and which give a group of analysts a sense of having a solid, accepted and acknowledged basis with which to work when facing such complex dynamics as those that arise when we work with different couples. We could say that, insofar as a group believes in, for example, the existence of shared unconscious phantasy, it establishes a belonging to a community, whether it is called the Tavistock or the Link or Object Relations, similar to what happens with couples. This is why it is not an easy task to leave a concept aside, or even question it, when talking about psychoanalysis and couples, since the concept stands for the reality and identity of the group, just as being in love is supposed to be part of the identity of the couple.

It was only lately that the psychic effects of being part of a relationship came to be recognized as a new source in the constitution of subjectivity. This represents a very important change in psychoanalytical tradition, which has mainly focused on studying the inner world, the internal reality and the world of object representations. Now, external reality – the other in the relationship – was making its way into the corpus of psychoanalytic theory and practice.

"The link" had not appeared initially in the vocabulary of couple psychoanalysis. Bion had theorized the notion in classical psychoanalysis stressing the importance of the capacity of the object, the mother, to contain and digest anxieties and make them thinkable for the baby (alpha function). Although he refers to what happens with the object, he also alludes to the relationship that the baby has with the mother as a person. Bion describes the different types of links that mould the relationship with an internal object and with the mother, and stresses the importance of the capacity to tolerate the absence of the object, which constitutes the first step towards thinking, i.e. symbolization.

From a different perspective, link theory has underlined the importance of considering the effects of the "presence" of the object and not only its absence. The presence of the other and its psychic effects in the constitution of the mind of the subject – the other of the link – had been underestimated by just considering the other, the object, as a character, an inhabitant of the unconscious fantasy in the internal world – and I believe had been given scarce relevance until these new developments.

The link is an unconscious structure and, because of its virtual nature, it cannot be apprehended by the senses but only through its effects in symptoms, dream-life, transference or slips of the tongue. The unconscious is the locus from which meanings emanate, or from where meaning is born. Working with couples and families has reinforced the need to keep this abstract dimension of the unconscious in mind when referring to what is produced in the in-betweenness of the relationship, so as not to confuse the observational dimension of the interaction with the production of meaning born from the fact of being part of a relationship. Link theory stresses this virtual dimension referring to it as the source of unconscious meaning that "stamps" the relation and that does not belong to either participant but rather to the fact of being together.

What is the link model endeavouring to describe?

Psychoanalysis has a wide and rich tradition grounded in a metapsychology of repetition: instincts, drives, repetition compulsion, trauma, après coup, transference, dream-life and infantile sexuality. Even love has been understood by means of theoretical tools anchored in the idea of repetition. Too little account has been taken of the role of the new – that is, of inscriptions arising within the fabric of human relations.[1]

The extraordinary discoveries by Freud of infantile sexuality, the conceptualizations on narcissism and the Oedipus complex have enlightened many aspects of human life, including object choice. Adulthood is rooted in childhood, and so, Freud remarked, was one's love object choice. Everyone is subjected to repetition from the past, which, at best, can be transformed through new versions of the same.

But since couples and families have been studied, it has been increasingly assumed that subjects are not only determined, as Freud suggested, by early infantile sexuality and historical experiences. Now one can consider the inclusion of the human being in a web of significant others after childhood that constitutes a new source of subjectivity.

The contributions of anthropology to the understanding of kinship in primitive cultures seen in Lévi-Strauss's *Structural anthropology* (1958, p. 2) have suggested that there are universal principles to the formation of families that apply to modern couples and families as well. This has contributed to an understanding that, for marriage to be more than a mere social ritual, a symbolic (unconscious) operation is needed: the alliance. The alliance implies a rupture from the families of origin that, as a consequence, establishes a new order, with its own legality that creates something new. Marriage does not necessarily imply that the alliance as a symbolic operation has actually taken place. What link theory argues is that the alliance cannot be conceived of as simply a repetition of the past, but rather as a new invention with its emotional effects of discontinuity with the preceding time. From this perspective, when this is achieved, couples invent a new origin, a new beginning, a new history, a new institution.

Another aspect of link theory stresses that just as the "internal child" must not be confused with the child in analysis, so it is important to distinguish the internal-object world making up an internal couple or family, from the couple or family link observed and treated. Thus, the patient is the link itself – not a sum of individuals but a patient different and distinct from an individual or singular patient. The basic term used here is "The Link", which is defined as an unconscious structure, the specific psychic reality that is constructed by the encounter of two or more subjects who are determined by a relationship of presence, different from the internal object projected on to an external object.

Consequently, the subject is moulded not only by their relationship with the body ego and the drives, but by the link with the other and with the social background. The subject is sustained within the sense of belonging inherent in the link, which differs from the sense of identity intrinsic to the ego, although both constitute the construction of subjectivity.

Each subject is not only linked to another subject but also to the set itself, being it a couple, a family, a group, or an institution. Despite their unstable character, such groups perceive themselves as if they were stable. To put it in other words, it can be said that the set is precisely the illusion that the encounter with the other is stable and lasting. This is why there is a need to represent it; as if by having a representation this instability can be caught, fixed, denying its evanescent quality by believing in the continuity of the set. We often find this need to represent the couple in the way in which couples speak of themselves – "we are this", "we never do this or that", or "we always like to". This need to have a picture or a definition of who they are is a way of representing in a fixed way their togetherness. Alain Badiou (2006) suggested that chance is always at the beginning. The great challenge of couples consists in transforming the ephemerality of the beginning into a duration. Following Badiou's idea, I assume that the transformation of the ephemeral into something experienced as lasting is achieved through the representation of the togetherness that provides a sense of identity to the collective "we". As we know, identity, even if it is imaginary, creates a sense of continuity to the ego of the couple.

The narcissistic foundation of togetherness

Couples have the need to represent their link and to assume that this representation is shared by both of them. The "we" that is built up from this representation stands for the couple's identity. Partners love this representation of their togetherness. Moreover, the togetherness is a result of the falling in love of the partners, as well as with this representation. This is a narcissistic love, but it is still love, and foundational for the couple.

Since the sense of belonging to the couple provides identity – a sense of existence – this representation of the link is very strongly defended and needs to be felt as shared so as to keep the sense of belonging. The couple link is nothing but an emotional experience, fleeting as all emotional experiences are; but this evanescent quality is not easy to bear, and needs to be fixed by representing it, to capture – or to try to capture – its evanescent nature.

This is also why misunderstandings or differences are felt as catastrophic for the relationship, as a serious problem that the partners often work to eliminate by convincing the other of the correctness of their own thoughts or positions. This is a reason why similarities or complementarities are searched for and idealized and why, when this representation cannot be held, love seems to have disappeared.

Where does this representation of the "we", of the "togetherness", of the plural come from? In every modern couple, there is a narcissistic foundation; this mythical foundation is created by the experience of falling in love and, it is placed in the past, supposedly when the partners met in a special encounter. This narcissistic love foundation has important effects on couples' functioning.

This original narcissistic myth – which is an individual one and unconscious – gives birth to the sense of togetherness and provides a representation that is supposed to be shared between the partners; it leads to the feeling of existence and identity within the link, the sense of a "we", a feeling of "belonging". This is an initial experience of love in couples, a narcissistic love, the love of the representation of the togetherness that has been created by the magic of the encounter that is supposed to be shared.

This illusory belief – the belief in a belief assumed to be shared – is also the source of couples' ideals. Among these ideals, the expectation of full understanding is central and is equated with love. Consequently, suffering or having conflicts is felt by the partners as evidence of the loss – or the threat of loss – of their identity as a couple, of the representation of the couple, and thus of the couple itself. This loss is felt as the vanishing of love. Discontent arises as a consequence of the disillusion of the illusion which was supposed as shared.

People not only suffer from being on bad terms with the partner, but that pain is enhanced by feeling that a failure has occurred, that something is lost when the assumed reciprocity in understanding collapses and suddenly the other appears to be somebody completely alien, sometimes hated and rejected. The failure in perfect attunement and understanding is experienced as a threat to the oneness and a collapse of love.

When this happens, the representation of the togetherness as being one changes, but it could make room for a new experience where togetherness can be held without a sense of oneness, recognizing the partner as another subject.

This is another dimension of love, much more complex, but also evanescent as every emotional experience is.

There are constant fluctuations between illusory fusional states (narcissism) within the link and the capacity to contain the otherness of the other (object love). When the other as another subject can be recognized, they are no longer a threat but somebody to be known, capable of arousing a curiosity that leads to new creative developments. The central premise here is that couples continually fluctuate between varying degrees of differentiation and otherness, with otherness not originally present in the constitution of the bond. If we accept that, at the beginning, falling in love involves the creation of a narcissistic unit, then the recognition of the other as a separate subject is not given from the outset. Rather, it is through the ongoing elaboration of disillusionment with the initial fusional or complementary unit that the possibility of recognizing otherness emerges. Put differently, couples oscillate between narcissistic love and object love within the relationship, and both are equally necessary and important.

Couples make big efforts to deny differences between themselves because sameness and/or complementarity are very idealized and provide narcissistic food.

When love seems to have vanished: infidelity

Love is neither a univocal word in ordinary language nor within the specificity of a psychoanalytic one. As we know, love is not the same when it is meant as parental love, a couple's love, love towards God, an ideal or a friend.

In *Instincts and their vicissitudes* (1915), Freud describes loving as the expression of the whole sexual current of feeling. He remarks that the attitudes of love and hate cannot be used for the relationship of instincts to their objects but are reserved for the relationship of the total ego to objects. In his reasoning, he underlines that employing the word love can be appropriate only after there has been a synthesis of all the component instincts of sexuality and the primacy of the genitals and in the service of the reproductive function (Freud, 1915, p. 138). However, the above-mentioned text was written before Freud had developed his second topography, where he described the unconscious part of the ego. Following Spivacow (2016), it seems more accurate to define love as a relation of the subject – and not the ego. Love involves the subject as a whole, which means that it includes aspects of the conscious and the unconscious. Love and desire are distinct, and they can follow different paths. Love pertains to the domain of the subject, while desire to the realm of drives. However, we know that when we say that the ego loves its object, there is a link between the loved object and the fact that it is one within the series of objects that had provided sexual satisfaction, even if we mean narcissistic pleasure.

There could be many ways to refer to love and whether love is enough to keep a couple alive. All you need is love? The famous song by the Beatles is a kind of declaration of principles, although we know it is quite romantic and idealistic.

It is common for people who suffer from infidelity in their marital life to believe that an episode of infidelity is evidence of a lack of love. In fact, the discovery of extramarital relations is a very common motive in couples seeking help with their relationship. It is not unusual for partners to engage in endless arguments about whether love is still there or not, since infidelity is usually experienced as the hallmark of the betrayal of love, although often the betraying partner argues that love is still there, and provides endless different explanations for the betrayal.

Infidelity can result from numerous tensions within couples, but it reflects an incapacity to do something together with those tensions, conflicts or dilemmas. It causes strong upheavals and shocks, and it shakes both personal identity and the identity of the set. People feel they are no longer what they believed they were, the partner is no longer who they were believed to be, and they no longer have what they thought they had. This can feel to be a complete crisis with a traumatic quality.

In her paper on infidelity as a manic defence, Shelley Nathans (2023) focuses on the problem that one partner or both "may have with mourning past or impending loss and the consequent infidelity that may result from a manic attempt to replace depression or psychic pain with excitement". In addition, enlisting a Kleinian theoretical background, Nathans underlines unresolved oedipal and pre-oedipal issues with triangulation that could structure an infidelity crisis. Yet, in her ideas there is no reference to the vanishing of love, something that partners usually argue about. Moreover, when referring to difficulties in mourning losses, she means individual losses that could not be processed and that might have caused turbulences within the couple.

Nathans' ideas are valuable, but I would bring here an additional perspective to elucidate what many couples face. Here I will turn to theoretical tools stemming from the link model that I described above.

I assume that infidelity usually takes place when the representation of the couple's togetherness cannot be held and cannot be recovered after its temporary, unavoidable evanescence. This is the loss I am stressing here; it is not an individual biographic loss but a link one. This would entail the collapse of the representation that sustains the "we", given that the narcissistic love towards the representation of the togetherness is no longer believed to be shared. The magnitude of the crisis can be explained because of the identifying power of the link that the partners have, not only towards each other but also to the representation of the set – the couple – that they created; both are sources of self and joint identity, no matter how illusory these might be. The collapse of the representation of togetherness is equated with the collapse of the identity. When this is at stake, instead of working through this loss within the couple, one partner may try to recover the lost love towards a togetherness outside the relationship, via an affair.

When the former representation collapses because of the rupture of the whole, the "we" (the identity of the couple) collapses and is experienced as a failure. It is assumed to mean the disappearance of love, no matter that we know that it is a narcissistic love. "If you'd loved me you wouldn't have done this."

The collapse of the experience of togetherness when differences appear is powerful; it is a collapse of the identity of the set. Hence, it demands that the partners do something with that which is not part of the togetherness, with that of the other that had not been previously included in the couple because it was unknown, rejected or denied. It demands psychic work to recover the sense of identity of the couple.

This may lead to new ways of experiencing the other. One way, the most sophisticated and emotionally challenging, is making room for the other as someone to be known as another subject, even as somebody not completely knowable. When this happens, there might be an initial experience of bewilderment but if there is a capacity to process the narcissistic wound, it might lead to interest and curiosity towards the other, a state with less persecution, thus an expansion of the experience of what love is.

Conversely, if there is an intolerance of the loss of this representation of the togetherness and there is no more trust that it can be recovered, and the narcissistic wound is too painful to be contained, the couple itself might be felt as if it had disappeared. There is no longer a "we" and this can be a fertile ground for an infidelity. In this new affair, the couple's partner might create a new relationship where another togetherness can be experienced and recreated with this new lover, providing a new narcissistic love. In the affair, partners can recover a new togetherness to fall in love with, displacing the previous couple's one.

Often, infidelity is suspected within a couple without it happening. This is the case of couples where the alienness of the partner is unbearable and cannot be signified except as betrayal, as an infidelity. This was the case in John and Peter's relationship. Every time that Peter went out with his friends, it was experienced by John as a betrayal. He could not tolerate that his husband could have a life other than with him. It was experienced as if he had completely forgotten him. The end of their relationship always loomed large if a separate life event took place. The representation of their togetherness seemed too fragile, in spite of the intense love they felt for each other. The continuity of their couple was felt as permanently threatened not because of lack of love but because uncertainty was unbearable, and the unknown of the other was assumed as known and badly intended.

When Dan and Judith started couple therapy, Dan had recently learned that Judith had been cheating on him for over four years. Her lover had sent him a letter telling him about the affair, sharing and exhibiting photos of their sexual life and the trips they had done. He was shocked and angry and yelled at his wife endlessly. How could she do this to him? He had supported her studies and cared for the girls while she was busy dedicating time to her career. Although she recognized how supportive he had been over time, she nevertheless claimed that he was no longer the happy and funny guy she had met years ago but was now a grumpy husband and father.

Dan and Judith had met at work and were both dating other partners. They fell in love and kept this love as a secret relationship for a while. Dan was the first to leave his girlfriend while it took a bit longer for Judith to separate from her fiancé. They had promised each other that they would never cheat but instead, if something would go wrong, they would talk about it: no secrets, no cheating.

When the current affair was discovered, Dan felt betrayed and Judith could not overcome her guilt, and thus she allowed Dan to curse, mistreat her and blame her with terrible words without reacting. He obsessively "wanted to know everything" about the affair and pressed her to tell him what she did not want to; but at times, she gave in and told him intimate things that only triggered more violence from Dan. She could only say that she loved him and that in her fantasy, letting him be abusive was the evidence of her love towards him. They became a couple consisting of an abusive partner and a passive abused one, like the couple that they had endeavoured not to be and as they had experienced in their previous relationships. Not being that couple was the text underlying an unconscious alliance that had brought them together in the past and had kept them together as a loving couple. But now, that representation of their togetherness as a non-abusive couple had collapsed.

What I am trying to illustrate in this brief vignette is how the loss of the representation of their togetherness that was supposed to be shared (we are not a couple in which one is abusive and one is abused) vanished and their incapacity to experience a renewal of their link triggered infidelity. On the other hand, the couple that came to the consultation unconsciously reproduced the abusive/abused dynamic which should have been kept excluded from the link.

It is not unusual that when an affair occurs the partner would claim that they want to know everything, in what can be conjectured as a desire to recover the past representation of the togetherness where there was a phantasy of transparency within the couple, both knowing the other and themselves as a set, without secrets and treasuring blind trust. This belief in knowing each other disavows the unknown and unknowable of the partner; hence, when suffering the effects of infidelity what seems to be curiosity can also be understood as an attempt to recover from disillusionment.

If we return to the initial question posed by the Beatles' refrain – "All you need is love" – the analysis developed here suggests that love, although indispensable, is never enough on its own. Love is the mythic foundation, the moment of enchantment in which the couple imagines itself as one. But this illusion of fusional unity cannot sustain the couple across time. What gives consistency to the link is the capacity to elaborate disillusion, to process the inevitable failure of sameness, or complementarity, and to reconfigure togetherness in ways that make space for otherness.

From the perspective of link theory, what binds the couple is not only reciprocal love between two individuals, but the unconscious structure that emerges in the encounter itself. The couple is a psychic reality of its own, a third entity that exceeds the sum of its parts. The representation of togetherness – the "we" – is thus as crucial as it is fragile, offering a sense of belonging and identity while also being vulnerable to collapse when confronted with difference, conflict. When this representation disintegrates, as in cases of infidelity, it is often experienced not simply as the loss of love, but as the collapse of identity itself. The traumatic quality of such crises derives from the collapse of the set that sustained both individual and collective subjectivities.

The vicissitudes of love in couples can therefore be thought of as oscillations between narcissistic states, in which sameness and complementarity are idealized, and object-related states, in which the partner is recognized as another subject with their own opacity and unknowability. Both poles are necessary: narcissism provides the sense of belonging and the illusion of permanence, while object love introduces alterity, curiosity and the possibility of renewal. The psychic work required in couple life is precisely the continuous elaboration between these positions – the elaboration of loss and disillusion, and the transformation of fragility into new beginnings. Seen from this angle, love is both a foundation and a task, a source of cohesion and a demand for psychic work.

Thus, to the initial question – *Is love enough?* – the answer is paradoxical. Love is indispensable but it cannot by itself guarantee the survival of the couple. If "all you need is love", then it must be understood not as a simple romantic ideal, but as love intertwined with loss, with conflict, and with the ceaseless work of linking.

Note

1 The place given to fate and novelty, to taking place (*acontecer*), to mathematical speculations within Alain Badiou's philosophy have modelled the body of link theory, especially Puget and Berenstein's ideas (Badiou, 2006; Puget & Berenstein, 1989).

References

Badiou, A. (2006). *Being and event*. Continuum.

Dicks, H.V. (1967). *Marital tensions. Clinical Studies Towards a Psychological Theory of Interaction*. Karnac Books (reprinted 1993).

Freud, S. (1915). Instincts and their vicissitudes. In: J. Strachey (ed. and trans.), *The standard edition of the complete psychological works of Sigmund Freud* (1953–74), Volume 14. Hogarth Press, pp. 109–140.

Lévi-Strauss, C. (1958). *Structural anthropology.* Perseus Books Group.
Nathans, S. (2023). *More about couples on the couch.* Routledge, pp. 57–74.
Puget, J. & Berenstein, I. (1989). *Psicoanalisis de la pareja matrimonial.* Paidós.
Rougemont de, D. (1983). *Love in the Western world.* (M. Belgion, trans.). Princeton University Press. (Originally published 1939.)
Spivacow, M. (2016) *La pareja en conflicto.* Paidos.

Chapter 12

The evolution of love through psychoanalytic and Daoist perspectives

Tao Lin

Love is one of the most complex and profound phenomena in human emotional experience, permeating every aspect of life. It evolves from the initial state of contained undifferentiated oneness within the maternal body during the foetal stage to the pursuit of fulfilment in romantic love, the acceptance and creativity inherent in familial love and its transcendence into Da Ai (Great Love, 大爱) – a state of harmony with the Dao (道)[1] as envisioned in Daoist philosophy. Far from being merely an emotion, love is also a philosophical and psychological practice that bridges an individual's yearning for fulfilment with an awakening to the essence of life and the Dao, achieving unity with all existence through effortless action (Wu Wei, 无为).

Whatever form love may take, it inevitably intertwines with the theme of "sad beauty". Love is both exquisitely beautiful and poignantly melancholic: in romantic love, fleeting moments of fulfilment are accompanied by disillusionment, where beauty and sorrow are interwoven; in familial love, profound and enduring beauty emerges through the acceptance of sorrow and impermanence, while still striving for a sense of connectedness and completeness that echoes the longing for the contained oneness of the foetal stage. In contrast, Da Ai represents the ultimate transcendence, where the pursuit of individual wholeness is relinquished, and the self dissolves into the infinite flow of the Dao. In this state, one harmonizes with all beings, nature, and existence, embracing them with unconditional acceptance and achieving the unity of heaven and humanity (Tian Ren He Yi, 天人合一).[2]

This chapter explores the evolutionary path of love from narcissism to Da Ai by drawing on philosophical analysis, literary examples and psychoanalytical perspectives. It reveals how "sad beauty" runs through this journey, pointing to love's ultimate meaning – not merely compassion, but the unconditional acceptance of life in its entirety and the harmonious oneness with the Dao.

The origin of love

Freud believed that love is a way for individuals to attempt to fill an inner void through external objects. In his seminal work *On Narcissism* (Freud,

DOI: 10.4324/9781003518129-12

1914), he proposed two directions of libido flow: object libido, where an individual projects emotional energy onto external objects and achieves satisfaction through connection with them; and ego libido, where emotional energy is directed inwards to maintain the stability and integrity of the self.

In Freud's view (1914), "real happy love" is a unique state where the boundary between object libido and ego libido dissolves. This state allows the individual to experience a sense of unity between loving others and the self, as if returning to a primal state of "original fusion". While Freud primarily focused on the postnatal mother–infant relationship, his theory implies that love originates from an innate yearning to recreate the early experience of unity.

Building on Freud's theories, Klein (1935) further explored the mechanisms underlying the development of love. She posited that infants can only truly develop the capacity to love objects after entering the depressive position, a position characterized by the ability to integrate good and bad elements. This development hinges on several factors, including the infant's innate ego functions, life and death instincts, and the care-giving environment. For Klein, the internalization of "good object relationships" forms the foundation of the ego and enables love to emerge. However, like Freud, Klein confined her analysis to the postnatal stage.

Recent scientific research has provided new evidence supporting the idea of the foetal period as the origin of love. For instance, studies have shown that the mother's emotional state during pregnancy directly affects foetal brain development through hormonal transmission and the placental barrier (Field, 2011). This finding suggests that the origin of love may not begin with the postnatal mother–infant relationship but could instead trace back to the earlier relationship between the foetus and the maternal body.

I view the state of the foetus in the maternal body as a form of "contained undifferentiated oneness" (Lin, 2024) – a state of being held within a unified yet undifferentiated existence. Psychoanalytic theories often describe early relational experiences using terms such as "primal fusion", typically referring to the undifferentiated unity between the mother and infant in the postnatal stage. However, my use of oneness extends this concept to the foetal stage, emphasizing the existential and philosophical dimensions of this state. While primal fusion often connotes dependency or enmeshment within the mother-child dyad, oneness captures a broader sense of harmonious oneness that resonates with Chinese philosophies, particularly the Daoist vision of unity between self and the Dao.

I have described this state of oneness as follows:

> We might question whether the embryo can perceive sensations such as warmth, safety, stability, hunger, or thirst. These sensations arise from differentiation. The embryo may exist in an infinite state – infinitely small and large, beyond our three-dimensional concept of space – and undifferentiated, with no sense of life or death. Perhaps, for the embryo, there

> is no sense of safety or danger, no warmth or cold, no stability or instability, no in or out, and no hunger or thirst. Yet, the embryo is the origin of both mental and physical life, based on the unity of the mother and embryo as a single entity, a oneness contained by the mother. I term this state the "contained undifferentiated oneness".
>
> (Lin, 2024, p. 15)

In this state, the foetus experiences not only complete physiological support – such as oxygen, nutrients and warmth – but also an unconditional psychological nurturing that transcends the boundaries of life and death. This state of oneness is not merely an absence of differentiation; it is an existential state of absolute safety, balance, and harmony, akin to the Daoist ideal of effortless unity (Wu Wei). It represents the original prototype of love, offering a sense of completeness and interconnectedness that becomes humanity's deepest longing. Within Daoist philosophy, this primordial harmony mirrors the natural flow of the Dao, where all beings exist in a state of mutual interdependence and oneness.

However, the rupture of birth disrupts this state of perfection. The transition from the contained oneness of the maternal body to the differentiated world marks the first experience of separation. This disruption, though necessary for the development of individuality, pushes the individual out of a harmonious oneness into a fragmented reality. In Daoist terms, this moment signifies a divergence from the natural flow of the Dao, where the individual becomes conscious of separation and begins to seek reconnection. It is this rupture that initiates the lifelong pursuit of love – a quest to recreate the oneness that was experienced in the womb.

In this context, the distinction between fusion and oneness becomes particularly meaningful. While the rupture of birth may lead to a longing for fusion as a psychological reconstruction of lost wholeness, the concept of oneness offers a broader and more profound understanding. Oneness transcends mere dependency or enmeshment, embodying a state of effortless harmony and balance that unfolds naturally throughout life. From a Daoist perspective, oneness is not a static return to the past, but a dynamic alignment with the Dao – a state of attunement where self and the Dao flow as one. In this way, oneness serves as both the origin and the ultimate realization of love.

The pursuit of contained undifferentiated oneness underpins the trajectory of love throughout life. From this perspective, the postnatal mother–infant relationship, as discussed in psychoanalytic theories, can be seen as a continuation, compensation or buffering of the rupture caused by birth – the interruption of the oneness experienced in the womb. The foundational theories of Bick, Winnicott and Bion do not represent the origin of this dynamic but rather elaborate on how postnatal maternal functions strive to restore or extend the primal state of oneness.

Bick's (1968) theory of the "primary skin" encapsulates the infant's need for psychological containment, a continuation of the womb's physical and emotional holding. The "primary skin" acts as a substitute for the physical envelopment experienced in utero, providing the infant with a sense of cohesion that mitigates the trauma of separation. Similarly, Winnicott's (1960) concepts of the "holding function" and the mother's "preoccupation with her infant" emphasize the maternal role in creating a stable environment that not only nurtures the infant but also serves to replicate the unconditional unity of the prenatal state.

Bion's (1962) "containment theory" builds on this foundation, illustrating how the mother's capacity to emotionally contain the infant's raw feelings contributes to the re-establishment of a sense of oneness. Bion introduces the concept of the "alpha function", where the mother's ability to symbolize and metabolize emotional experiences aids the child in developing their own capacity to think, reflect and manage emotional states. This function, while crucial for psychological growth and independence, can also be understood as part of the ongoing effort to recapture the lost oneness of the prenatal experience.

Collectively, these theories highlight that the maternal role in the postnatal period is not merely about fostering independence or promoting psychological development. Rather, it is deeply rooted in the existential task of reconstituting, however partially, the sense of contained undifferentiated oneness that forms the original prototype of love. This perspective integrates the primal origins of love with the psychoanalytic focus on maternal functions, situating the journey of love as a lifelong pursuit to reconcile the rupture of birth with the longing for oneness.

From the moment of birth, individuals continuously strive to re-create the experience of "contained undifferentiated oneness" – the original prototype of love. Based on this perspective, I will explore the evolution of couples' love from romantic love to familial love, as well as the ultimate form of love: Da Ai.

- *Romantic love*: an illusion of perfect contained undifferentiated oneness, shattered by reality.
- *Familial love*: expanding the pursuit of oneness through acceptance, shared creation, and a broader vision of connection.
- *Da Ai*: achieving contained undifferentiated oneness through effortless harmony with the Dao.

Across its evolutionary stages – romantic love, familial love and Da Ai – the theme of sad beauty weaves a profound narrative. In romantic love, it emerges in the fleeting sweetness of illusion and the inevitable sorrow of disillusionment. In familial love, it is found in the balance between imperfection and the hope of shared creation. Finally, in Da Ai, it reaches its pinnacle as the sorrow of relinquishing ego-driven desires transforms into a serene acceptance of impermanence and harmonious interconnectedness with the cosmos. Rooted in Daoist philosophy, Da Ai transcends the self and achieves effortless alignment with the Dao, where longing and loss dissolve into the ultimate harmony of oneness. This unifying aesthetic reveals the profound tension and harmony between longing, loss and love's ultimate transcendence.

Couple's love

Couple's love is one of the most profound forms of human emotional connection. It originates in the idealization and projection inherent in romantic love and transcends disillusionment to evolve into familial love. Romantic love pursues the completeness of primal oneness, embodying a strong narcissistic quality, while familial love sustains the depth and meaning of love through acceptance and creation following disillusionment. From the perspective of psychoanalysis to cultural studies, couple's love illustrates a developmental path from the "ideal illusion" to "mature reality".

Romantic love: an illusion of perfect contained undifferentiated oneness, shattered by reality

Romantic love is deeply rooted in the individual's pursuit of the contained undifferentiated oneness experienced during the foetal stage. From a psychoanalytic perspective (Freud, 1914), love is a narcissistic process of projection, whereby the individual projects unintegrated parts of their inner self onto an object, thus experiencing a sense of "completeness" through the relationship with that object. Freud suggested that men often seek partners modelled after their internalized image of the mother. While Freud's view primarily relates to the idealization formed during the oedipal stage, I propose that this search is ultimately driven by a deeper longing for the contained undifferentiated oneness experienced in the foetal state. This state represents the original prototype of love.

In my view, romantic love attempts to recapture this primal state of completeness, evoking an illusion of wholeness that transcends the boundaries of individuality. This longing, however, carries within it an inherent fragility. The illusion of primal oneness is inherently at odds with reality, where the complexities of life and the individuality of the partner inevitably disrupt the fantasy of perfection. Romantic love, therefore, oscillates between the sweet allure of imagined completeness and the sorrow of disillusionment. The tension between these two states gives rise to what can be described as the "sad beauty" of romantic love.

The Yin-Yang dynamics

Additionally, Freud (1905) proposed that humans are inherently bisexual. When combined with the concept of Yin and Yang in Chinese philosophy (Needham, 1956; Wu Zongguo, 1990), this bisexuality can be understood as a unified state of Yin and Yang. At the beginning of life, the individual's Yin-Yang characteristics exist in a state of undifferentiation. However, as sexual characteristics develop and psychological individuality emerges, this internal unity is disrupted, creating a gap between the psychological and physical aspects of Yin and Yang.

Taking men as an example, the "Yang" aspect of their psyche can align with the "Yang" aspect of their physical body, forming a complete "Yang". However, because the male body lacks the physical embodiment of "Yin" (represented by the female sex), the "Yin" aspect of their psyche tends to drift out of balance. This internal tendency towards imbalance inclines individuals to seek the "missing half" in the external world as a way to return to harmony.

Through a relationship with a woman, a man attempts to establish a connection between the "Yin" of his psyche and the "Yin" of the woman's physical body, thereby creating a complete "Yin". This process ultimately leads to the harmonious oneness of Yin and Yang, achieving a natural alignment between body and mind. The complete oneness of Yin and Yang, along with the resulting harmony of body and mind, evokes a sense of returning to the contained undifferentiated oneness experienced in the foetal stage. However, this state remains an illusion of completeness, as it reflects a longing rather than the effortless alignment (Wu Wei) found in the Daoist ideal of ultimate harmony.

This sense of oneness is inevitably disrupted by the realities of individuality and separation. Romantic love, though intoxicating in its illusion of harmony, is inherently fragile, as it is vulnerable to the disillusionment arising from the complexity and impermanence of human relationships.

Sad beauty in romantic love

This delicate balance between the imagined perfection of romantic love and its inevitable disillusionment finds poignant expression in Chinese literature.

The Tang Dynasty poet Cui Hu's "On the Southern Village of the Capital" encapsulates this duality through its vivid imagery and emotional depth:

> Last year, on this very day, within this door,
> Her face and peach blossoms blushed together, more and more.
> But now, her face – who knows where it may be?
> The peach blossoms still smile at the spring breeze with glee.
> (Cui Hu, Tang Dynasty)

According to *Essential tales of poetry* (Benshi Shi) by Meng Qi (Tang Dynasty), after failing the imperial examination in Chang'an, Cui Hu wandered alone during the Qingming Festival and happened upon a manor by chance. He knocked on the door to ask for water, and a beautiful young woman answered. Though they did not speak, a deep and unspoken connection arose between them in that fleeting moment. The following year, during the Qingming Festival, Cui Hu revisited the manor but did not see the young woman. Moved by sorrow and longing, he composed this poem on the spot.

The emotional tension of this poem lies in the contrast between the first encounter, where "her face and peach blossoms blushed together", symbolizing the illusory perfection of romantic love, and the later lines, where her face is nowhere to be found, yet "the peach blossoms still smile at the spring breeze with glee" revealing the sorrow of disillusionment. This sense of "sad beauty" is not only reflected in the individual's lament over loss but also underscores the inherent fragility of romantic love: it constructs an illusion of returning to the primal contained undifferentiated oneness. Yet, this illusion is inevitably shattered when confronted with reality.

However, people are more inclined to preserve romantic love in its idealized beauty rather than allow the grind of reality to diminish its brilliance. This is evident in the touching love story inspired by the poem: the young woman, pining for Cui Hu, fell gravely ill. When Cui Hu visited for the third time, she was on the brink of death. Yet, miraculously, upon hearing Cui Hu's heartfelt call, she awakened, and the two were finally united as a couple.

Although this tale may not be factual, it deeply reflects humanity's attachment to the illusion of perfection. In the face of loss and impermanence in reality, people long for the fleeting beauty of "her face and peach blossoms blushing together" to become eternal, as if frozen outside the bounds of time.

The Chinese tale of Liang Shanbo and Zhu Yingtai provides another striking illustration of romantic love's interplay of illusion and disillusionment (Idema, 2010). Zhu Yingtai spent three years as a classmate of Liang Shanbo, during which their shared experiences nurtured a deep bond of affection. However, bound by societal norms, Zhu Yingtai is forced into an arranged marriage, leading to Liang Shanbo's untimely death. In the story's climactic moment, Zhu Yingtai visits Liang Shanbo's tomb, where it miraculously splits open, allowing her to leap inside. The two lovers are then transformed into butterflies, flying together forever.

Their transformation into butterflies after death grants their love an eternal quality, symbolizing a return to the primal oneness that transcends earthly confines. The shared tomb and the imagery of the butterflies evoke a state of unity beyond the constraints of reality – a poignant rebellion against life's impermanence.

The transformation of Liang Shanbo and Zhu Yingtai into butterflies is not merely a romantic ideal; it symbolizes the deeper human longing for eternal meaning. Romantic love, despite its inherent sorrow, becomes a vessel for transcending the finite, granting love a timeless resonance.

Romantic love as a stage in love's evolution

Romantic love does not fail because of its disillusionment; rather, this disillusionment marks an essential stage in the evolution of love. The idealized pursuit of wholeness, rooted in the primal oneness of the foetal stage, cannot withstand the complexities of reality. Yet, it is through the mourning of this loss that individuals begin to move towards deeper forms of connection.

The "sad beauty" of romantic love lies in its ability to illuminate the tension between illusion and reality, beauty and sorrow. It is this very tension that propels individuals towards greater self-awareness and prepares the foundation for familial love. Romantic love, in its fleeting perfection and inevitable disillusionment, serves as both a mirror of humanity's longing and a gateway to love's higher dimensions.

Familial love: expanding the pursuit of oneness through acceptance, shared creation and a broader vision of connection

Familial love represents the evolution of romantic love, a sublimation that integrates the longing for wholeness into broader dimensions of shared creation, acceptance and life's temporal journey. While familial love does not entirely transcend the yearning for the contained undifferentiated oneness experienced during the foetal stage, it transforms this pursuit into a shared relational framework, encompassing partners, family and collective aspirations. This evolution reflects a growing capacity to reconcile the imperfections of reality while retaining an unconscious drive for the sense of unity and security symbolized by primal oneness.

The transition from romantic love to familial love often begins with the disillusionment of romantic idealization. As partners awaken to the reality of each other's imperfections, they are invited to let go of unattainable ideals and reconstruct a deeper emotional connection rooted in acceptance and collaboration. This transformation does not signify a loss but rather a progression: by embracing the imperfections of reality, partners discover a new sense of security and stability within their relationship. The longing for primal oneness, now extended beyond the self, shapes the foundation of familial love.

Morgan's (2001, 2019) concept of the "couple state of mind" underscores this transformation. In this state, the relationship itself becomes an independent entity, offering containment, stability and emotional nourishment to both partners. The couple's shared attention and care for this "third entity" enable them to transcend self-focused projections, nurturing their bond and allowing it to become a resilient support system in their lives.

Morgan's (2005, 2019) theory of the "creative couple" further complements this perspective by highlighting the dynamic, evolving nature of familial love. Familial love does not conform to rigid societal norms or fixed patterns but thrives through shared exploration and the creative construction of meaning. In this process, couples collectively navigate challenges, demonstrating emotional resilience and adaptability while building a shared future.

Dana Birksted-Breen's (1996) concept of the "penis-as-link" emphasizes the dual role of connection and separation in relational dynamics. The "link" not only facilitates emotional and physical intimacy but also provides a structural framework for the relationship, enabling partners to maintain their individuality while building a shared bond. This balance of connection and separation resonates deeply with the essence of familial love, where partners navigate the boundaries between self and other, integrating their individual desires into a unified relational system.

Niulang and Zhinü: a timeless allegory of familial love

In Chinese culture, the folk tale of Niulang and Zhinü (Ying Shao, 195 AD, Eastern Han Dynasty) beautifully illustrates the essence of familial love. The story tells of Niulang, a kind and diligent orphan, who meets Zhinü, a celestial weaver maiden who secretly descended from heaven. The two fell in love at first sight, married and lived a happy life together.

However, when heaven discovered Zhinü's act of descending to the mortal world, celestial soldiers were sent to forcibly take her back, separating her from Niulang. Determined to follow her, Niulang used the hide of a divine ox to fly to heaven in pursuit. Yet, the Queen Mother of the West (王母娘娘, a goddess in Chinese mythology) created the Heavenly River (the Milky Way) to separate them, keeping them on opposite shores. Despite this separation, the Heavenly Emperor allowed the lovers to reunite once a year on the seventh day of the seventh lunar month. On this day, countless magpies from all directions gather to form a Magpie Bridge with their bodies, spanning the vast Milky Way and connecting Niulang and Zhinü. This annual reunion of the star-crossed lovers has become a cherished symbol of love and longing.

In this tale, the river, created by the Queen Mother of the West, symbolizes both the constraints of reality – societal, cultural and existential – that interrupt the idealized oneness of romantic love, and the boundaries necessary for maintaining individuality. However, the Heavenly Emperor's allowance for an annual reunion on the Magpie Bridge offers a poignant metaphor for connection within separation.

The Magpie Bridge serves as a dynamic link between Niulang and Zhinü, highlighting the structural and emotional function of connection in familial love. Their love persists not despite the separation but because of it, with each reunion deepening their bond. This cyclical alternation between connection and separation mirrors both Morgan's "couple state of mind" and Birksted-Breen's "penis-as-link". Familial love thrives within this delicate tension, allowing partners to grow individually while remaining connected through a shared vision.

The imagery of the Heavenly River and Magpie Bridge also resonates with Morgan's emphasis on the collaborative creation of relational meaning. Just as Niulang and Zhinü sustain their bond through limited yet profound reunions, couples in familial love construct their relationship by integrating the realities of separation and connection. The Magpie Bridge becomes a symbol of emotional resilience and creative attachment, allowing familial love to transcend the confines of romantic idealization.

A contrast to fragility: flying together through adversity

In Chinese culture, the proverb "夫妻本是同林鸟，大难临头各自飞" ("Husband and wife are like birds of the same forest; when adversity strikes, they fly apart") offers a striking counterpoint to the resilience demonstrated by Niulang and Zhinü. This saying metaphorically reflects the fragility of relationships when confronted with life's challenges. While couples may share a common "forest" of family and union, their bond often fails under the weight of adversity, revealing an attachment to self-interest, which is rooted in unresolved narcissistic tendencies, rather than a unified relational mindset.

In contrast, familial love in its mature form transcends such self-preserving tendencies. By cultivating the "couple state of mind", couples learn to approach their relationship as a source of containment and support. This relational system not only nurtures their emotional bond but also provides a framework for facing life's challenges together.

The poignancy of sad beauty in familial love

The intertwining of sorrow and beauty is a recurring theme in familial love. Familial love embraces the impermanence and incompleteness of reality, yet this acceptance carries a trace of sorrow, as it requires letting go of the attachment to immediate wholeness. However, this sorrow is not a negative force but a deepening of emotion. The story of Niulang and Zhinü vividly embodies this intertwining of beauty and sorrow: their love is tinged with sadness due to their separation, but it also radiates a poignant brilliance through their commitment and creative connection.

This delicate balance between connection and separation is profoundly captured in the classic love poem "Striking the drum" (Bei Feng – Ji Gu) from *The Book of Songs* (n.d., translation mine):

> Through life and death, in separation and union,
> With you, I made this vow.
> Holding your hand,
> Together we shall grow old.

The opening lines, "Through life and death, in separation and union", vividly echo the themes explored earlier, including penis-as-link, the couple state of mind, and the Magpie Bridge in the Niulang and Zhinü legend. This poignant statement encapsulates the essence of familial love: a commitment that transcends not only the physical realities of union and separation but also the existential boundaries of life and death. It symbolizes the enduring relational framework that allows partners to remain connected even amid the impermanence of life.

Unlike romantic love's yearning for unattainable perfection, familial love transforms this longing into a sustained commitment to co-create a meaningful life. The phrase "Holding your hand, together we shall grow old" beautifully illustrates this commitment, revealing familial love's capacity to weave individual and collective aspirations into the shared journey of life. It integrates the sadness of imperfection into a deeper beauty, bridging the gaps between the individual and the collective, the transient and the eternal.

The bridge towards Da Ai

Familial love acts as a vital bridge, not only connecting romantic love to Da Ai but also fostering the emotional depth and relational harmony necessary for aligning with the Dao. However, this does not imply that familial love, in its literal or traditional sense, is the sole pathway to Da Ai. Rather, it is the psychological capacities nurtured within familial love – such as embracing impermanence, reconciling individual and relational needs, and transcending ego-driven desires – that form the foundation for naturally attuning with the Dao, the essence of Da Ai.

Ultimately, the pathway to Da Ai is not defined by the specific form love takes but by the spiritual and emotional transformation it entails. Whether through familial relationships or alternative profound experiences, the key lies in transcending self-centredness and entering a state of effortless harmony with the Dao. Familial love provides a natural setting for this transformation, offering an accessible opportunity to cultivate the emotional maturity essential for achieving Da Ai. In transcending individual desires and relational boundaries, Da Ai embodies the ultimate realization of oneness, where love evolves beyond the personal and flows seamlessly into the infinite interconnectedness of existence.

Da Ai achieving contained undifferentiated oneness through effortless harmony with the Dao

Da Ai represents the ultimate transcendence in the evolution of love – a state of profound harmony where the individual moves beyond self-centred desires and aligns effortlessly with the Dao. It is not an isolated phenomenon but emerges as the culmination of earlier forms of love. Romantic love, with its yearning for oneness, and familial love, which balances connection and separation, lay the emotional and psychological groundwork for Da Ai. However, while these earlier forms are often constrained by personal relationships and ego-driven longings, Da Ai transcends these limitations, embodying an expansive harmony that reflects the infinite interconnectedness of existence.

The distinction lies in the transformative journey from "I seek to be oneness" to "I am one of the oneness". Da Ai moves beyond the confines of self-interest and attachment, into a realm of effortless acceptance (Wu Wei) and harmonious interconnectedness. It is not merely an extension of romantic or familial love but a profound transformation – a higher dimension where love transcends the fulfilment of desire and achieves unity through oneness. In this state, love becomes a force that dissolves boundaries rather than reinforces them, that accepts the natural flow of existence rather than seeks to control it.

From a Chinese Daoist perspective, Da Ai finds its resonance in the concept of the unity of heaven and humanity (Tian Ren He Yi). Daoism emphasizes living in harmony with nature, following the spontaneous flow of life (Ziran, 自然), and releasing attachments to utilitarian pursuits. Zhuangzi's (*Xiaoyao You*, Zhuang Zhou, 1961) notion of Xiaoyao (逍遥), often translated as "spiritual freedom" or "carefree wandering", illustrates the transformative journey towards Da Ai. In this state, individuals achieve profound alignment with the Dao – the root of all things, giving birth to, nurturing and transforming all beings. This alignment is achieved through Wu Wei, or effortless action, where nothing is forced, yet everything is accomplished. It reflects a transcendence of narrow self-interest, an embrace of life's inherent impermanence, and a deep recognition of the interconnectedness of all existence.

Zhuangzi's parable of the great Peng[3] (鹏) and the small bird Jiao Liao (鷦鷯) vividly illustrates this transformative journey. The great Peng, a mythical bird of immense size, soars 90,000 li above the Northern Darkness (Bei Ming, 北冥), carried effortlessly by the winds. Its majestic flight symbolizes transcendence, freedom and alignment with the Dao. In contrast, the small bird flutters within a confined world, clinging to immediate concerns and mocking the Peng's journey as unnecessary and absurd. The small bird represents attachment to familiarity, habit and narrow perspectives, while the great Peng exemplifies the expansive freedom and harmony achieved by transcending finite attachments and embracing the Dao.

This allegory resonates deeply with the essence of Da Ai. Like the great roc's journey, Da Ai requires individuals to release narrow attachments, transcending self-centred desires, to embrace life's infinite interconnectedness. However, this transition is not without sorrow. Letting go of personal desires and confronting life's impermanence necessitate profound acceptance, a process that inevitably evokes grief. Yet, it is through this grief that the beauty of Da Ai emerges – a reconciliation of human limitations with the infinite flow of existence. In Da Ai, sorrow and transcendence co-exist, reflecting the Daoist ideal where unity is achieved not by denying impermanence, but by harmonizing with it.

Zhuangzi's own life offers a profound illustration of Da Ai in practice. When his wife passed away, Zhuangzi surprised his students by beating a drum and singing joyously. Explaining his actions, he said (Zhuang Zhou, 1961; author's translation):

> From nothingness to existence, from existence to life, and from life to death – this is merely the natural cycle of life. Now that she has peacefully returned to the heavens and earth, if I were to mourn and cry, I would be ignorantly defying the Dao.

Zhuangzi's response transcends personal grief, embodying the harmony and interconnectedness inherent in Da Ai. His actions demonstrate that Da Ai does not eliminate sorrow but transforms it into a serene acceptance of impermanence and a deeper alignment with the Dao. By relinquishing attachment to personal loss and perfection, Zhuangzi exemplifies the boundless care and effortless harmony that characterize Da Ai. This state reflects the Daoist ideal of unity with the Dao, where individual sorrow dissolves into the infinite flow of existence.

In the context of Daoist thought, contained undifferentiated oneness provides a foundation for understanding Da Ai. Unlike earlier stages of love, which unconsciously strive to re-create the primal oneness of the foetal state, Da Ai represents the natural realization of oneness with the Dao. It is not about returning to an undifferentiated state but about attaining a state of harmonious oneness, where the individual transcends self-centredness to effortlessly align with all beings, nature and existence. In this state, longing dissolves into unity, and separation becomes a means of connection rather than division.

Even for those who do not follow the conventional path of familial relationships, I believe the seeds of capacities essential for Da Ai – such as acceptance, egolessness[4] and an unbounded, effortless love – are often sown in early relational experiences. Without these foundational capacities, it would be challenging, if not impossible, to transcend self-centeredness and align with the Dao. Thus, Da Ai does not reject earlier forms of love but transcends and transforms them, reconfiguring their emotional foundations into a boundless state of harmony. In this way, the longing for oneness is reconciled within the infinite flow of the Dao, achieving a serene and eternal alignment with existence.

Sad beauty, as embodied in Da Ai, does not disappear but ascends to a higher dimension. It arises from the sorrow of confronting impermanence and the limitations of human existence. Yet, this sorrow is not a source of despair but a gateway to profound beauty – a serenity born of accepting life's transience and harmonizing with the infinite flow of the Dao. This beauty is not found in perfection or permanence but in the reconciliation of human finitude with the boundless, dynamic balance of the universe.

Zhuangzi's teachings and allegories vividly illustrate the transformative power of Da Ai, inviting individuals to transcend the confines of self-interest and align with the Dao. Like the great Peng's boundless flight, Da Ai is the ultimate expression of harmony and freedom – a state where sadness and beauty are not opposites but complementary forces, reflecting the infinite interconnectedness of all existence. In this state of effortless unity and profound acceptance, the essence of love achieves its highest form, dissolving individual boundaries and merging into the eternal flow of life.

Case illustration: the evolution from romantic love to familial love

Anna and Mike, both in their late 30s, sought couple therapy after repeated conflicts had strained their once seemingly perfect relationship. They described the early days of their relationship as "a dream come true", marked by passion, mutual admiration and a sense of absolute completeness. However, over time, unresolved conflicts and external pressures began to fracture this idyllic state, leaving them feeling disconnected and hostile towards each other.

The beginning: romantic idealization

Anna and Mike met at a mutual friend's party. Both reported feeling an almost mystical connection from the moment they started talking. "It was like I had found my missing piece", Mike said in the first therapy session, and Anna described their love as "effortless and magical, as though we were meant to be".

In the initial months, they experienced what can be described as a state of primal oneness. They saw each other as perfect complements, fulfilling their emotional voids and creating a sense of wholeness. This phase was characterized by intense passion and a profound sense of security, reminiscent of the foetus–maternal oneness during the early stages of life.

However, this romantic idealization masked the deeper dynamics of narcissistic projection. Anna, who had grown up feeling neglected, unconsciously sought in Mike an omnipresent nurturer, someone who would always put her needs first. Mike, on the other hand, sought in Anna an image of perfection that aligned with his internalized longing for unconditional approval. Their love, while beautiful, was deeply intertwined with an unconscious desire to re-create the illusion of contained undifferentiated oneness.

The crisis: the collapse of the illusion

As their relationship progressed, reality began to intrude. Financial stress and the pressures of balancing careers eroded the harmony they had once enjoyed. They began to argue frequently, often over seemingly trivial matters, that escalated into intense conflicts. "He doesn't listen to me. It's always about him," Anna complained in one session. Mike, in turn, felt increasingly resentful, saying, "I can never meet her expectations. Nothing I do is good enough."

During this phase, their relationship reflected the proverb, "夫妻本是同林鸟，大难临头各自飞" ("Husband and wife are like birds of the same forest; when adversity strikes, they fly apart"). Each partner retreated into self-preservation mode, prioritizing their own needs and perspectives. They blamed each other for the relationship's breakdown, unable to see the relationship itself as a shared bond requiring mutual care and responsibility or to feel contained by it.

This phase revealed the collapse of the illusion of romantic love. Their initial feelings of completeness gave way to disillusionment, leaving them feeling exposed and vulnerable. The therapist observed that their mutual blame reflected an unresolved grief over the disruption of their earliest experience of contained oneness, a yearning for wholeness that had shaped their relational patterns but remained unacknowledged.

Therapeutic process: mourning and the depressive position

In therapy, Anna and Mike sat in silence for a few moments after an emotional conflict between them. The tension in the room was palpable, yet neither of them seemed ready to break it. The therapist gently reflected, "It seems like both of you were seeking something deeper in that moment – perhaps a sense of being fully seen and cared for."

Anna hesitated, her gaze dropping to the floor. After a long pause, she spoke softly. "I think … I've always felt like Mike just doesn't get me. Like, no matter how much I try to explain, he's not listening." Her voice faltered, as if she were unsure whether to keep going.

Mike shifted uncomfortably in his seat. He glanced at Anna, then down at his hands, which were clenched together. "And I feel like no matter what I do, it's never enough," he said, his voice tinged with frustration and defeat. "I just end up feeling like a failure."

The therapist allowed the weight of their words to settle in the room. After a moment, he spoke with warmth and steadiness. "It sounds like both of you are carrying some very heavy feelings – Anna, the longing to be truly heard, and Mike, the fear of not being enough. What happens when these feelings come up between you?"

Anna turned slightly towards Mike, her expression softening but uncertain. "I get angry," she admitted, her tone quieter now. "I push him away before he can let me down again."

Mike glanced at her, his brow furrowing slightly as if considering her words. After a moment, he nodded. "And I shut down," he said quietly. "Because I feel like whatever I say will make it worse."

The therapist leaned forward slightly and said, "These reactions – anger, shutting down – make sense given what you've both been through. Anna, it seems that when you feel unheard, it brings up a deeper hurt from your past. And Mike, when you feel like you're failing, it touches something deeply vulnerable within you as well."

Anna's eyes welled up with tears. She hesitated before speaking, her voice breaking slightly. "When I was a kid, I felt invisible. My parents … they were always too busy. I used to think if I were just better – quieter, smarter – they'd notice me."

The room grew quiet again. Mike's gaze lingered on Anna, his expression shifting from defensiveness to something softer. After a while, he exhaled deeply, the sound carrying the weight of unspoken emotions. "And I … I always had to be the strong one growing up," he said, his voice barely above a whisper. "There was no room to be vulnerable, no one to lean on."

The therapist nodded gently, giving them space to sit with their words. "It seems like these old feelings – of being invisible, of having to hold everything together – are playing out in your relationship now. But what I'm noticing is that, in this moment, you're both staying with those feelings rather than turning away."

Anna wiped her tears with the back of her hand, glancing at Mike with a mixture of hesitation and relief. "I guess … I've been blaming him for something that isn't really his fault," she said slowly. "It's just … hard to let go of that anger."

Mike looked at her, his expression tender but serious. "I never realized how much you were holding inside," he said, his voice steady but filled with regret. "I'm sorry I made it worse. I was so busy trying not to fail that I forgot to just … listen."

The therapist responded, "It sounds like you're both beginning to see each other differently – not as perfect or infallible, but as two people who are trying their best despite the weight of what you've carried."

In subsequent sessions, the therapy focused on creating a space where Anna and Mike could mourn not only their unmet needs but also the loss of their romantic illusions. As Anna allowed herself to feel the sadness of her childhood neglect, her anger towards Mike began to dissolve. She expressed her sorrow without blame, creating room for connection rather than distance. Similarly, as Mike explored his own vulnerabilities, he found compassion for both himself and Anna, realizing that their struggles were not about failure but about navigating the complexities of being a person.

Through this shared process, Anna and Mike began to experience moments of connection that felt more authentic and grounded. They were no longer clinging to an idealized version of their relationship but instead embracing its imperfections.

With the mourning of the lost illusion came a shift towards what Klein (1935) described as the depressive position. Anna and Mike began to show concern not only for themselves but also for each other. They acknowledged their mutual contributions to the relationship's challenges and expressed genuine care for the wellbeing of their partner. For the first time in years, Anna described feeling "a sense of peace" in their relationship, while Mike shared that he felt "more connected and less defensive".

The therapist observed that this shift marked the emergence of familial love. Their relationship evolved from a projection-driven dynamic to one characterized by acceptance, collaboration and shared responsibility.

As Anna and Mike continued therapy, they grew more adept at navigating the challenges of daily life together. They developed what Morgan (2001, 2019) describes as a "couple state of mind", wherein the relationship itself became a shared, third-party entity that could contain and hold their emotions, particularly during moments of conflict or difficulty. Instead of reacting with blame or defensiveness, they learned to turn towards this shared space, finding in it a source of stability and containment.

This shift also allowed them to observe their relationship as something distinct from themselves, providing a new level of awareness. In times of difficulty, they could step outside their immediate reactions to view their relationship more objectively, while also reflecting on their own roles within it. This capacity for reflection helped them identify patterns, acknowledge vulnerabilities, and nurture a more compassionate understanding of both themselves and each other.

Through this growing awareness, Anna and Mike began to approach their challenges collaboratively, recognizing that their relationship was not just a sum of two individuals but a dynamic entity requiring mutual care and attention. They expressed excitement about their future, speaking of plans to have a baby and support each other's goals.

However, familial love is not an endpoint reached overnight; it is a dynamic, evolving process that requires continual effort and emotional growth. Along the way, Anna and Mike experienced moments of uncertainty and occasional setbacks, as old patterns and vulnerabilities surfaced. Yet, their growing couple state of mind and their capacity to embrace imperfection provided them with the resilience to navigate these challenges.

Through their shared commitment to nurturing the relationship, they began to see these fluctuations not as failures but as opportunities for deeper connection and mutual growth. Their relationship transformed into a space that could hold both their individual needs and collective aspirations. This ongoing journey of familial love, though imperfect and at times challenging, laid a foundation for a mature and enduring partnership – one that embraced the complexities of life while fostering a sense of shared purpose and hope for the future.

Conclusion

Anna and Mike's journey illustrates the transformative progression from romantic idealization to familial love. By mourning the loss of their illusions and embracing imperfection, they moved beyond self-focused patterns to cultivate a deeper bond rooted in shared aspirations and care. Familial love represents an expansion of focus, integrating individual and collective needs while fostering collaboration and acceptance. Their story highlights love as an evolving process, one that creates a foundation for enduring and dynamic partnership.

Summary

This chapter explores the origins, transformation and ultimate transcendence of love, tracing its roots to the contained undifferentiated oneness experienced during the foetal stage. Love begins as a longing for oneness, yet the idealization within romantic love inevitably leads to disillusionment, revealing the fragility of perfection and the transient nature of human relationships. Familial love, while still grounded in the longing for oneness, deepens this pursuit by embracing imperfection, fostering connection and creating shared meaning through relational harmony.

Ultimately, Da Ai transcends narcissistic desires and self-centred attachments, representing the highest realization of love. It embodies the Daoist principles of Wu Wei (effortless action) and Tian Ren He Yi (unity of heaven and humanity), achieving a profound alignment with the Dao. In Da Ai, love evolves beyond personal longing and relational boundaries, reconciling human finitude with the infinite interconnectedness of existence. This state of harmonious unity offers not only true fulfilment but also spiritual transcendence, reflecting the boundless flow of life and the eternal harmony of the cosmos.

Notes

1 Dao (道), often translated as "The Way", is the fundamental principle of all existence in Daoist philosophy. It is the root of all things, giving birth to, nurturing and transforming all beings, while remaining beyond form and definition.
2 "Unity of Heaven and Humanity" (Tian Ren He Yi) is a Daoist concept that emphasizes the profound harmony or oneness between humans and the Dao, where individuality dissolves into a state of interconnectedness with all existence.
3 The Peng is a gigantic legendary bird in the Zhuangzi, associated with transformation, vastness and soaring freedom.
4 Egolessness, a concept central to Zhuangzi's philosophy, refers to the transcendence or dissolution of the ego, where the individual moves beyond self-centredness and personal identity and experiences a state of profound freedom and harmony with the Dao.

References

Bick, E. (1968). The experience of the skin in early object-relations. *The International Journal of Psychoanalysis*, 49, 484–486.

Bion, W.R. (1962). *Learning from experience*. Heinemann.

Birksted-Breen, D. (1996). Phallus, penis and mental space. *International Journal of Psychoanalysis*, 77: 649–657.

Book of Songs (*Shijing*) (n.d.). 《诗经》的经典爱情诗《邶风·击鼓》Bei Feng –Ji Gu [Striking the drum]. In: *The Book of Songs*. Translation by author.

Cui Hu (Tang Dynasty). 崔护. (唐代). 题都城南庄. 诗歌出处: 《全唐诗》第五卷。On the southern village of the capital. *The complete Tang poems*, Volume 5.

Field, T. (2011). Prenatal depression effects on early development: A review. *Infant Behavior and Development*, 34 (1), 1–14.

Freud, S. (1905). *Three essays on the theory of sexuality*. In: J. Strachey (ed. and trans.), *The standard edition of the complete psychological works of Sigmund Freud* (1953–74), Volume 7. Hogarth Press, pp. 123–246.

Freud, S. (1914). *On narcissism: An introduction*. In: J. Strachey (ed. and trans.), *The standard edition of the complete psychological works of Sigmund Freud* (1953–74), Volume 14. Hogarth Press, pp. 67–102.

Idema, W.L. (ed. and trans.). (2010). *The butterfly lovers: The legend of Liang Shanbo and Zhu Yingtai: Four versions, with related texts*. Hackett Publishing.

Klein, M. (1935). A contribution to the psychogenesis of manic-depressive states. *The International Journal of Psychoanalysis*, 16: 145–174.

Lin, T. (2024). The mind of the Dao: Origin of creative thinking in psychoanalysis – A transcultural approach. *International Journal of Psychoanalysis Open: Open Peer Review and Debate*, 10: 1–26.

Meng Qi (Tang Dynasty). 孟棨(唐代). 《本事诗》 *Benshi Shi* (*Essential Tales of Poetry*).

Morgan, M. (2001). First contacts: The therapist's "couple state of mind" as a factor in the containment of couples seen for initiation consultations. In: F. Grier (ed.), *Brief Encounters with Couples*. Karnac Books, pp. 17–32.

Morgan, M. (2005). On being able to be a couple: The importance of a "creative couple" in psychic life. In: F. Grier (ed.), *Oedipus and the couple*. Karnac Books, pp. 9–30.

Morgan, M. (2019). *A couple state of mind: Psychoanalysis of couples and the Tavistock Relationships model*. Routledge.

Needham, J. (1956). *Science and civilisation in China*, Volume 2: *History of Scientific Thought*. Cambridge: Cambridge University Press.

Winnicott, D.W. (1960). The theory of the parent-infant relationship. *The International Journal of Psychoanalysis*, 41, 585–595.

Wu Zongguo. (1990). 《中国传统哲学概论》. 北京: 中国社会科学出版社。(*An introduction to traditional Chinese philosophy*). China Social Sciences Press.

Ying Shao (Eastern Han Dynasty). 应劭�东汉�著. 《风俗通义》。*Fengsu Tongyi* (*Comprehensive meanings of customs and habits*).

Zhuang Zhou (1961). 《庄子·逍遥游》. 战国时期. 收录于《庄子集释》, 郭庆藩注, 中华书局 Xiaoyao You (Free and easy wandering). Included in: *Zhuangzi Jishi* (*Collected annotations on Zhuangzi*), annotated by Guo Qingfan. Zhonghua Book Company.

Zhuang Zhou (1961). 庄周. (1961). 《庄子·至乐》. 战国时期. 收录于《庄子集释》, 郭庆藩注, 中华书局 Zhile (Supreme happiness). Included in: *Zhuangzi Jishi* (*Collected annotations on Zhuangzi*), annotated by Guo Qingfan. Zhonghua Book Company.

Chapter 13

Somewhere There's a Place for Us …

A cross-cultural approach to psychoanalytic psychotherapy with intercultural and interracial couples[1]

Perrine Moran

My aim in this chapter is to think about difference, and more specifically about love and difference, as my focus is on couples and couple therapy. Difference is a topic that touches a deep chord in me, partly because of the wave of fear and hatred of difference we are witnessing in the world today, partly because it relates to my personal life experience, and partly because of my work as a couple psychotherapist.

Difference, in my opinion, is on the side of life. Our very first experience is of suddenly existing with a body that is separate and different from the one in which we came into being. When we develop, when we learn, we become different from that which we were and if difference is not embraced, growth is stunted. The ordinary expression "What's the difference?" is revealing. It implies that if there is no difference, then it does not matter; it is all the same; we might as well give up. Difference is precious. Yet, difference is also frightening. It triggers the anxieties attached to otherness, it provokes envy and shame. Cultural difference can be what attracts two individuals to one another. Yet, it can also be invoked to explain their disagreements and conflicts.

My title refers to a song from one of the most beautiful and moving artistic representations of difference, West Side Story (1957, 1961, 2021) – an American story that has lost none of its relevance. The protagonists belong to different and opposing camps: the Puerto Ricans and the poor Whites, all victims of social inequality, and sworn enemies. The song *Somewhere …* (Sondheim, 1956) evokes the characters' belief that their love can transcend the social and psychological barriers enclosing their world, that their togetherness is strong enough to fight the separation that others try to force onto them. They dream of finding a haven where difference and prejudice would no longer be obstacles to being together. In the 1961 film version, Maria and Tony sing the song as a duet, taking turns and uniting, their voices – his low and hers high – marking both their difference and their togetherness.

Couple therapists deal with couples' conflicts over difference and differentiation every day. Helping partners to find a balance between togetherness

DOI: 10.4324/9781003518129-13

and separateness and accept the other while preserving the self, forms an essential part of the work. The specific concerns that intercultural couples present add a social dimension to this. Being aware of the impact of cultural differences on the couple in order to distinguish between what is intrapsychic, what is interpersonal, and what is, culturally, transgenerationally transmitted, and examining how all levels are intrinsically linked and how they interact with one another, are crucial. Because students from a variety of cultural backgrounds wish to train, and more and more couples from backgrounds that are other than Western come for help, the need to reflect on ways of integrating the transmission of couple psychoanalytic theory with an awareness of the possible relativity of some of its tenets and the need for openness and adaptability in the application of its concepts are paramount. Already, the development of attachment theory and the broader perspective offered by contemporary psychoanalysis on such fundamental concepts as the Oedipus complex, along with recent work relating to intercultural therapy and issues of difference and race (Davids, 2011; Lowe, 2014; Alleyne, 2022), are making psychoanalytic theory more immediately relevant in a wider set of circumstances. Concepts must evolve and change, as does society, while the essence of the approach – in the case of psychoanalysis, the belief that working with the unconscious can be mutative – must be preserved. The French analyst Jacques Lacan said that the unconscious was structured like a language. He drew a parallel between the processes it uses to manifest itself – condensation and displacement – and the stylistic figures of speech of metaphor and metonymy. Is it possible that this language, into which a White, middle-class, Austrian, Jewish physician provided such extraordinary insight more than a hundred years ago, could be better understood today if its different idioms were given greater consideration? What if different myths, for example, could better illustrate the workings of the unconscious in different cultures, as suggested by David Hewison in his comparison of the parent–child myths of Oedipus and the Indian god Ganesh (Hewison, 2007)? How can we be both flexible and vigilant, so that we move forward without losing what we believe to be an exceptionally rich and productive understanding of the human mind?

Thinking about difference opens up a vast area of reflection. In what follows, I would like to explore the part that intercultural differences play in love relationships and the difficulties intercultural and interracial couples present, and the extent to which psychoanalytic psychotherapy is able, or not able, to help resolve these difficulties. The expression "intercultural" covers many possible configurations. For the purpose of this chapter, I shall focus exclusively on partners who have chosen to be together despite, or perhaps because of, their difference.

Facilitating mutual comprehension and building bridges is central to our therapeutic task. In 2016, Tavistock Relationships organized a conference that considered object relations and link theory perspectives on couples and families. Link theory is a development of psychoanalytic thought that originated in South America and is well established there as well as in France. During the conference, the tension between similarity and difference in what presenters from different countries offered was tangible and stimulating. In a spirit of continued and, I hope, productive curiosity, I shall include in my thinking here a cross-cultural comparison between some of the concepts in object relations and in link theory as they are, or can be, applied to work with couples, with particular reference to the writings of René Kaës.

Before delving into this, I would like to tell a brief story about myself, as I am a product of an intercultural relationship. I was born and raised in Paris, France, by a French father and an English mother. At home, my parents, my brother and I switched from one language to the other all the time. My grandparents on both sides were Polish Jews, first-generation immigrants. They all originally came from the same *shtetl* (small town) in Poland and had fled the pogroms at the end of the nineteenth century. Some of the villagers had emigrated to France and some to England, and they had kept connections. Those who stayed in Poland moved to Warsaw and were all exterminated during the Second World War. My paternal grandparents were tailors, my maternal grandfather was a barber. At some point in the very early 1930s, my father's sister, in Paris, had been sent to my mother's family in London to learn some English. In return, my mother had then been sent to France to stay with my aunt, and that is how my parents met. They fell in love, but were very young and for several years theirs was a long-distance relationship. Eventually, they were married in France. My brother was conceived just before my father joined De Gaulle and the Free French in England, and my parents were separated again, this time by the war. By the time I was born, 12 years later, my parents had settled down and moved to a very posh area of Paris, the 16th arrondissement. They loved it there – the residential feel of it reminded my mother of England, and my father, a doctor, was understandably proud, as the first member of his family to be educated and join the middle class, to be able to keep us there. Most of our neighbours came from established and wealthy Catholic families. They owned their flats as well as homes in the country where children spent their holidays. We rented our flat and when we went on holiday, we always stayed in hotels. This was partly because my father had zero business sense, and never thought of investing rather than spending, and partly because my mother wanted to be able to pack a suitcase and leave at a moment's notice, rather than be attached to a property, the way her relatives in Warsaw had been. My parents seemed to feel totally at home in this aristocratic environment. They were "different", and they did not seem to care. But I did. I could not define what it was, but outside of our flat, I felt totally out of place. I felt we did not belong. I was brought up without any reference to religion. My paternal grandparents would come over on Sunday, speak Yiddish to each other, and I would help my grandma make *kneidler* (dumplings) in the kitchen, but I had no idea what any of it meant. I did not know the difference between Polish and

Yiddish. I had no idea that I was Jewish. My mother was very overprotective and she did not hesitate to lie if she felt it was safer for me not to know the truth. She knew that being Jewish was dangerous. When I started to attend primary school, she told me that if anyone asked me what my religion was, I should say, "My mother is English and I'm a non-practising Protestant – *protestante non pratiquante*". For some reason, I did not ask any questions. I must have felt that it was best not to. Children, who did not see me at mass on Sundays or at catechism, did ask me about my religion, and I said what my mother had told me to say. Unfortunately, what my mother did not know, was that in those days, just before the Beatles and the promotion of London to European capital of rock music and cool fashion, little French children were taught in school that the English had burnt their national heroine Jeanne d'Arc at the stake. This was a very vivid image that stuck in the imagination and my connection with England was not viewed favourably. One little girl said to me in the playground, "My mummy says that your mummy is stupid and she can't even speak properly". My mother did have a strong English accent that she kept till the day she died, and despite her efforts to protect me, I was ostracized precisely because of her. There was no escaping difference.

Being bilingual, language has always played a particularly important role in my life. I have spent, and still spend, a lot of time translating or interpreting in a wide range of circumstances. Although I can switch with ease from one language to the other, I have never found the experience of thinking in two languages particularly comfortable. In fact, it is sometimes disturbing. Lacan, who cultivated a very mannered style, stated that when you say something differently, you are actually saying something different. I would add that you sometimes feel like you are somebody different. In a presentation, Mary Morgan (2016) said that the polysemic nature of words played a part in the difficulty that all couples find in understanding one another. An illustration of this is the moment in the award-winning film *Past Lives* (Celine Song, 2023) when Arthur, a White American writer married to Nora, who is South Korean, points out that she dreams in a language he does not understand. In couples where one partner has had to learn the other partner's language, or both communicate in a third language that belongs to neither, the feeling of not being thoroughly understood, which is common to many couples, is amplified.

Language can also be an issue for intercultural couples if, for example, partners disagree about what language to speak with their children, or one partner refuses to learn the other's language. Other specific issues pertaining to intercultural couples are very real and need to be considered as such rather than interpreted exclusively as revealing of an unconscious conflict. Which country will the couple choose to live in? What if one partner gives up their country and the other does not? What if one partner cannot get a work visa and, contrary to the couple's wishes, is financially dependent on the other?

What about the very real condition of homesickness and the feeling of mutilation that can come with exile? How do partners manage the demands of their families of origin? If cultural ideas on education are very different, how will they deal with conflicting wishes for their children? How do partners help their mixed-race child find his or her place in society? How do they and their therapist recognize and deal with internalized unconscious racism and xenophobia?

One issue that has to be addressed is the difference between intercultural and interracial couples. Alyssa Pereira defines the word race as a social, and therefore cultural, construct which "very generally speaking ... involves shared physical characteristics, especially skin color, and a shared ancestry or historical experience" (Pereira, 2020). Based on this, one might regard the notion of "interracial" as included in that of "intercultural". Yet the specificity of race issues must be considered because of the weight of prejudice.

Partners of different races (as defined above) might come from different countries, with different cultural values. Looking back to their origin, they undoubtedly do. But they might also have both been born and raised in the same country, have the same nationality, speak the same language, have attended the same schools, and have a similar socioeconomic and professional status. Yet despite all that makes them "the same", history, experience and the colour of their skin also make them different. The idea that some humans are superior to others has always been around. It is at the root of Islamophobia, sexism, ageism, nationalism, anti-Semitism, racism and all forms of genocide. Colonization legitimizes it, with devastating consequences. Taken to its extreme, it leads to the belief that there is such a thing as a pre-existing human essence and that it is not shared by all – that presenting Semitic characteristics (which are or are not recognizable) or having the wrong colour skin (which is inescapable) is a sign of sub-humanity. History leaves deep external and internal traces in all of us. It contributes to the formation of unconscious beliefs. According to Ron Britton:

> *Belief* is an ego activity which confers the status of psychic reality on to existing mental productions (phantasies), thus creating *beliefs.* These beliefs may be conscious or unconscious, but cannot be relinquished without becoming conscious. Whether they are conscious or unconscious they have *psychic consequences.*
>
> (Britton, 1995, p. 20)

The sedimentation of ideas that we might, at one level, vehemently reject has to be borne in mind if it is to be overcome.

When choosing a partner from a different culture or race, there is undeniably at some level a wish to differentiate oneself from one's background. Partners may feel that they have more in common with someone who comes from a totally different background, than they do with their family of origin.

This may well be the case. However, lack of familiarity with one's partner's background, preconceptions about what their cultural identity implies, and possible linguistic differences, can enable phantasies about who that partner is to get in the way of seeing who they really are. The risk is then that, when reality sets in, the normal process of disillusionment that all couples experience may be amplified and, in some cases, become insurmountable. Or, as Nina Cohen (1992) suggests, the unconscious choice of a partner may originate in the need to define one's identity as different, because one finds it difficult to become a separate individual within one's family of origin. The potential problem with this is that the need to define oneself through one's difference from, or opposition to, another is often repeated in time within the couple, particularly when partners become parents. New and old roles and dynamics can get confused, and the new family become a threat to one's sense of self, just like the family of origin once did.

What I would like to explore, through the use of vignettes, is the efficacy and limitations of our theoretical tools in dealing with these issues. To what extent, for example, do the concepts of unconscious partner choice, shared phantasy and projective system enable us to understand and help intercultural couples? Is the very set-up we offer – the sharing of an intimate relationship with a stranger – simply incomprehensible and unacceptable to some?

As a therapist working with patients from different cultures, one has to be particularly sensitive to the way therapy might be perceived. A Chinese patient, Wen, related how her English girlfriend had once locked herself in the bathroom because she felt nauseous. At first, Wen had not understood why she would not let her in to help. In her country, that was what you did if someone was ill. But then she realized that her partner felt it would be humiliating to be sick in front of her. Wen said she felt the same way about talking about herself in front of me. It was private and it was humiliating to do it in front of anyone.

Kim and John

Kim and John had met at the laboratory where they worked. She was Vietnamese and he was a divorced Irishman, father of two, her senior by ten years. She had agreed to follow her husband into therapy because their arguments were getting more frequent and explosive, particularly after his sons' visits. However, to her, the concept of talking to a therapist was baffling. In Vietnam, she said, people talked to their friends or worked things out for themselves, and had no need for this process that, like Wen, she felt to be humiliating.

Her English was poor, and a lot of the early sessions seemed to be exercises in a form of translation. He would say something to her. She would misunderstand. I would try to paraphrase and get the message across to her. She would respond and I did the same in reverse. I think I was offering this as a model in the hope that they might learn to try and understand each other rather than row and lose control. Eventually, I understood that actually, communicating verbally was the last thing they wanted. They had picked each other precisely because they could not communicate, only act and use one another. In their projective system, she held all the passivity he had suffered from in his abused childhood, he held all the rage and violence she felt compelled to keep inside. One of the difficulties in working with them was that in Kim's view everything was cultural. Whenever they disagreed about anything, she said, "In my culture, we don't see things like that". This was often true but, backed by the beliefs and values of a whole nation, she also felt that her way was the only way. Questioning this felt like an attack. Trying to get to what was "her, individually", as separate from "her, as part of a cultural entity", went totally against her way of thinking. Any attempt to look at things from John's point of view threatened her sense of identity. He, on the other hand, felt provoked by her otherness and justified in his fury.

John related how, when he was eight years old, his father had said something particularly cruel and humiliating to him during a family outing. For once, his mother had taken his side and told her husband to be quiet. John had felt vindicated, and he was clearly moved by the memory, but Kim was shocked. In "her culture", she said, standing against a father in front of his son was totally wrong, in any circumstance. I immediately felt incensed by Kim's lack of empathy towards her partner, and intensely critical of a culture that puts rules before care and insists on showing respect to a sadistic grown man rather than protecting a vulnerable child. The inner racist in me stood in judgement, blinding me to the fact that my countertransference was reflecting not only John's experience but also Kim's, as a victimized child and as an adult in a set-up that felt totally alien to her. The degree of conviction in Kim's statement had triggered an equally closed-minded reaction in me. I had been seduced into her "cultural theory", and lost touch with the internal processes at play. In a paper that examines the "power relationships" in the therapy of an interracial couple in post-Apartheid South Africa, Rika van den Berg writes that "racism may be viewed as the product of an interaction between the internal and the social world" (2007, p. 121). She illustrates the way social stereotypes impacted on the therapy, and concludes that "[e]ffective analytic practice requires the integration of social and psychoanalytic theory and ongoing self-analysis" (van den Berg, p. 131).

John and Kim's shared unconscious phantasy and shared defence was that they could be together so long as they could avoid really knowing one another. Their unconscious partner choice was paradoxically dictated by the –K wish to not know or be known by their partner, and I too, on this occasion, had turned away from knowing them.

Helping both partners access the frightened, enraged child in themselves helped them see it in the other. Progressively, terror sometimes gave way to compassion. The way they spoke to each other changed and became more fluid, their voices alternating and no longer needing my translation. Gradually a dialogue was established, which was the first step towards building a safe space where difference and intimacy would be tolerable.

Despite Kim's initial resistance, part of her felt relieved at having someone hear what she had to say, and when our couple work ended, she decided that she would seek individual therapy, possibly with a therapist who shared her culture.

Link theory

Returning to theory, one could draw a parallel between Kim and John's resistance to understanding one another and Lacan's determination to make his audience and readers work hard to understand his ideas. As he saw it, only a cryptic style could reflect the elusive nature of the subject of his writing. Part of his legacy to contemporary French thought in general has been to encourage the use of a convoluted way of expressing ideas. In my opinion, this has at times helped to hide the absence of ideas. At other times, the complexity and richness of the concepts make fighting one's way through what, at first, feels like a forest of entangled words and sentences worth the effort, as is the case with the writing of René Kaës.

I think link theory is particularly relevant to work with intercultural couples because of its emphasis on the dynamic between the relationship to one's internal objects and the relationship to one's external objects. As Christopher Clulow writes:

> [in link theory] intergenerational histories and traumas, as well as current socio-political and cultural environments may be gathered into the transference and become the object of analysis … Unbounding the scope of factors that influence transference relationships to include a wider field of intersubjectivities, and viewing these as jointly constructed by patient and therapist, increases the complexity of analytic work. It cautions against being too confident in our understanding of clinical experiences without heeding the contexts in which that understanding occurs.
>
> (Clulow, 2017, p. 345)

In his work on group analysis, Kaës distinguishes three psychic spaces: one that relates to the individual, another to the intersubjective links between the members of a group, and a third to the group as a whole. Kaës points out that this opens the way to an extension of psychoanalysis beyond its traditional one-to-one dimension. He postulates the existence of several topologies of the unconscious, based on what happens between the three psychic spaces – how they impact on and, to use the French terminology, "interfere" with one another, rather than on how they function internally and separately (Kaës, 2016). This, to me, resonates with the way we conceive couple psychoanalytic work, in which we constantly navigate between issues relating to the partners' individual histories and psychological make-up, issues relating to the dynamic partners have established between one another and between them and the therapist, and issues relating to the couple that the partners may or not succeed in creating; all three realms being in constant interaction with each other and with the social and historic reality that surrounds them.

Applying the concept of "interference" to clinical practice with couples, the Argentinian link therapist Isidoro Berenstein suggests that as well as transference, one should work with "interference". He writes:

> Interference is not about working through, as in the transference, but about making room for the other as a different subject. It is about the couple members' ability to produce something new and different, instead of *reproducing* what each carries from childhood and what he or she has brought to the couple. This, too, is a therapeutic tool.
>
> (Berenstein, 2012, p. 576)

The concept of "interference" offers an enriching perspective and possibly innovative techniques in couple therapy. Once again, it resonates for me with what has been written about the need to be separate and accept the other's otherness in order to be in a relationship and find the means to form what Mary Morgan (2005) calls "a creative couple".

Ndeye and Youssouf

Ndeye and Youssouf were a Black, French-speaking, African couple with whom I worked in Paris. Ndeye came from Senegal and Youssouf from Mali, and they had emigrated as children. They were now in their early 20s and the issue they presented was that cultural differences between their two countries of origin were making them unable to agree on anything.

Their relationship had, at first, been very happily fusional: it was both of them against the world. To use Janet Mattinson and Ian Sinclair's terminology, they had been "babes in the woods" together (Mattinson & Sinclair, 1979). However, since the birth of their child, now aged one year, everything had changed. Youssouf felt his parents should be in charge of their son's education while he and his wife continued to prioritize each other. But Ndeye had become a mother intent on not repeating the bad parenting she felt she had received, and Youssouf had lost his place at the centre of her life. Suddenly, his parents could do no wrong and Ndeye could do no right. She thought this was a result of family pressure and different cultural views on parenting. Unfortunately, I was not able to explore this with both partners together as Youssouf never returned after the first session. Like many other African couples, Ndeye and Youssouf regularly attended large, extended family advisory meetings, in which the couple's intimate life was discussed, and this was as far as Youssouf was willing to go. There was something too deeply alien in the set-up I offered (the three of us in a fairly sterile consulting room, with me, a White, middle-class woman who sat and listened rather than advise them on what to do) for him to fathom how the process could possibly help. While I totally understood, I found this very frustrating. However, something about this set-up – perhaps the very fact that it was "different" – appealed to Ndeye and she and I continued to work together.

Ndeye was left with the difficult task of negotiating how to live within three cultures: that of her family of origin, that of her husband, and that of the country in which she lived. For example, the French ban on girls wearing headscarves in schools, which affected some of her young relatives, was a disturbing event that she had to consider from different angles. Much of our work together had to do with helping her to accept otherness without losing herself. She stopped punishing herself for not being the person others expected her to be. She became more able to state her views clearly and consequently to elicit an understanding response from her husband. Ndeye and I also had to learn to accept each other's otherness. I frequently had to remind myself to put aside my views and principles, to help Ndeye formulate her own, and to swallow hard not to suggest she ask her mother-in-law, aunts, uncles, and her own mother to stop telling her to obey and please her husband, and just walk out the door. I think that possibly she sensed this, and that the fact that I could think what I thought yet respect where she was coming from was important to her. What I had to offer as a psychoanalytic couple psychotherapist could not reach Youssouf. However, it did speak to Ndeye, and working with one partner ultimately helped the couple.

Shared unconscious phantasies and unconscious alliances

Other concepts appear with variations in object relations and link theories – for example, shared unconscious phantasies and defences on the one hand and unconscious alliances on the other. Comparing such complex concepts would in itself warrant a separate study. What follows presents an initial overview.

Shared unconscious phantasies have to do with the meaning that being in a relationship has for each partner and with the image partners have of what constitutes an ideal couple relationship (Hewison, 2014). These images are coloured by each partner's early relationships, particularly in the dyadic and oedipal phases, which provide models for later adult relationships. According to Helen Tarsh and Elaine Bollinghaus, "the unconscious hope of most couples as they look to the future is that this new partnership can rework their past emotional experiences more favourably" (Tarsh & Bollinghaus, 1999, p. 125). In a healthy relationship, this shared hope unites the couple whose projective system ensures that their unconscious goal is sustained. Defence mechanisms such as splitting and projective identification, which are present to a variable extent in all couple relationships, are put to good use to maintain a balance within the couple. An unconscious agreement might, for example, enable one partner to project their own feared competitiveness on to their ambitious partner, who might in turn invest in the other their own wish to be looked after. In this instance, the projective system, on which rests the unconscious trust in the couple's ability to repair the past, can be compared with what Kaës refers to as an "unconscious alliance":

> I call unconscious alliance a trans-subjective psychic formation constructed by the subjects of a link in order to strengthen in each of them certain processes, certain functions or certain structures from which they derive such benefit that the link which connects them has a decisive value for their psychic life.
>
> (Kaës, 1994, p. 369)

For Kaës, unconscious alliances exist intrapsychically, between internal objects (Kaës, 2009) as well as intersubjectively. In society, the subjects of a link – such as the partners in a couple – have to form alliances in order to strengthen and preserve the relationship they need to fulfil their desires. Alliances provide agreement and are constructive. However, even in the case of predominantly productive alliances, difference and disagreements have to be ignored or cast aside in order to avoid conflict and discord. According to Kaës, "alliances unite and exclude" (Kaës, 2009, p. 2). Intrapsychically, this entails the repression of thoughts and representations. Intersubjectively, alliances can be based on denial and a shared unconscious "negative pact".

In the couples who present for therapy, the wish to repair past dysfunctional relationships is often blocked by a shared unconscious phantasy that all couple relationships are ultimately disastrous and that intimacy is dangerous. In this case, the conscious wish to sustain a relationship is accompanied by the unconscious fear that its fulfilment would be catastrophic. The projective system then becomes a shared means of defending against the conscious wish to be a couple, and against recognizing the negative unconscious phantasy. According to Douglas Woodhouse, the shared defence is an "unconscious agreement between the partners to maintain mutual misperceptions as a defence against the recognition of their underlying problems" (Woodhouse, 1965, p. 5). Francis Grier illustrates this process in an extract from a case study of a couple who

> relied on an unconscious agreement, almost a contract, that each would let the other down just when it mattered most, so proving the point for each of them that their closest objects were absolutely not to be depended on, or, more accurately, could be trusted to betray them.
>
> (Grier, 2011, p. 25)

The idea of an unconscious agreement to maintain a status quo, which might at a manifest level be dysfunctional, is close to the concept of the particular type of unconscious alliance that Kaës refers to as "the negative pact":

> By this I mean that which, in any trans-subjective set, is fated, in an unconscious agreement, to being repressed or negated, denied, disavowed, rejected, encapsulated: the function of the pact is for a link to be organised and maintained between the complementary vested interests of those who are linked by it … This cost of the link is the very thing which must be kept quiet between those who are linked by it, in mutual vested interest, in order to satisfy the double interrelated economy of the individuals and of the chain to which they belong.
>
> (Kaës, 1994, p. 368)

A negative pact might apply to a country, a class, an institution. In its determination to reject reality, it can lead to such phenomena as historical negationism (Kaës, 2009, p. 7). In relation to couples, it is close to the concept of "shared unconscious beliefs" (Morgan, 2010). The "negative pact" – such as the one struck by Kim and John – is what we try to unpick in the therapeutic process, both from our outside third position, and from the inside, as we struggle repeatedly to extricate ourselves from it.

Unconscious alliances refer to the systems put in place to ensure the maintenance of a shared interest. "Shared phantasy is based on the projective and introjective systems of each of the couple. The spouses are doing something to each other" (Hewison, 2014, p. 28). While shared unconscious phantasies belong to the couple, unconscious alliances pertain to a wider realm. From this perspective, object relations and link theories can be seen as complementary. An object relations approach relates the pact that exists within the couple's psychic formation to the negotiation of former stages of development (mother–infant and oedipal in particular) and the partners' consequent ability or inability to produce a containing and creative couple. Link theory helps to remind us of our own participation in the pact that we establish with patients, and of the social context in which couples form and therapeutic work takes place.

Bashirah and Michael

Bashirah and Michael were an interracial couple in their 30s, who came for help because Bashirah would not commit to a long-term relationship even though she wanted to have a baby, and this was making Michael feel insecure and unsettled. Michael, a secondary school teacher, came from a White, middle-class, English background. His childhood had been uneventful, but he had an older sister compared with whom he felt he had always paled into insignificance. Bashirah, an artist who specialized in Batik, had come from Ghana with her parents when she was a few months old. Her parents' relationship had been volatile, and they had struggled financially. When she was a teenager, her father left. She rebelled, got in with very much the wrong crowd and got into a lot of trouble. Eventually, she pulled herself together, finished school and studied art. She agreed that she and Michael should live together for a few years if they had a child, but she was adamant that the relationship would not last and that one day she would leave and they could then have joint custody of the child.

Bashirah felt very guilty for "selling out" and betraying her class and her race by choosing a White partner. The feeling of alienation and of not being truly understood by one's partner, which is not uncommon in couples who come from different social classes, is frequently amplified in intercultural and interracial couples. For some, the attraction and attachment are strong enough to overcome the feeling. For others, help is needed to understand the partner choice that was made. Bashirah was presenting the social, cultural and racial difference between them as an unsurmountable obstacle to the relationship. And indeed, it was an obstacle. Some work was done on both partners' rescue and revenge phantasies, which were connected to their racial difference. In addition, Bashirah, whose internalized parental model was poor, had been repeatedly let down by those to whom she had made attachments. She was therefore understandably averse to letting herself become emotionally dependent on anyone. I believe that one of the unconscious factors – though not the only one – that had made her choose a White partner, was that in her mind this would ultimately bring the relationship to an end. It gave her an escape route. By choosing a partner with whom she felt it was wrong to stay, she was protecting herself against dependence and commitment. This, of course, is only part of a much more complex picture that cannot be adequately related here, and which involves not only Bashirah's, but also Michael's, conflict over dependence, and the negative pact they had established to keep this shared conflict "quiet". Naming their fear of dependence eventually helped both partners to get in touch with something they shared, and to recognize other more positive and creative elements of the partner choice. In the case of Bashirah and Michael, who had both grown up and been educated in this country, the model of therapy offered was easily accepted and ultimately productive. On the one hand, the specific cultural element that Bashirah put forth as a reason for the relationship to be doomed had to be considered at face value and addressed; on the other, it was also helpful to view it as the form in which a latent fear of dependence was manifesting itself.

Reflections

In this chapter, I have explored the use and limitations of couple psychoanalytic psychotherapy with intercultural and interracial couples. The integration of aspects of link theory to an object relations approach has offered a different perspective, the aim of this addition being to encourage a creative intercourse between concepts that originate in different cultures.

Difference was central to the couple dynamic in the three couples referred to above. For Kim and John, the cultural and racial difference and internalized stereotypes served as an excuse for remaining at a distance and not taking the risk of knowing the other or letting the other know oneself. In this case, couple therapy helped both partners be less afraid of the very early needs and states of mind that still governed their behaviours and assisted the couple towards overcoming their fear of truly knowing one another. For Ndeye, cultural differences in response to the arrival of a child catapulted what had been a merged couple all the way to the other end of the spectrum. Though couple therapy with both partners could not take place, Ndeye's ability to use individual therapy to consider her couple through a new lens ultimately facilitated a coming together of the couple. For Bashirah and Michael, difference was paradoxically what kept the couple together as it served as an insurance against long-term commitment. Couple therapy helped the partners get in touch with their fear of intimacy and access the deep desire for connection and togetherness that they unconsciously were defending against.

All couples dream of building something together, and perhaps that dream is strongest in intercultural couples who are not repeating models, but trying to invent between them a new space in which the desire to be together is stronger than the differences that stand in their way. Confronting opposing external, as well as internal, forces is a struggle. Awareness of the former is crucial to our ability, as psychoanalytic couple psychotherapists to help our couples with the latter.

In *West Side Story*, a beautiful Puerto Rican woman, Maria, and a White, New York gang member, Tony, fall in love and are defeated by the forces opposing their intercultural union. But the song I refer to in my title remains, and so does the hope for all intercultural and interracial couples who embrace the challenge of making their alliance stronger than any internal or external opponent, that "somewhere" they will find a time and place that is right for them, and for us, that perhaps we can help them on their way.

Note

1 "Somewhere There's a Place for Us… : A cross-cultural approach to psychoanalytic psychotherapy with intercultural and interracial couples" is, with the kind permission of Karnac Books Limited, an adapted reprint of an article published in *Couple and Family Psychoanalysis* (2017), *7*(2): 153–167. A shorter adapted version was published in *Love Songs. Listening to Couples* (2025), Chapter 5, pp.59–72, Bicester: Karnac.

References

Alleyne, A. (2022). *The burden of heritage: Hauntings of generational trauma on Black lives.* Karnac Books.

Berenstein, I. (2012). Vinculo as a relationship between others. *Psychoanalytic Quarterly,* 81: 565–577.

Britton, R. (1995). Psychic reality and unconscious belief. *The International Journal of Psychoanalysis*, 76: 19–23.

Clulow, C. (2017). Before, between, and beyond interpretation: Attachment perspectives on couple psychoanalytic psychotherapy, *Psychoanalytic Inquiry, 37: 5*, 343–354.

Cohen, N. (1992). Same or different? A problem of identity in cross-cultural marriages. *Journal of Family Therapy*, 1: 177–199.

Davids, F. (2011). *Internal racism: A psychoanalytic approach to race and difference.* Palgrave Macmillan.

Grier, F. (2011). Psychotic and depressive processes in couple functioning. *fort da*, 17 (1): 11–29.

Hewison, D. (2007). The power of our attachment to theory – or Oedipus meets Ganesh. In: M. Ludlam and V. Nyberg (eds), *Couple attachments. Theoretical and clinical studies.* Karnac Books, pp. 171–188.

Hewison, D. (2014). Shared unconscious phantasy in couples. In: D.E. Scharff and J.S. Scharff (eds), *Psychoanalytic couple therapy. Foundations of theory and practice.* Karnac Books, pp. 25–34.

Kaës, R. (1994). Psychic work and unconscious alliances in therapeutic institutions. *British Journal of Psychotherapy*, 10 (3): 361–371.

Kaës, R. (2009). *Les alliances inconscientes.* Dunod. [Reprinted Dunod, 2014]. My translation.

Kaës, R. (2016). Link and transference within three interfering spaces. *Couple and Family Psychoanalysis*, 6 (2): 181–193.

Lowe, F. (ed.) (2014). *Thinking space. Promoting thinking about race, culture, and diversity in psychotherapy and beyond.* Karnac Books.

Mattinson, J. & Sinclair, I. (1979). *Mate and stalemate.* Tavistock Institute of Marital Studies.

Morgan, M. (2005). On being able to be a couple: The importance of a "creative couple" in psychic life. In: F. Grier (ed.), *Oedipus and the couple.* Karnac Books, pp. 9–30.

Morgan, M. (2010). Unconscious beliefs about being a couple. *fort da*, 16 (1): 36–55.

Morgan, M. (2016). Unpublished presentation at British Association for Counselling and Psychotherapy Conference on Private Practice, 24 September 2016.

Past Lives (2023). Film. Celine Song (Director). USA and South Korea.

Pereira, A. (2020, July 31). "Race" vs. "ethnicity": Why these terms are so complex. https://dictionary.com/e/race-vs-ethnicity/ (last accessed on 14 February 2024).

Sondheim, S. (1956). Somewhere (there's a place for us). Leonard Bernstein Music Publishing.

Tarsh, H. & Bollinghaus, E. (1999). Shared unconscious phantasy: Reality or illusion? *Sexual and Marital Therapy*, 14 (2): 123–136.

van den Berg, R. (2007). An impasse in power relationships: An intersubjective view in a South African socio-cultural context. In: M. Ludlam and V. Nyberg (eds), *Couple attachments. Theoretical and clinical studies.* Karnac Books, pp. 121–132.

West Side Story (1957). Musical. Lyrics by S. Sondheim, music by L. Bernstein. First staged at 1681 Broadway, New York.

West Side Story (1961). Musical. Film directed by R. Wise and J. Robbins. USA.

West Side Story (2021). Musical. Film directed by S. Spielberg. USA.

Woodhouse, D. (1965). Introduction. In: K. Bannister and L. Pincus (eds), *Shared phantasy in marital problems: Therapy in a four-person relationship.* Tavistock Institute of Marital Studies, pp. 5–7.

Chapter 14

Open and polyamorous relationships

Many loves, or the mad hatter's tea party!

Damian McCann

Introduction

Within the context of intimate relationships, there are many and competing narratives about the nature of these partnerships and the value attached to them. For instance, the centrality of the primary couple, the dyad, rooted in romantic love, sits in opposition to more open and polyamorous relationships, since these relational configurations appear to challenge both normative and mono-normative assumptions concerning the legitimacy of couple relating. Fern (2020) suggests that in Western society, romantic relationships are fraught with prescriptions and restrictions that inhibit non-traditional expressions of love. She goes on to say:

> As the landscape of romantic love continues to expand and monogamy is no longer the only possible course of action that a relationship can take, our societal notions, as well as our psychological models of love and partnership, also need to grow and include relationship structures beyond the monogamous norm.
>
> (p. 4)

This chapter is concerned, therefore, with interrogating the nature of open and polyamorous relationships, particularly regarding the question and place of love within these relationship formations.

In thinking about relationships more generally, incorporating references to emotion, romance, love, intimacy, sex, passion, etc., we might wonder how these ingredients combine to create the basis of a trusting and enduring developmental coupling and the extent to which this is also available to those in open and poly relationships. Kernberg (1976), for instance, suggests that "The capacity to fall in love is a basic pillar of the relationship of the couple" since it implies the potential for in-depth object-relating, integrating, as he says, the linkage of idealization with eroticism. However, the thrust and focus of this endeavour has historically been applied almost exclusively to the closed monogamous heterosexual union, with alternatives being viewed with suspicion or treated with derision, since they

DOI: 10.4324/9781003518129-14

appear to fundamentally challenge the notion of emotional and sexual exclusivity as well as the structural nature of monogamy.

A further complication in attempting to expand the field of vision is the split between the monogamous couple, associated with a deeper sense of intimacy (Spence, 1997) and "specialness" (Jamieson, 2004), which is often contrasted with the somewhat poorer and less responsible models of relating in open and polyamorous relationships (Conley et al., 2013). In fact, Barker (2018) in their chapter on "Rewriting the rules of monogamy" captures this thinking when they say that pairing off and getting married are viewed as "an inevitable, natural, normal and healthy part of development over the lifespan" and that "relationships outside of the couple are only considered in the context of cheating and infidelity and the damage this can do" (p. 96). Therefore, notions of love, romance, intimacy and so on, associated with the romantic ideal, are often overlooked or questioned in more open forms of relating, something that I wish to examine more fully in this chapter.

Monogamy and non-monogamy

Reflecting further, high divorce rates and the practice of secret non-monogamy among supposed monogamous couples indicates that all is not well in the assumed normative model of coupling. Yet, this shadow side of closed monogamous coupledom is often downplayed in contrast to more open forms of relating, especially when considering the value and nature of such relationships. I have also come to understand that at least some of the sources of unhappiness and discontent that lead partners to look outside their closed relationships reflect the rationale given by those already engaging in open and polyamorous relationships, e.g., the recognition that it is not possible to have all of one's needs met by a single partner; the desire for something new and exciting; and an incompatibility in sexual needs within closed relationships.

Yet, when sex, love and emotion are not solely directed towards one's partner and lived out and contained in one place, the danger of only seeing this as infidelity does little to promote the cause of polyamory or to embrace the meaning of ethical non-monogamy. At the same time, we must also understand that the decision to look outside the primary couple may not always be viewed as something liberating, since it can represent the actualization of splits within the individual and couple's shared unconscious organization being lived-out with a third (Scharff, 2014). Kernberg (1991) also links this behaviour to unresolved oedipal conflicts, which he believes are a major cause of invasion of the couple's sexual boundaries and a vehicle for the expression of dissociated aggression from many sources. Indeed, Kernberg draws attention to the indissoluble nature of the interaction of libido and aggression and of love and hatred as important determinants in the nature of the emotional relationship of the sexual couple.

We therefore cannot ignore the possibility that for some individuals and couples wishing to open their relationships, this may be a symptom of possible unresolved issues from childhood or a breakdown in the current relationship that is being managed through non-monogamy. Some might say that it constitutes a form of acting-out, since it could be viewed as an attack on intimacy associated with the challenges of maintaining a long-term couple relationship. Certainly, in my own work with couples over many years, I have come to understand the complexities associated with opening relationships as well as the unspoken power dynamics at play between partners. For instance, when reflecting with one man, who had regular secret affairs while married to his wife, he freely admitted that he would not like it if she were to sleep with other men (or other women, for that matter). And, if a recent YouGov poll (YouGov, 2016) is anything to go by, when asked "What would be your ideal relationship" only 10 per cent of respondents opted for non-monogamy, and barely 5 per cent indicated that they would be tolerant of their partner's wish to engage in sexual activities with someone else. With this as the backdrop, it seems incumbent to understand properly the arguments for opening one's relationship and for embracing polyamory, and particularly those arguments that highlight the more positive and loving aspects that hitherto have been absent from thinking. This is especially important given that some believe non-monogamy to be the fullest expression of love and sexuality (Fosse, 2021; Fern, 2020).

Non-monogamy is essentially the practice of having more than one partner and although it takes a variety of forms, e.g., open relationships and polyamory, a fundamental distinction concerns the question as to whether the non-monogamy is secret or consensual. Consensual non-monogamy is a term that is used for the practice of simultaneously having multiple sexual or romantic partners. Fern (2020) suggests that people who practise consensual non-monogamy value transparency, consent, open and honest communication, personal responsibility, autonomy, compassion, sex positivity and freedom for themselves and others. She goes on to suggest that love is not possessive or a finite resource and that it is not unusual for individuals and partners to be attracted to more than one person at the same time or to express that love, intimacy and sexual attraction in a variety of ways. It is also worth noting that researchers have found similar levels of commitment, longevity, satisfaction, passion and love in those practising consensual non-monogamy when compared with those in monogamous relationships. Fern (2020) goes on to suggest: "Many non-monogamous people have secure, loving and healthy relationships with multiple partners" (p. 7).

Open and polyamorous relationships – same or different?

Open relationships

In essence, open relationships refer to a form of dyadic couple relationship that is open to partners having sex with others. For instance, within gay male couple relationships this openness usually takes the form of the men in a primary relationship cruising (either together or separately) for sex with other men. The sexual encounters tend to be brief, although sometimes there may be longer-term sexual friendships. For instance, Pawlicki & Larson (2011), who conducted a small-scale qualitative study of eight gay men in open relationships, suggest that "While participants reported varying levels of emotional connection to sexual partners outside their primary relationship, partners viewed their primary relationship as the strongest sources of comfort, reliability and security in interpersonal relationships" (p. 53).

However, in the same way that sexual infidelity in monogamous relationships constitutes a crisis for the couple, emotional infidelity within an open relationship may be just as devastating. Furthermore, the splitting of sex and emotion that often accompanies the decision to open an existing couple relationship, is something that can feel both challenging and alien to many. That said, the decision to open one's primary relationship commonly appears to be rooted in a dissatisfaction with and incompatibility in sexual needs, although some of the men I have seen in my practice wanted an open relationship from the beginning. Nevertheless, Bonello (2009) suggests that sexual variety is often a motivating factor for most couples who choose non-exclusive relationship arrangements. And, whilst for some it provides freedom from outmoded patterns of psychosexual relating as well as an important means of managing discrepancies in sexual desire, for others it appears to enhance the sex and intimacy within the committed relationship (Bergstrand & Williams, 2000; Spears and Lowen, 2010). Barash & Lipton (2001) even suggest that passionate love may be rekindled when partners venture outside the primary relationship.

Returning to the Pawlicki & Larson's (2011) study, participants viewed sex with outside partners as mainly recreational, sex for strictly physical gratification, and one participant in comparing sex and love, spoke of "*sex as an act*" whereas "*love, on the other hand, is what you feel in your heart*". However, given the basis of open relationships, and particularly the need for transparency, it seems that there is a greater emphasis on the strength and security of the primary partnership. This is especially important, given the need when venturing out to hold not just one's partner in mind but also to hold the couple's relationship in mind. In my own experience of working with some gay male couples grappling with issues relating to the decision to open their relationships, I found this especially so. They would appear to compete or manically engage with outsiders in a way that came to threaten the security of the primary couple relationship itself.

Another source of tension in open relationships is related to a partner feeling that, in order to preserve the primary relationship, they must agree to their partner's wish or demand to open their dyad. In his autobiography, Michael Cashman talks of the discovery that his partner was having sex with other men, although he had also engaged in secret non-monogamy himself. When things came to a head and the couple considered parting, Paul, the partner, agreed to remain on the condition: "... there have to be changes. I don't want a monogamous sexual relationship. I want more" (Cashman, 2020, p. 186) and Cashman says: "I looked at him, and I knew there was nothing I could say" (p. 186). The couple agreed to a set of rules that would help them navigate their open relationship with an insistence from Paul that they had to be honest with one another. Cashman goes on to say that

> I finally admitted to myself that I didn't want to lose him. I loved him. He made me feel safe and wanted, so I would do whatever it took to have him in my life. I know the difference between love and sex.
>
> (Cashman, 2020, p. 187)

A somewhat different outcome from Cashman's story occurred with Larry and Peter, a long-standing gay male couple with successful careers and a home that reflected their shared interests. On the face of it, they appeared to have a collaborative and committed relationship, although they had come to therapy because of the discovery that Larry had been having sex outside their relationship. Peter felt betrayed as he had assumed that they were in a monogamous relationship, and so he was looking to therapy to help them restore their link.

From the outset, Peter made it clear that he was serious about leaving Larry unless he was willing to be monogamous. This all-or-nothing feel to the presentation struck at the heart of the couple's ongoing struggle and represented a fundamental split and developmental challenge to their partnership. For instance, Larry felt that the couple relationship had been stagnating for some time and highlighted the fact that they had not had sex together for several years. He said that when he had tried to talk about this, Peter would become defensive. Nevertheless, these snatched conversations seemed to bring them closer for a time, but it did not actually result in them making love. Larry also said that despite having sex outside their relationship that he was willing to explore possibilities within the relationship if Peter was open to this. Peter, however, was only concerned about extracting an agreement from Larry that he would not have sex outside the relationship. Larry felt that Peter was missing the point and was keen to continue the conversation, since he wanted to address their difficulties and to recapture something more satisfying and fulfilling.

Couples in this situation are often faced with an unbearable choice – do they separate, or can the sexual infidelity be worked through? Clearly Peter's hard line on monogamy at any cost and his failure to engage with Larry's complaint about the absence of sexual intimacy within their couple relationship resulted in Larry looking outside. Even in the context of therapy Peter continued to maintain his stance that Larry was wrong to look outside. Despite the therapist's attempt to think with the two men about the impasse regarding sex, Peter refused to be drawn and instead continued to punish Larry for turning away from him towards other men. The therapy ended when Peter decided to move out of the couple's home and Larry sought therapy on his own with another therapist to help him process the loss of the relationship.

Polyamory

Contrasting open relationships with polyamory, we begin to see a greater emphasis on love and connection. In fact, Klesse (2006) suggests that love is central to the discourse of polyamory, which may not be too surprising given that the literal translation of polyamory is "multiple loves" (*poly*, many; *amor*, love). Being polyamorous therefore implies an ability to be sexually and romantically involved with more than one person at any given time, although some who identify as poly may not strictly hold to this criterion (Fosse, 2021; Fern, 2020; O'Connor, 2019). Furthermore, it seems that most polyamorists use the term "partner" to refer to their multiple relationships, although the idea of intimate friendships (both sexual and non-sexual) also form part of the discourse, which is why Klesse (2006) believes that polyamory blurs the boundaries between sexual and non-sexual partnerships and friendships. Furthermore, the emphasis on love in polyamory often sits together with a de-emphasis on sex. Given that polyamory is less about how many people one is having sex with and more about allowing love to determine the appropriate form of connection, Klesse (2006) believes that it is essential that we release our attachments to conditioned beliefs about love, sex and intimacy, and commitment.

The term polyamory was coined in 1990 by Morning Glory Zell-Ravenheart, and the words polyamory, polyamorist and polyamorous officially entered the *Oxford English Dictionary* in 2006. According to Wikipedia, polyamory defies a single definition and instead structures and lifestyles may be complex and varied. For instance, the somewhat hierarchical model consisting of a primary partnership plus one and/or others, referred to as one's secondary partner(s), has broadened and shifted towards non-hierarchical polyamory, in which all parties involved have a more equal status. Hierarchical or not, polyamorous constellations fluctuate

> with new partners added, marriages fall away, primary partners become secondary, tertiary partners become primary, hierarchical arrangements become non-hierarchical, a relationship of three can become six and then go down to four, some partners have sex, some do not. People who would never imagine being in a relationship with one another become metamours – becoming directly involved with their partner's other partner.
>
> (Fosse, 2021, p. 2)

Moreover, some polyamorists conduct their relationships over long distances, only ever seeing their partners once or twice a year.

Perhaps for some, and especially for those holding more traditional notions of partnering, where the stability and longevity of the couple relationship represents its most valued attributes, the landscape outlined above can feel mind boggling and alien, something akin to the "mad hatter's tea party".

Some may even suggest that polyamorists are only really engaging in part object-relating, or that it represents a manic attempt to deal with the constraints or demands of an enduring couple relationship since, to them, it seems impossible to share love with so many people. Yet, within polyfidelity one witnesses a commitment to keeping the sexual activity within the group (Lano & Perry, 1995) and to establishing boundaries around the group that protect the integrity at its centre. Therefore, within poly relationships there may also be stability and longevity, alongside love, intimacy, honesty and transparency. In fact, some make claim to polyamory being a superior form of relating, requiring more personal autonomy, self-awareness and responsibility as well as equality and negotiation within relationships (Anapol, 2010; Easton & Hardy, 2009).

The above notwithstanding, the arrangements within polyamory may raise questions or concerns for couple therapists thinking only in terms of dyads or holding an uncertainty as to who or what constitutes the couple in open and polyamorous relationships. And, although Morgan's invaluable ideas concerning "*a couple state of mind*" and the "*creative couple*" (Morgan, 2019) apply equally well to open and poly relationships, since they reflect a way of relating, I still worry that the emphasis on couple in both of these concepts may result in some therapists unwittingly re-inscribing the notion of dyads when thinking about open and poly relationships. This is especially important when considering the non-hierarchical form of polyamory, where there is an absence of a primary couple. How then do we think about these relationships and do our models of practice for working with couples more generally help us navigate the intricacies that exist within these relational configurations? Perhaps, we should also be incorporating theoretical ideas from both group analytic and systems thinking, to help us in our thinking and practice with open and polyamorous relationships.

A further tension for those unfamiliar with polyamory is perhaps the need to pin things down, something that runs counter to those practising polyamory, where the emphasis is much more on keeping options open and in having less definition, precisely to create greater room for manoeuvrability. For instance, it has been suggested that polyamorists are suspicious of romantic love, simply because of the ways in which it has functioned to limit women's choices, and Klesse (2006) also draws attention to splitting within the field regarding open relationships and polyamory where one is pitted against the other in terms of value and acceptability. To some extent this only serves to re-inscribe the binary notion of mono-normativity being a better and healthier version than polyamory, resulting in the work that needs to be undertaken to fully understand and embrace the nature and value of open and poly relationships being avoided. An example of this kind of splitting concerns the notion that those in open relationships are over-sexed and promiscuous, whereas polyamorists are not, prompting Klesse (2006) to suggest that such thinking renders polyamorists vulnerable to being appropriated by normative and assimilationist ideologies. Frank and DeLamater (2009) also suggest that the "bifurcation between relationship styles (monogamous or 'alternative') can flatten out important differences in practice, belief and experience" (p. 9). It is worth noting that within the poly community some have coined the term relational anarchy and relationship queer for a more deliberately non-possessive style of relationship rooted in the idea of mutual freedom, trust and continual negotiation.

At this point I would like to introduce some case scenarios with the intention of broadening the perspectives on poly relationships presented so far.

Case scenarios

The struggle to establish a polycule[1]

Amy and Richard are an unmarried couple who had been together for three years when Amy began talking about opening their relationship. This came about because Amy had become infatuated with Lily who she met at night school. Amy identifies as bisexual, something that Richard always knew and accepted, although until Amy met Lily the couple's relationship had been closed and monogamous. New relationship energy is something that is talked about within poly relationships, and whilst being a natural aspect of all intimate relationships, it has, nevertheless, the potential to be a disruptive force for existing relationships within the poly network. Initially, Amy conducted her relationship with Lily separately from her couple relationship with Richard, but as things began to settle Amy had a desire to integrate Richard into her relationship with Lily. All three partners got on well when they met, but in the meantime, it seems that Richard had reconnected with an old school friend, Jemma, who he met at a school reunion. This became a source of stress for Amy, since she loved both Richard and Lily and her version of polyamory was being frustrated by a hierarchical model of a primary couple with two possible satellites, since Richard was conducting his friendship with Jemma along separate lines. Meanwhile, Lily, although she liked Richard, had no desire to be intimate with him and Amy together and, try as she might, Amy was essentially in two separate relationships with Richard and Lily, who themselves had become each other's metamor, i.e., friends of their partner's partner with no romantic or sexual interest.

Fern (2020) suggests that non-hierarchical polyamory exists without the imposition of a pecking order, and where each relationship can grow into what it naturally wants to be. However, Amy's version of what she had confirms the earlier notion of there being no single definition of polyamory and even a blurring of the boundaries between hierarchical and non-hierarchical polyamory. For instance, if we take the model of the primary plus one (or more), a person's primary relationship would sit at the top of the pecking order, since primaries usually cohabit, share resources and make decisions together. Yet, with Amy, we see her living separately with both partners, sharing space with both partners together and separately, and trying in some way to manage for herself Richard's friendship with Jemma. In non-hierarchical polyamory, multiple simultaneous relationships exist without the need to impose hierarchies, where each relationship is allowed to grow and develop in a variety of ways. However, this also raises questions concerning the amount of time and energy that goes into maintaining multiple relationships and within the field there is an acknowledgement that polyamory necessitates the spreading of resources and particularly that of time.

Giddens (1992) suggests that there has been a long-term shift towards the ideal of the democratic egalitarian relationship between the sexes and that a love relationship and partnership should be a matter of personal choice and not constrained by tradition and arrangement. In this way of thinking, people commit to a relationship only in so far as it fulfils their needs and, furthermore, it offers a more pragmatic concept of love, based on equality and mutual trust, and a willingness to let go when it is no longer working.

"Three into two won't go"!

Hugo, Diana and Amber are a throuple[2] of seven months' standing. They met online when Hugo and Diana welcomed Amber into their partnership. Although the relationship had been going well, Amber had at times questioned her place within the throuple, as Hugo and Diane's pre-existing couple relationship seemed to unbalance the symmetry of the three-way partnership. For instance, Hugo and Diane were invited to a friend's wedding and there was much discussion about including Amber or not in the invite, as well as talk about the ways of introducing her to others if she did attend.

In fact, there had already been much consideration concerning the presence of Amber in their lives particularly since Hugo and Diane have a seven-year-old daughter, Alice. It seems that they had been expressing concern about the potential reactions of family, friends and outsiders and whether they would be sympathetic and supportive of Hugo and Diane's lifestyle choice. Anapol (2010) also draws attention to the real-life consequences for the children of poly parents being vulnerable to discrimination from teachers and authorities, since they may view poly relationships with suspicion or even concern. For instance, she suggests "parents must decide how and when to integrate visitors into the family and what, if anything, to say to the children about the new lover who is now sharing Mommy and/or Daddy's bed" (Anapol, 2010, p. 129). It seems that poly parents are careful in talking to others and particularly officials about their lifestyle, for fear that it may trigger unwanted attention or even safeguarding concerns. There may also be unwarranted anxieties about sexual abuse, concerns about partners separating and the impact on children, or sensitivities in the children themselves about having to explain to friends about their family set-up. Yet, Sheff (2014), who has researched poly families over many years, believes that the children of poly parents are equally if not more emotionally healthy than their peers and, like children growing up in same-sex family households, are generally more accepting of relationships than children in families with heterosexual and mono-sexual parents.

The same anxieties as those relating to children, may also prevail within the workplace, since the disclosure of one's poly status and lifestyle may attract negative attention or even compromise one's position within one's employment. This notwithstanding, some polyamorists report more positive outcomes from family, friends and work colleagues, suggesting a more hopeful reading of their situation (Fern, 2020).

At the heart of Hugo, Diane and Amber's throuple is a further consideration concerning the question of the establishment of a secure base. It is understood that in adulthood, relational-object constancy promotes trust, and that connections and bonds that are established will endure even when partners are apart. However, Amber finds herself questioning where she really belongs within the throuple, particularly as she joined an existing established couple and family unit and is beginning to feel something of an outsider. Hugo and Diane are trying their best to make Amber feel welcome inside their home and inside their family unit. However, they are now faced with Amber's wish to look outside the throuple with a view to finding another partner, the idea being that she could possibly integrate that individual into her relationship with Hugo and Diane, although this is not at all certain.

It has been suggested that attempting to open one's relationship when one's attachments are insecure, has the potential to disrupt not just the relationship(s) but also one's sense of self. Fern (2020) believes that unlike monogamous relationships where there is an assumption of security, consensual non-monogamy (CNM) is a relationship structure that is inherently insecure.

> In CNM, we don't have the security of knowing that the partner is with us because they see us as the best, one or only partner out there for them. Instead, we often have to figure out how to fit together alongside pre-existing structures and commitments with other partners.
>
> (Fern, 2020, p. 138)

Inevitably, at least to begin with, partners like Amber, looking outside the throuple or polycule, become less accessible and even less committed, until things become clear and begin to settle. Hugo and Diane, however, did not welcome this new development with Amber wanting to look outside. Instead, they were keen for the three of them to think together, possibly within a therapeutic context, in order to address the insecurities within their relationships and to find a container for the feelings that were in danger of spiralling out of control and of being acted-out.

The flattened hierarchy

For the past two years, Gary, Jasmine and Nancy have been living together as equals, sharing space, sharing friendships and sharing love. Recently, Jasmine has felt some insecurity, since Gary has been spending more time with Nancy and Jasmine is feeling neglected. When she tries to share her feelings with Gary, he appears unsympathetic, accusing her of being possessive, and dynamically her anxieties seem to push him further away. The resulting conflict between Jasmine and Gary appears to be unsettling the fragile balance of the relationships within the polycule and Nancy is beginning to resent Jasmine's wish to have more of Gary. Unfortunately for both, Gary has accepted a job offer that will entail international travel, and he has been talking about seeing other women while he is away.

Much has been made of the existence of jealousy within polyamory, and whilst it is certainly the case that jealousy exists, as indeed it does at times within closed and monogamous relationships, work must be undertaken by those identifying as polyamorists to establish relational security. For instance, particular focus is placed on creating appropriate boundaries that balance security and freedom, and that also attend to feelings of insecurity and jealousy. Fosse (2021) believes that daring to love entails opening oneself to the uncertainties of love while also trusting that those we love will be available to us when we need them. Unfortunately for Jasmine, she is now faced with the prospect of possibly losing the kind of relationship she once had with Gary, since he appears to be rebalancing his priorities, However, those in poly relationships have greater freedom to explore the possibility of new loves and perhaps of negotiating the integration of these additional partners into their existing poly networks. Indeed, greater emphasis is placed on discussing the boundaries of sexual involvement with others, conducted in the spirit of avoiding hurt and averting betrayal (Fosse, 2021). That said, jealousy may be a natural and inevitable aspect of all relationships, especially when a person feels that they are losing the ones they love.

Despite efforts to avoid or to attend to jealousy, it does, nevertheless, have the potential to unsettle or call into question the sense of security and comfort within poly relationships. Yet, those in poly relationships have introduced a creative concept "compersion" to help navigate and even neutralize the corrosive quality of jealousy within intimate relationships. Compersion, which has its roots in compassion, is essentially a feeling of joy that comes from celebrating another's positive experiences, thereby transcending jealousy. The term was coined in the early 1990s by the Kerista polyamorous community in San Francisco to refer to a feeling of total joy and happiness in response to a loved one having a positive romantic experience. It is even suggested that compersion can help a partner or partners become more empathetic towards one another and may increase the potential for partners to feel more connected.

One view is that the goal of working through jealousy is to attain compersion, but for the partnerships in all the above-mentioned case scenarios, this is proving something of a challenge. Ultimately, the outcome of the work will depend on the openness of the partners to explore and work through the feelings stirred up by existing partners looking outwards for new/other partners or, for that matter, trying to incorporate new partners into the existing relationships. In some respects, the claustro-agoraphobic dilemma may be helpful to our understanding of the shifts in closeness and distance that appear to be operating within these relationships. After all, it would be unsurprising if feelings did not run high when faced with the prospect of losing one's attachments or adjusting to new attachments that threaten the balance of the co-existing relationships. These and other considerations regarding the developmental challenges facing those within poly relationships rely on the therapist and the therapeutic setting being robust enough to attend to the complexities involved. For that reason, I will now turn my attention to the clinical implications of working with those in poly relationships.

Some clinical considerations

Weitzman (2006), found that 38 per cent of poly people who were in therapy chose not to mention this to their therapist and, of those who did, many experienced negative responses. A more recent study by Grunt-Mejer and Lys (2022), who examined current and prospective psychotherapists' attitudes towards different relationship types, found that participants demonstrated a tendency to pathologize those engaged in consensual non-monogamy, based on the assumption that it would be harmful to relationships. This is perhaps not so surprising given the possibility of therapists' having negative reactions when working with difference. Masters (2008) highlights the fact that when, for example, gay patients describe their sexual activities in sessions, it can create a host of countertransference responses regardless of the gender or sexual orientation of the therapist. "At times we may find ourselves intrigued, disgusted, envious, and, yes, even sexually excited" (Masters, 2008, p. 376). By the same token, therapists may secretly feel lost or find themselves questioning or even disapproving of open or poly relationships although actually working with such clients or patients in their practice.

There is a certain irony in the shift from closed monogamous relationships to more open and polyamorous relationships, relying as they do on openness and transparency, when the profession itself appears to be so closed and protective of its space. An example of this concerns the question of self-disclosure and the possibility of greater transparency regarding the therapist's feelings in working with open and poly relationships, as well as a client's or patient's own curiosity about their therapist's position regarding their situation. I wonder how many therapists would feel confident opening themselves to this challenge, especially if it falls outside the comfort of their therapeutic paradigm? To some extent, this also relates to the question concerning one's training (the extent to which trainees are exposed to and confronted with difference), as well as one's ongoing continued professional development. For instance, it has been suggested that the therapist's conscious and unconscious beliefs, emotional reactions and internal motives are as important to examine as are a client's beliefs, feelings and conflicts regarding opening their relationship or in managing the challenges inherent within polyamory.

Essentially, when confronted with lifestyles different from their own, therapists may struggle to navigate the complexities inherent in working with poly and open relationships. With that in mind it may be helpful to consider frameworks that address this challenge from different perspectives. For instance, Falicov (1996), in her paper "Learning to think culturally: A comparative framework", suggests that a growing number of training programmes are exploring avenues to include cultural diversity issues, which I hope is also true when working with gender and sexuality. In her paper, Falicov reflects on what she calls the "Universalist" position (the idea that we are all more alike than different – representing a denial of difference) with a "Particularist" position (which emphasizes the uniqueness of all couple and family relationships – suggesting that it is all about difference), while pushing for a "Multi-dimensional" position (which reflects the complexities involved and encourages an openness to exploring those differences).

Fine (1994), also in regard to thinking about difference from the perspective of "othering", believes that we can interrupt "Othering" by working what she refers to as the hyphen between self and other. This would, for instance, include examining with others the validity of one's own representations of them, listening to others' accounts of us as a way of exposing the operation of "Othering", listening to members of the powerful group in order to hear the ways in which they construct others, and developing opportunities for dialogue between us and others. However, although all of this touches on gaps in knowledge, or the ability to speak to differences that exist within the work, technically it can be challenging and even exposing to let clients or patients know that we do not understand, or that we are not familiar with a certain term, or indeed to question aspects of their presentation that may be of concern to us. The surprised reaction I received when I first came upon the term "metamor" and asked what it meant, speaks to the sensitivity surrounding the existence of gaps in knowledge and the way that this plays out in the therapeutic encounter.

Whilst to some extent I am touching here on the question of transference and countertransference within the therapeutic endeavour, the process of "Othering" suggests a more active engagement with the self and other than one with which psychotherapists may feel comfortable. It also implies a more external and perhaps concrete perspective on the construction and meaning of relationships surrounding difference, something that may be at odds with a paradigm that is more inward looking and where the self of the therapist is less available to scrutiny. To some extent, confidence when working with difference lies in one's own experience of that difference, as well as the extent that one's training has helped in the active engagement with difference. Despite my own largely positive couple psychoanalytic psychotherapy training, the couple format that most dominated the curriculum, the literature and indeed the clinical discussions was, unsurprisingly, the closed monogamous heterosexual dyad. This may also be reflected in intake processes and the arrangement of one's clinical space where there is a chair for the therapist and a sofa or two chairs for the couple, representing a more mono-normative approach to practice. I have also been struck by accounts of couple therapists being thrown off balance when they were expecting a couple to arrive for the initial appointment and found themselves confronted with four individuals on their doorstep forcing them to scrabble around to alter the arrangement of the consulting room to accommodate the foursome.

A further consideration in working with polyamory is that concerning the question of who to invite to an initial consultation and how to think about this with those making the initial enquiry. For instance, returning to the case of Amy, one might wonder if it would be more helpful to meet with Amy on her own in the first instance to get a better understanding of the situation. However, by inviting Amy for the initial consultation, although we may get a better understanding of "her" situation, we may be left wondering what Richard or Lily's thinking or experience might be. Ultimately, we should probably leave it for Amy to decide who should attend, assuming she is the one who is making the referral – but this means we are already engaged in a decision that may have an impact on the polycule and on the absentees. Similarly, if we were to push to see Amy and Richard together, given that they constitute the primary couple, are we then in danger of denying the importance of Lily or, for that matter, Jemma, who also has a place in the system? Furthermore, it is also important to consider the question of dual relationships and indeed conflicts of interest where a therapist may find themself working with an individual who identifies as poly, and the same therapist, without knowing it, is also working with another individual who is part of the network and who is expressing deep concern about the other client or patient that the therapist has just seen. How should this be thought about and managed when that therapist becomes aware of the situation involving their two individual patients/clients?

Conclusion

In this chapter I have considered the place of love in open and polyamorous relationships. The structural nature of closed monogamous relationships provides an obvious backdrop for understanding the nature of couple-relating. Yet, those whose relationships do not fall within this tight corridor of relational formations are at best overlooked and at worst viewed as inferior or pathological. My hope is that in opening our eyes to the rich tapestry of relating associated with open and poly relationships, we can begin to see the value also of these affiliations.

As Giddens (1992) suggests, there has been a long-term shift towards the ideal of the democratic egalitarian relationship between the sexes, and a love relationship and partnership should be a matter of personal choice, not constrained by tradition and arrangement. This would include recognizing that the wish to open themselves and their relationships to others has the potential for growth and love. Too often the emphasis on sex associated with open relationships does little to illuminate the importance of these casual encounters and indeed attachments that may flow from them. Furthermore, open and poly relationships may be more elided than first thought, especially since there are obvious overlaps that no longer keep them in different camps. Here I am thinking about the primary plus one model where an outsider who was brought in for sex becomes an important presence in the couple's relationship but in a way that falls short of it being a throuple. This also militates against the tendency to pin things down in a way that limits the richness and complexity.

The complexities built into an open and polygamous relationship points to the need for a greater awareness and openness in the therapist, so as to fully engage with and understand the conscious and unconscious processes at work. According to Nichols and Shernoff (2007), therapy will only be effective when ideas of normality and pathology are critically explored and deconstructed, and when the therapist has examined their own biases. The extent to which therapists are equipped to meet this challenge relies largely on their capacity to think about and work with difference and, to that end, training, supervision and continued professional development play an important part in attending to the developmental needs of the therapist.

Notes

1 A "polycule" is a connected network of people in polyamorous (consensual non-monogamous) relationships, acting as a "molecule" of interconnected partners rather than just a pair.

2 A "throuple" is a romantic relationship between three people.

References

Anapol, D. (2010). *Polyamory in the 21st century: Love and intimacy with multiple partners.* Rowman & Littlefield Publishers.

Barker, M. (2018). *Rewriting the rules: An integrative guide to love, sex and relationships.* Routledge.

Barash, D. & Lipton, J. (2001). *The myth of monogamy: Fidelity and infidelity in animals and people.* W.H. Freeman.

Bergstrand, C. & Williams, J.B. (2000) Today's alternative marital styles: The case of swingers. *Electronic Journal of Human Sexuality*, 3 (10).

Bonello, K. (2009). Gay monogamy and extra-dyadic sex: A critical review. *Counselling Psychology Review*, 24: 51–65.

Cashman, M. (2020). *One of them: From Albert Square to Parliament Square.* Bloomsbury Publishing.

Conley, T., Moors, A., Matsick, J. & Zeigler, A. (2013). The fewer the merrier: Assessing stigma surrounding consensually non-monogamous romantic relationships. *Analysis of Social Issues and Public Policy*, 13, 1–30.

Easton, D. & Hardy, J. (2009). *The ethical slut: Polyamory, open relationships and other adventures.* 2nd edition. Ten Speed Press.

Falicov, C.J. (1996). Training to think culturally: A multidimensional comparative framework. *Family Process*, 34 (4): 373–388.

Fern, J. (2020). *Polysecure: Attachment, trauma and consensual nonmonogamy.* Thorntree Press.

Fine, M. (1994). *Working the hyphens: Reinventing self and other in qualitative research.* In: N.K. Denzin and Y.S. Lincoln (eds), *Handbook of qualitative research.* Sage Publications, pp. 70–82.

Fosse, M.J. (2021). *The many faces of polyamory: Longing and belonging in concurrent relationships.* Routledge.

Frank, K. & DeLamater, J. (2009). Deconstructing monogamy: Boundaries, identities, and fludities across relationships. In: M. Barker and D. Langridge (eds), *Understanding non-monogamies.* Routledge.

Giddens, A. (1992). *The transformation of intimacy: Sexuality, love and eroticism in modern societies.* Stanford University Press.

Grunt-Mejer, K. & Lys, A. (2022). They must be sick: Consensual nonmonogamy through the eyes of psychotherapists. *Sexual and Relationship Therapy*, 37 (1), 58–81.

Jamieson, L. (2004). Intimacy, negotiated nonmonogamy and the limits of the couple. In: J. Duncombe, K. Harrison, G. Allan and D. Marsden (eds), *The state of affairs: Explorations in infidelity and commitment*. Lawrence Erlbaum Associates.

Kernberg, O.F. (1976). *Object-relations theory and clinical psychoanalysis.* Rowman & Littlefield Publishers.

Kernberg, O.F. (1991). Aggression and love in the relationship of the couple. *Journal of the American Psychoanalytic Association*, 39 (1): 45–70.

Klesse, C. (2006). Polyamory and its "others": Contesting the terms in non-monogamy. *Sexualities*, 9 (5): 565–583.

Lano, K. & Perry, C. (1995). *Breaking the barriers to desire: Polyamory, polyfidelity and non-monogamy – new approaches to multiple relationships.* Five Leaves Publications.

Masters, S. (2008). Homosexuality and psychoanalysis. iii: Clinical perspectives. *Journal of Lesbian Mental Health*, 12 (4): 373–378.

Morgan, M. (2019). *The couple state of mind: Psychoanalysis of couples and the Tavistock Relationships model.* Routledge.

Nichols, M. & Shernoff, M. (2007). Therapy with sexual minorities queering practice. In: S.R. Leiblum, (ed.), *Principles and practice of sex therapy.* Guilford Press, pp. 379–415.

O'Connor, M. (2019). Polyamory: A romantic solution to wanderlust? *European Journal of Psychotherapy and Counselling*, 21 (2): 1–14.

Pawlicki, P. & Lawson, P. (2011). The dynamics and conceptualisation of non-exclusive relationships in gay male couples. *Sexual and Relationship Therapy*, 26 (1): 48–60.

Scharff, D.E. (2014). Working with affairs. In: D.E. Scharff & J.S. Scharff (eds), *Psychoanalytic couple therapy: Foundations of theory and practice*. Karnac Books, pp. 254–268.

Sheff, E. (2014). *The polyamorists next door: Inside multiple-partner relationships and families*. Rowman & Littlefield Publishers.

Spears, B. & Lowen, L. (2010). *Beyond monogamy: Lessons from long-term male couples in non-monogamous relationships*. http://thecouplesstudy.com/wp-content/uploads/BeyondMonogamy_1_01.pdf.

Spence, H. (1997). Sex and relationships. In: W.K. Halford and H.J. Markham (eds), *Clinical handbook of marriage and couples intervention*. John Wiley & Sons, pp. 73–101.

Weitzman, G. (2006). Therapy with clients who are bisexual and polyamorous. *Journal of Bisexuality*, 6 (1/2): 137–164.

YouGov. (2016). *Young Americans are less wedded to monogamy than their elders*. https://yougov.com/en-us/articles/16622-young-americans-less-wedded-monogamy.

Chapter 15

Love as a containing function in later years – or its victim

Christopher Vincent

Shakespeare famously asserted that love is a strength that can be drawn upon to negotiate and survive the challenges and losses that life presents, which I take to include those faced by couples as they navigate old age. As Shakespeare put it, "Love is not love which alters when it alteration finds ... it is an ever-fixed mark and looks on tempests and is never shaken" (Shakespeare, 1973, Sonnet 116). This interpretation of what Shakespeare meant is a powerful and contentious idea that asks us to consider many interrelated questions about love itself, what we mean by old age, the distinctive opportunities and stresses experienced by couples at that time of life, and how couple psychotherapists have responded to them.

An account of love in later years, or at any point in the life cycle, is difficult because of love's elusive subjectivity and variability that, arguably, the artist conveys better than the psychotherapist attempting to analyse and deconstruct the experience (see Ludlam, 2020). However, if conveying the phenomenology of love is best left to the poet, songwriter, film producer and others, social scientists and psychoanalysts have written about the conditions that promote love, and how love adapts to ageing.

It is also true that unpacking what we mean by "later years" or "old age" is almost as difficult a task as understanding the nature of love. Some would say that old age is a state of mind rather than an identifiable stage in the life cycle and, in holding this view, are often reacting against some of the negative stereotypes associated with the labelling of old age. Chronology provides the most straightforward definition and 65, once the general age for retirement, is used in the United Kingdom's national statistics as the point where old age is given a lower limit. If we take 65 as a starting point, we know from the 2021 census figures that men on average can expect to live a further 14 years to 79 and women a further 18 years to 83 (Office of National Statistics, 2024).

Life expectancy at birth in the developed world has approximately doubled in the past two centuries (Barker, 2011) and this trend will result in an expanding elderly population. Between 2022 and 2047, the 12 million persons of state pension age in the UK will increase by 25 per cent, the largest increase of any life stage (Office of National Statistics, 2025), creating massive

DOI: 10.4324/9781003518129-15

challenges for mental health services and the part that couple psychotherapy plays within them.

Different frameworks have been used to study this burgeoning section of the population. These include biological ageing, sexual ageing and psychological ageing, the last of which covers such matters as changes in cognitive functioning and affect regulation (Ryan and Coughlan, 2011). Studies within these fields confound the notion that old age is all about decline and loss and provide a more nuanced and complex picture of ageing and the experience of partnerships in later years.

What does the couple therapist need to know about ageing?

An important source of our knowledge about ageing comes from the personal experience that psychotherapists draw upon as they seek to attune to the cognitive and emotional experience of their clients. Many of us will have had or, maybe, are still having experience of our parents, relatives and friends ageing and dying. Knowledge acquired from this part of our lives is idiosyncratic, reflecting a partial window into the ageing process. For some, the knowledge will focus on the upsides of individuals and couples ageing whilst others will be more familiar with the downsides, which might include growing physical and mental frailty, increasing dependence on social support, managing the last phases of life and living with the consequences of being bereaved.

Alongside the knowledge of what happens to older people, will be a growing understanding of how our relationships with them change. How close or distant will your relationship be? To the extent that you are drawn in, how are family boundaries redefined and oedipal settlements revisited? How do you manage a progression of losses both before and after death? An added difficulty for the younger and generally fitter therapist is how to identify with challenges that have not yet been encountered. De Beauvoir (1977, p. 315) quotes Goethe as saying "Age takes hold of us by surprise", and she goes on to claim "Old age is particularly difficult to assume because we have always regarded it as something alien, a foreign species: Can I have become a different being while I still remain myself?". For me, this question is answered when I look in the bathroom mirror each morning and see my late father's outline.

The second sources of knowledge will derive from both social research and clinical studies, which have produced an increasing amount of data about the ageing populations in advanced Western societies, countering de Beauvoir's assertion, when writing 50 years ago, that society has adopted a conspiracy of silence about ageing. Much of this knowledge is demographic and conveys the experience of ageing in broad brush strokes, aggregating experience in clustered ways. In doing so, there is a danger that general findings conceal wide variations and say little about the implications these variations have for understanding how they translate into lived experience and their effects on couple relationships.

Nonetheless, there are, in my research and clinical experience, four headline findings that are helpful to note. These findings refer to (1) the quality of life in later years, (2) the impact of losses resulting from bereavement, (3) the increasing impact of ill health, and (4) the shifts some couples must make to become "carer" and "cared for".

The first headline, the quality of life in later years, is positive. There is good evidence to show that, compared to other phases of the life cycle, early old age is a relatively happy period offering opportunities for older people to embrace new projects and interests. Contrary to many stereotypes, research consistently finds that older adults maintain a positive attitude about sex (Garner & Bacelle, 2004) and report the importance of continuing sexual activity with their partners (AARP Survey, 2005; Vincent, 2002).

Reviewing the literature on social relationships in adulthood, Luong and colleagues (Luong et al., 2011) concluded that older adults generally experience more satisfying and positive social relationships than their younger counterparts. They suggest that this level of wellbeing is the result of several factors including time horizons shortening, regulating and reducing social relationships to those that are most significant and successfully adopting strategies to avoid conflict with others. While this may be true for a general cohort of people, we also know from clinical experience that the shortening of time horizons in later life and a reduction in the numbers of significant relationships can, for some couples, be associated with heightened anxiety and a reduced quality of life. Nonetheless, a UK study (Office of National Statistics, 2016) undertaken between 2012 and 2015 interviewing 300,000 adults found that respondents between ages 65 and 79 had the highest average levels of personal wellbeing across all age groups, but this finding fell away after the age of 75 when increased levels of loneliness were found. These findings are consistent with studies that show that being in a partnership, overall wellbeing, and better mental and physical health are all positively correlated (Schwarzbach et al., 2014; Waite & Gallagher, 2000; Wilcox et al., 2003).

The second headline is that loss of a partner through bereavement is a common experience of couples in the seventh decade. Approximately 60 per cent of the 12 million over-65s in the UK register themselves as being in either an opposite-sex marriage or a civil partnership, and for this group the median age for women losing their partner is 75 and for men is 78. These figures do not account for the remaining 40 per cent of the elderly, many of whom will have informal partnerships and may also suffer bereavement in their lives at around the same time. Loss of a partner though bereavement is a final separation preceding which many couples' relationships will have experienced important changes in distance regulation. Retirement of one or both partners can propel partners closer together (Mattinson, 1988), while changes in the lives of children, grandchildren and older parents may all exert pulls and pushes that can divide or unite partners in early old age. For those couples who benefit from any additional closeness that comes at this time of life, bereavement may be all the harder to bear.

The third headline to note is that, whether living alone or with a partner, advancing old age sees the increased prevalence of long-term ill-health conditions. In the UK, 86 per cent of people 85 years and over have at least one long-term adverse ill-health condition, an increase of 12 percent above those in the 65 to 74 age category (Age UK, 2023). This gradual increase in the prevalence of different illnesses as the population ages is found in other advanced economies (Eurostat, 2020). The most common illnesses include hearing loss, deteriorating sight, arthritis, chronic pulmonary disease, diabetes, depression and dementia (World Health Organisation, 2022), all of which can impact on couples' quality of life.

The fourth headline arising from these health statistics is to note that many older couples have to negotiate the transition whereby one partner takes on the role of carer and the other, that of being cared for. This transition can be triggered by many health conditions but is an especially common occurrence for couples contending with dementia. In the United Kingdom there are approaching 1 million people with diagnosed dementia looked after by a similar number of unpaid carers many of whom will be long-term partners (Alzheimer's Research UK, 2024). The asymmetry in couple relationships that then follows can have profound emotional and practical significance for those affected and is only beginning to be researched and understood (Ablitt et al., 2009; Clare, 2002; Vincent, 2019: Balfour & Salter, 2019).

What have couple therapists written about ageing?

The literature about therapy with older couples is not large – reflecting, in part, the relatively small numbers of older couples seeking therapy. Writing 20 years ago, Evans (2004) commented that the small numbers were likely to be the result of the then elderly generation being averse to seeking counselling or therapy when faced with relationship problems. Age UK (2019) reported 15 years later that the situation had not changed. Their researchers found that continuing low take-up was the result of senior citizens' reticence to seek therapy, coupled with the reluctance of mental health practitioners to recommend talking therapies and with family doctors more inclined to offer medication for depression and anxiety. Since the Covid epidemic, there has been an increase in the demand for mental health services overall, but it is not clear whether older couples have been part of this trend or whether the introduction of therapy online has benefitted older couples.

Many psychoanalysts working with individual patients have alerted couple psychotherapists to some of the dynamic opportunities and restrictions that old age brings. Three papers have been helpful to me in thinking about work with older couples. The first is the paper by Jaques (1965), "Death and the mid-life crisis", wherein Jaques drew on his clinical experience and the reported lives of eminent literary and artistic figures, to argue that mid-life sees the gradual emergence of an internal pressure to make sense of one's own death and that to make headway with this task requires both celebrating what has been achieved in life and mourning what has been missed or lost. This reckoning of life-to-date means coming to terms with ambivalent feelings and marks a shift from a paranoid-schizoid to a depressive position. The second paper that struck chords was Coltart's (1991) "Analysis of an elderly patient" in which she makes the claim that, because psychic defences have been in place for many years, the therapist has to settle for limited gains. As she put it, "competent psychic defence systems ... cannot be expected to steal away and silently vanish for ever" (p. 93). In the context of couple work this is an important observation and leads on to the possibility that, if defences cannot be changed fundamentally, processes of mutual understanding and acceptance between partners might become important. The third paper to mention is that by Martindale (1989), "Becoming dependent again: The fears of some elderly persons and their younger therapists". In this paper Martindale makes the point that, for many elderly people, failing health can stimulate fears of becoming dependent, evoking primitive anxieties from early childhood that become difficult for younger therapists to work with in the transference. He makes the point that, for therapists to appropriately attune to the experience of dependent older clients, they must process their feelings and experience towards their own parents who, contemporaneously, may be failing in health and becoming dependent. These possible developments in the therapist's private life are the sort of triggers that stimulate the mid-life reflections about the meaning of death and loss that Jaques argued for in his paper.

Within the couple psychotherapy field, Andrew Balfour has for many years written about and actively researched how couples in later life can be offered therapeutic help (Balfour, 2017; Amos & Balfour, 2007; Balfour & Salter, 2019). and his most recent book (Balfour, 2025) brings together his research findings, his thoughts about the ageing process and the ethics of assisted dying. His thinking draws on many sources to support his contention that to live and love well in old age requires coming to terms with the losses associate with ageing and the finality of death. In doing so he has found Klein's theories crucial for the central role they afford to the role of containment in managing loss. In his paper, "Growing old in mind and body" (Balfour, 2017), Balfour, together with the ensuing commentary by Russell (2017), provide an important exploration of what therapeutic change means in the context of couples ageing. Unlike Jaques who, in his seminal paper, explicitly excluded a consideration of ill health in his thinking about death, Balfour and Russell place bodily deterioration in the forefront of their discussion, thereby, helping the reader think about living in the present with all the challenges that failing health brings. Balfour emphasizes the importance of therapeutic containment which allows couples

> [a] place to think, to process experience, to mourn losses … (so that) couples are not driven to retreat or recoil from one another … but are equipped instead with a tolerance that allows for contact and accompaniment through the process of late life and dying.
>
> (Balfour, 2017, p. 242)

This formulation is particularly helpful because it speaks to the love that follows from tolerating differences rather than emphasizing what changes in behaviour and character structure might look like. Russell concludes her commentary by cautioning against too great a reliance on depressive position functioning. She makes the point that for children "symbol formation must make its way slowly against concreteness but in old age, symbol formation gives way to concreteness as language gives way to the sensorium which is once again our gateway to the world" (Russell, 2017, p. 252). In her reference to the "sensorium", she is referring to the parallels between the earliest physical interchanges between mother and baby and the importance of bodily experience in old age – such as touch, smell, physical comfort, reduction in pain – as the conduits through which intimacy and care can be shared or given.

What has psychoanalysis had to say about love?

Freud wrote a lot about love, but his drive theory placed limitations on explaining love that is not connected to instinctual gratification. According to his drive theory, mental life is a reflection of and limited to a biological process that goes through a series of developmental stages. As he put it in his paper "Instincts and their vicissitudes", "an instinct appears … as the psychical representative of the stimuli originating within the organism and reaching the mind" (Freud, 1915, p. 118). At each stage, libido (or instinct) seeks satisfaction through engagement with an object or person. In early life this will be the infant's mother but will extend to others over the lifetime and will include the infant's own body in the narcissistic stage of early development or later when physically ill. Should the wish for drive satisfaction become thwarted, anger and hatred towards the frustrating object will be elicited contributing to the important idea that love and hate are binary opposites.

> The love that we long for is, therefore, in constant danger of dissolution from our own, and the other's propensity for destructiveness. This battle (between love and hate) defines the human condition in the Freudian and Kleinian view of human nature and it logically follows on that it will colour and threaten our capacity for love.
>
> (Brown, 2005, p. 27)

So, Freud's conception of love is that it begins with narcissism and progresses through a series of developmental stages culminating in mature genital sexuality. In this model there is little room to consider how libido fluctuates and often diminishes as individuals age, and how couples manage these developments together. In fact, Freud avoided tangling with the dynamic challenges facing the middle-aged and elderly believing that psychoanalysis was only effective for those of younger years.

The move away from drive theory opened the possibility for love to be thought about as a relational need operating independently from instincts. Erich Fromm pursued this possibility in his book, *The Art of Loving* (Fromm, 1995), which was written for the general reader and, perhaps because of that, has been disregarded by the professional world (McLaughlin, 2019). The title refers to Fromm's claim that loving is an active process and one that one learns about and can get better at as an adult – even if the foundations for loving are laid down in the earliest stages of childhood development when the capacity to recognize "I" and "other" is formed. He argues that mature love is comprised of four basic elements. These are care, responsibility, respect and knowledge. By care Fromm means the active concern for the life and growth of those we love; by responsibility he means the readiness, when needed, to act on behalf of those we love; and by respect he means the concern that the other person should grow and develop as they are and not for the lover's self-interested purposes. His fourth element, knowledge of the other person, is not given priority over the first three but is, in my view, a necessary condition for the first three to operate. Unless you know your partner very well it is impossible to care appropriately, to be emotionally responsive at the right time, and to respect their autonomy. I also suggest that there are some times when knowing another is, in itself, a form of love. These moments, which otherwise might be described as empathic understanding or "being with", occur at all stages in life but are particularly important in later years when old age presents problems and stresses that have to be borne rather than acted upon, remedied or cured.

However, what is meant by knowing another in the context of a loving relationship is itself a complex and elusive phenomenon. Developmentally, the foundations for knowing another and being known are formed in early infancy through the mother enjoying a succession of attuned vocal, musical and bodily interactions with her baby (Pickering, 2020). The knowledge that the mother imparts through these different behaviours gives shape to the baby's experience that, over time, the baby can come to recognize as their own. In this loving process the mother demonstrates the qualities Fromm describes: care must be timely and given in ways that respect the baby's autonomy as a separate being. From this process the child internalizes the first prototype of a loving couple relationship where they begin to appreciate that their independence as a separate being is contingent upon the capacities of another separate being. The child now has an experiential world comprising their own subjectivity and a recognition that other people have theirs, a realization reinforced by observing others interrelating in ways that may exclude them (Britton, 1998).

There is a tension for any parent between fostering the child's capacity to think and feel for themself on the one hand and imposing "knowledge" onto or into the child on the other hand. For this reason, the mother's understanding or knowledge has to be conveyed in ways that allow the child to apply playful curiosity to what is offered (Stokoe, 2023).

> What the mother does, in the best of all worlds, is to read accurately the cues of her baby and to respond in ways that are in tune with the baby's internal state but not in ways that replicate it. When her responses are in tune with the infant's gestures they have been described as "contingent" but what she also does is to mark (differentiate) her responses, so that a distinction is drawn between what belongs to her and what belongs to her baby.
>
> (Clulow, 2014, p. 50)

If these conditions apply, the child's curious and creative response may give the mother new understanding about their world and, thus, an enriched and enriching relationship between parent and child can develop. However, if the mother's knowledge lacks being marked or differentiated and is felt to be imposed, the child may develop a fused relationship where their autonomy is not respected or encouraged; if the mother's responses lack contingency and are not attuned, the child will feel misunderstood and will tend towards isolation and emotional avoidance.

This model of parent–child interaction is one that we carry forward into adult partnerships where interaction is now between two autonomous and separate individuals and offers insight into what Morgan calls the creative couple. She means by this a relationship in which both partners are able "to think together in a way that they could not do each on their own" (Morgan, 2019, p. 184), and in order to achieve this outcome she and Stokoe (Morgan and Stokoe, 2014) argue that, like the infant, each partner must mobilize their curiosity, a process that requires tolerating uncertainty about what one's partner's thoughts might be. The state of uncertainty being referred to requires the withdrawal of projections based on narcissistic rather than creative illusions (Colman, 2014; Fisher, 1998; Pickering 2022; Friend, 2013). Even so, because one's partner is a separate, autonomous individual, knowledge of what goes on their mind is necessarily incomplete and cannot be controlled. With this in mind, Fisher (1999) writes about "giving the object its freedom" (p. 280) and, in the same vein, Kernberg (1998) observes that, however much lovers may know about each other's bodies, their minds are impenetrable and, thus, ultimately mysterious.

The adult-to-adult partnership differs from the parent–child partnership because adults are able to choose one another in a way parents and children cannot and the "blind" idealization that features so strongly when falling "in love" allows for an unconscious bond to exist alongside conscious thoughts and feelings. When couples come to therapy and declare that they do not understand the distress they create together, it is highly likely that the unconscious elements in their personal chemistry, which have been functional up to that point, are now causing problems. For couples in later years, the normal balance of their relationship may be upended by many factors, but I have chosen to illustrate the impact of ill health through a clinical case for the reasons already discussed. In the case I describe, ill health in one partner created great anxiety that drove the couple into very angry arguments; the meaning of illness challenged the unconscious fit between the couple which had operated reasonably well for over 30 years. Exploring the background to this anxiety helped them regain some degree of calm and mutual understanding, which in turn lessened their destructive arguments. The case material has been heavily disguised.

Daytime sleepiness and fear of dependency

Kate and Richard sought couple therapy at the suggestion of Kate's individual therapist who had been helping Kate with anxiety. This centred a lot on her multiple health conditions, including sleep apnoea, which produced bouts of sleepiness during the day and prevented her being able to drive her car safely. It was apparent to her therapist that there was also a couple problem because Kate reported getting into very bitter and angry arguments with her husband.

When they first consulted me, Kate and Richard were both in their early 70s but looked older and, generally, unhappy. Kate tended to talk for both of them conveying her wish for help and her obvious distress. Richard, by contrast, was reserved and difficult to engage but he communicated his pent-up anger and frustration powerfully by tapping his knees with his hands and finding it difficult to be comfortable in his chair.

They had been married for nearly four decades and had three adult children who lived away and were caught up with their own lives to a degree that reinforced a sense of Richard and Kate being somewhat isolated as a twosome. Their life together had been largely happy until the last few years when Kate's health problems and Richard's financial worries gradually increased. He had over the years built up a portfolio of investments and savings that he managed on his own, but which were producing poor returns and causing great worry for him. They were seriously thinking that they would need to have a more modest lifestyle with a move to a smaller house and a less expensive car.

When I asked them to talk about their childhood backgrounds, they each gave me what I came to understand as pithy and concise formulations of their shared problems. Kate told me her childhood had been happy and could not think of anything to add. She then remembered that her mother had insisted that should one of her friends give her a present, she must respond by giving back one of equal value. Richard gave me a much fuller picture of his parents where his mother was the dominant partner. He described her as being unfulfilled and insisted he worked hard so that, as an adult, he would not have to live in social housing. I noted these comments early on in the work, but it was only as the therapy unfolded that I began to appreciate their full emotional significance.

I came to understand that what they told me spoke to a shared unconscious fear that had two elements. The first was that their parents insisted that they should be independent individuals who were not to be indebted to anyone else (Kate's situation) and must survive through hard work (Richard's situation). The second element was that how one was seen by others was of huge importance. Were Kate not to have responded with a present equal in value to the one she was given and had Richard lived in social housing, enormous shame would have befallen them. These two elements began to emerge as key dynamic themes in the two years of weekly joint couple therapy.

There were two subjects that provoked painful rows. The first was ignited when Kate was a passenger in their car, which she claimed Richard drove angrily and very fast. Her difficulty in staying awake reinforced her sense of being a helpless passenger in his hands. She thought they would crash and die in a road traffic collision. She was quite terrified and had no trust in Richard at those times. The second flashpoint was trying to jointly decide on selling their large house and moving to somewhere smaller. Kate encouraged this move, but Richard would come up with all sorts of reasons against moving – alternatives were not in the right areas, he could not bear to sell off unneeded furniture, the gardens were too small … and the excuses seemed endless – but, in parallel, Richard spoke about their growing financial problems. He presented as someone with a problem he would not allow anyone else to solve.

I came to like this couple a lot. They offered graphic details of their problems, and I was acutely conscious of the shame that they would feel if I did not address underlying anxieties with sensitivity.

The material that was most powerfully charged was connected to the car journeys because these would precede our sessions and would instigate arguments when we met. Kate's inability to stay awake and her fear that they would both die in a crash was conveyed vividly. In recounting these journeys to see me I acknowledged how frightened Kate was and how angry Richard became, and I made the more general point that they were telling me that Kate being dependent on Richard was terrifying for her and made Richard very angry. This interpretation made in a variety of ways seemed helpful to them and freed up the difficulties they had in talking about moving to a smaller house. When discussing a potential house move, the tables were somewhat reversed because Kate was in favour of the move and Richard found it hard to take on board her wishes and advice. In these exchanges, I was able to weave in links to Richard's childhood fears of being seen to be living in shame-inducing, low-grade housing and how he was unable to trust Kate's advice.

I think that the way I formulated my responses was both contingent and marked. It was not difficult to register their anxieties, and I offered my thoughts backed by varying degrees of emphasis and directness that enabled them to take in and use what I said. As a result, Richard and Kate came to a better understanding of each other's anxieties and formed an appreciative relationship with me. They finished after two years with the house problem unresolved and Kate's daytime sleepiness no better and no worse as far as I could tell. But they had fewer rows and finished expressing warm gratitude for the work we had undertaken. Whether Richard drove more carefully I could not judge, but I heard less about the journeys to see me.

Final thoughts and reflections

I started this chapter with a Shakespearean quotation about the power of love to surmount all obstacles in its way. It made me want to think about whether and how love surmounts the obstacles typically encountered by couples in old age and, if it does, whether and how couple psychotherapists can contribute to that process.

In thinking about old age, I write as an interested party. I am in my late 70s, married and aware that in selecting to characterize the challenges faced by older couples in general I am describing my own, but that is only to admit that my circumstances conform to the experience of other UK citizens of my generation living in material comfort. I have not considered the variations in experience associated with economic circumstances that show, for example, that there are marked variations in health status by ethnicity, wealth and geography. In the UK there is a marked difference between the levels of reported health in the north of the country and the more prosperous south (Centre for Ageing Better, 2024).

The invitation to think about love from a psychoanalytic perspective and to apply that understanding to couple interaction in later years has opened up new ways of thinking for me. In my professional work I have not been used to theorizing about love, content to focus upon the circumstances that make love possible. I realize that this theoretical neglect on my part begs a series of questions, not least, whether love is a constant as Shakespeare is asking us to accept. I think I remain uncertain; I am tempted by the Platonic notion that there is an ideal notion of love that we discover by aggregating all the instances of love together and from this distil its essence. These situations, which can involve both positive and negative emotions, often reveal a transcendent quality involving a measure of commitment that objective evidence cannot explain. As onlookers we might comment that love survives "in spite of everything", and we are left with a range of different feelings including puzzlement, warmth, admiration and, perhaps, envy. It is the memory of these moments that inclines me to believe that love does, indeed, possess enduring and unchanging transcendent qualities.

Set against this idea is the general idea that love means many things and does alter according to changing circumstances. Within an historical framework our understanding of love has been shaped by philosophical, religious and political changes that have redefined values underpinning family life and relationships between adults. Within a developmental framework, the changes brought about by ageing present stresses which strain the capacity to love and elicit new ways of showing love. I am thinking of the burdens that some carers have to manage when their partners deteriorate into long-term ill health. At such times the distinct losses encountered along the way call on partners to show a quality of love that, while it might not be unique to old age, is most often needed at that time. I am referring to the love that tolerates each partner's vulnerabilities, foibles and differences in a shared experiential world where each partner knows, consciously or not, that time is running out and that one will outlast the other. This idea of tolerance requires a form of knowing each other that has, as I have tried to show, parallels with the form of knowing that operates between mother and baby. There is, however, one major difference between the two scenarios, for while the resulting intimacy between mother and baby prefigures what is hoped to be a happily developing childhood, the intimacy between partners in old age prefigures death and bereavement. It takes a particular form of generosity to remain committed to a relationship you know will end, but, if couples can be helped to see that the dilemma is shared, perhaps the loss becomes a little less frightening and love can survive.

References

AARP (American Association of Retired Persons) (2005). *Sexuality at midlife and beyond.* AARP. https://www.aarp.org/research/topics/life/info-2014/2004_sexuality.html.

Ablitt, A., Jones, G.V. & Muers, J. (2009). Living with dementia: A systematic review of the influence of relationship factors. *Ageing and Mental Health*, 13 (4): 497–511.

Age UK (2019). *Later life in the United Kingdom.* http://www.ageuk.org.uk. Accessed 21 January 2026.

Age UK (2023). *The state of health and social care of older people.* http://www.ageuk.org.uk. Accessed 21 January 2026.

Alzheimers Research UK (2024). *Dementia statistics hub.* https://dementiastatistics.org/aboutdementia. Accessed 21 January 2026.

Amos, A. & Balfour, A. (2007). Couples psychotherapy: Separateness or separation? An account of work with a couple entering later life. In: R. Davenhill (ed.), *Looking into later life.* Karnac Books.

Balfour, A. (2017). Growing old together in mind and body. In: S. Nathans and M. Schaeffer (eds), *Couples on the couch: Psychoanalytic couple therapy and the Tavistock model*, Routledge.

Balfour, A. & Salter, L. (2019). Living together with dementia. In: A. Balfour, C. Clulow and K. Thompson (eds), *Engaging couples: New directions in therapeutic work with families.* Routledge.

Balfour, A. (2025). *Life and death: Our Relationship with ageing, dementia, and other fates of time*, The Library of Couple and Family Psychoanalysis. Routledge.

Barker, M. (2011). Ageing and attachment. In: P. Ryan and B.J. Coughlan (eds), *Ageing and older adult mental health*. Routledge.

Britton, R. (1998). Subjectivity, objectivity and triangular space. In: *Belief and imagination: explorations in psychoanalysis*. Routledge, pp. 41–58.

Brown, J. (2005). The compelling nature of romantic love: A psychosocial perspective. *Psychoanalysis, Culture & Society*, 10: 23–45.

Centre for Ageing Better (2024). *Health and Well-being*. https://ageing.better.org.uk/health-and-wellbeing-state-ageing-2023-4. Accessed 21 January 2026.

Clare, L. (2002). We'll fight as long as we can: Coping with the onset of Alzheimer's Disease. *Ageing and Mental Health*, 6 (2): 139–148.

Clulow, C. (2014). Attachment, affect regulation, and couple psychotherapy. In: D.E. Scharff and J.S. Scharff (eds), *Psychoanalytic couple therapy: Foundations of theory and practice*, Karnac Books.

Colman, W. (2014). The intolerable other. *Couple and Family Psychoanalysis*, 4 (1): 22–41.

Coltart, N. (1991). The analysis of an elderly patient. In: G. Junkers (ed.), *Is it too late: Key papers on psychoanalysis and ageing*. Karnac Books.

De Beauvoir, S. (1977). *Old age*. Penguin Modern Classics. Penguin Books.

Eurostat (2020). *Ageing, Europe: Statistics on health and disability*. https://ec.europa.eu>eurostat.statisticsexplained/indexphp?=AgeingEurope_statistics_on_health_and_disability#causes_of_death_among_older_people. Accessed 21 January 2026.

Evans, S. (2004). Elderly couples and their families. In: S. Evans and J. Garner (eds), *Talking over the years: A handbook of dynamic psychotherapy with older adults*. Brunner-Routledge.

Fisher, J. (1999). *The uninvited guest: Emerging from narcissism towards marriage*. Karnac Books.

Freud, S. (1915). *Instincts and their vicissitudes*. In: J. Strachey (ed. and trans.), *The standard edition of the complete psychological works of Sigmund Freud* (1953–74), Volume 14. Hogarth Press.

Friend, J. (2013). Love as creative illusion and its place in psychoanalytic couple psychotherapy. *Couple and Family Psychoanalysis*, 3 (1): 3–14.

Fromm, E. (1995). *The art of loving*. Thorsons Publishers. (First published by George Allen & Unwin, 1957.)

Garner, J. & Bacelle, L. (2004). Sexuality. In: S. Evans and J. Garner (eds), *Talking over the years: A handbook of dynamic psychotherapy with older adults*. Brunner-Routledge.

Jaques, E. (1965). Death and the mid-life crisis. *International Journal of Psychoanalysis*, 46: 502–514.

Kernberg, O. (1998). *Love relations; Normality and pathology*. Yale University Press.

Ludlam, M. (2020). Three musical love letters. *Couple and Family Psychoanalysis*, 10 (1): 1–13.

Luong, G., Charles, S.T. & Fingerman, K.L. (2011). Better with age: Social relationships across adulthood. *Journal of Personal Social Relationships*, 28 (1): 9–23.

Martindale, B. (1989). Becoming dependent again: The fears of some elderly persons and their younger therapists. *Psychoanalytic Psychotherapy*, 4 (1): 67–75.

Mattinson, J. (1988). *Work, love and marriage: The impact of unemployment*. Duckworth.

McLaughlin, N., (2019). The triumph of the psychosocial perspective: Lessons from the rise, fall and revival of Erich Fromm. *Journal of Psychosocial Studies*, 12 (1–2): 9–22.

Morgan, M. (2019). *A couple state of mind: Psychoanalysis of couples and the Tavistock Relationships model.* Routledge.

Morgan, M. & Stokoe, P. (2014). Curiosity. *Couple and Family Psychoanalysis*, 4 (1): 42–55.

Office of National Statistics (ONS) (2016). *Measuring national well-being: At what age is personal well-being the highest?*ONS website statistical bulletin. Released 2 February 2016. https://ons.gov.uk/peoplepopulationandcommunity/wellbeing/articles/measuringwellbeing/atwhatageispersonalwellbeingthehighest.

Office of National Statistics (ONS) (2024). *National life tables: Life expectancy in England and Wales:2021–2023*. ONS website statistical bulletin. Released 23 October 2024. https://www.ons.gov.uk/government/statistics/national-life-tables-life-expectancy-in-england-and-wales-2021-to-2023–2.

Office of National Statistics (ONS) (2025). *National Population Projections: 2022 based.* ONS website statistical bulletin. Released 28 January 2025. https://ons.gov.uk/peoplepopulationandcommunity/populationandmigration/populationprojections/bulletinsnationalpopulationprojections/2022based.

Pickering, J. (2020). Harmony of the spheres: Musical elements of couple communication. *Couple and Family Psychoanalysis*, 10 (1): 42–58.

Pickering, J. (2022). Through a glass darkly: Bion, unknowing, and the couple. *Couple and Family Psychoanalysis*, 12 (2): 130–148.

Russell, L. (2017). Discussion of "Growing old together in mind and body". In: S. Nathans and M. Schaeffer (eds), *Couples on the couch: Psychoanalytic couple therapy and the Tavistock model.* Routledge.

Ryan, P. & Coughlan, B.J. (2011). *Ageing and older adult mental health: Issues and implications for practice.* Routledge.

Schwarzbach, M., Luppa, M., Forstmeier, S et al. (2014). Social relations and depression in later life: A systematic review. *International Journal of Geriatric Psychiatry*, 29, 1–21.

Shakespeare, W. (1973). Sonnet 116. In: *William Shakespeare Sonnets.* Heron Books.

Stokoe, P. (2023). Curiosity vs. beliefs: The battle for reality and what this means for relationships and development. *Couple and Family Psychoanalysis*, 13 (2): 196–211.

Vincent, C. (2002). Health challenges for older women: Some implications for sexual health. *Sexual and Relationship Therapy*, 17 (3): 241–253.

Vincent, C. (2019). Illness, couples and couple psychotherapy, *British Journal of Psychotherapy*, 35 (44): 628–641.

Waite, L. & Gallagher, M. (2000). *The case for marriage.* Doubleday.

World Health Organisation (2022). https://www.who.int/news-room/fact-sheets/detail/ageing-and-health. Accessed 21 January 2026.

Wilcox, S., Evenson, K.R. & Aragaki, A. et al. (2003). The effects of widowhood on physical and mental health, health behaviors and health outcome: The Women's Health Initiative. *Health Psychology*, 22 (5) 513–522.

Index

Note: Page numbers in *italic* indicate figures.

For Product Safety Concerns and Information please contact our EU representative GPSR@taylorandfrancis.com Taylor & Francis Verlag GmbH, Kaufingerstraße 24, 80331 München, Germany